mTOR Signaling in Ophthalmology

Kambiz Thomas Moazed

mTOR Signaling in Ophthalmology

Understanding the Essentials

Springer

Kambiz Thomas Moazed
New York, NY, USA

ISBN 978-3-032-05043-4 ISBN 978-3-032-05044-1 (eBook)
https://doi.org/10.1007/978-3-032-05044-1

This Springer imprint is published by the registered company Springer Nature Switzerland AG
The registered company address is: Gewerbestrasse 11, 6330 Cham, Switzerland

Preface

The mammalian target of rapamycin (mTOR) is a central node in cell regulation, impacting everything from cellular growth and metabolism to the intricate mechanisms of aging and disease. Its role in the eye, however, is an emerging field that promises to revolutionize our understanding of ocular health and disease. This book aims to bridge the gap between deep molecular biology and clinical ophthalmology by focusing on the profound effects of mTOR signaling in various parts of the eye.

The initial chapters of this book lay the foundational knowledge necessary to understand the complex biology of mTOR.

Chapter 1, "Molecular Biology of mTOR," introduces the structure, function, and regulation of the mTOR complexes, which are pivotal in integrating both intracellular and extracellular signals.

Chapter 2 expands on this by detailing the "mTOR Signaling Pathways," emphasizing how these pathways influence cellular processes such as protein synthesis, autophagy, and energy metabolism.

Chapter 3, "mTOR Effect on Eye Embryology," discusses how mTOR signaling facilitates the development of the eye, influencing cellular proliferation, differentiation, and survival from the earliest stages of embryogenesis. This chapter sets the stage for understanding the pathological conditions discussed in subsequent sections.

In Chaps. 4, 5, 6, 7, 8, 9, and 10, the book shifts focus to the pathophysiological aspects of mTOR in various ocular structures:

- In Chap. 4, we explore the "mTOR Effect on Conjunctiva," particularly in the context of Pterygium, a common ocular surface disease.
- Chapter 5 examines the "mTOR Effect on Cornea," with a specific look at its role in the development and treatment of Dry Eye Disease.
- In Chap. 6, the exploration continues with the "mTOR Effect on Anterior Segment," particularly in glaucoma.
- In Chap. 7, "mTOR Effect on Lens," we discuss the role of mTOR in cataract formation.

- The posterior segment of the eye is discussed in Chaps. 8, and 9 delves into the "mTOR Effect on Retina" and "mTOR Effect on Retinal Pigment Epithelium," respectively. Here, we explore how mTOR signaling impacts crucial cellular populations like retinal ganglion cells and the pathogenesis of diseases like Macular Degeneration.
- In Chap. 10, "mTOR Effect on Optic Nerve," we examine the role of mTOR in conditions such as ischemia or traumatic injury, offering insights into potential therapeutic avenues.

Chapter 11, "mTOR Effect on the Brain," stretches the discussion beyond the eye, highlighting the implications of mTOR signaling in neurodegenerative diseases, particularly Alzheimer's disease.

Finally, Chap. 12, "mTOR Alterations," discusses the pharmacological modulation of mTOR, primarily through agents like rapamycin. This chapter not only reviews the therapeutic potential of mTOR inhibitors but also cautions about the complexity and the need for precise targeting to avoid unintended consequences.

This book is written for researchers, clinicians, and students who are part of a multidisciplinary team striving to push the boundaries of ocular research into mTOR pathways. By the end of this journey, readers will have a comprehensive understanding of the multifaceted roles of mTOR in the eye and the brain, equipped with the knowledge to translate these insights into innovative treatments for ocular and neurodegenerative diseases.

We embark on this journey with hope and determination, believing that the intricate dance of mTOR within cells holds the key to unlocking new frontiers in the fight against eye diseases.

This preface is designed to give an overview of the book's content while also highlighting the importance of mTOR research in various domains of eye disease and beyond.

New York, NY, USA Kambiz Thomas Moazed

Pretext

Molecular biology is a rapidly evolving field of science, with many signaling molecules, their pathways and their specific terminology. It is important to get familiar with these abbreviations as they are crucial to understand these complex processes. The field of molecular biology plays a pivotal role in understanding the intricate mechanisms that underpin all biological processes. At its core, molecular biology provides insights into the molecular and atomic interactions that drive cellular functions and the organization of life itself. These interactions often occur through a complex network of signaling pathways that resemble a domino effect and a cascade where each molecular event triggers the next, leading to a broad array of cellular outcomes.

This cascading nature of molecular interactions is especially evident in the process of signal transduction, which is how the cells respond to external signals, converting them into internal cellular responses. Through signal transduction, cells can communicate, adapt, and coordinate their functions across the entire organism, which is essential for maintaining homeostasis, facilitating development, and responding to environmental changes. Understanding these molecular details not only enhances our grasp of biological processes but also informs medical and biotechnological advances. By dissecting how molecular machinery operates and interacts within the cells, researchers can develop targeted therapies for diseases, engineer biological systems for new applications, and create more effective biotechnological tools. Hence, molecular biology is foundational, not just in a scientific context, but also has its practical applications in health and industry.

Terms and Abbreviations The following are limited examples of molecular biology abbreviations with a brief description, according to their relevance to our discussions in all chapters of this book.

Atg13 (autophagy-related protein 13) Is a key regulator of autophagy that interacts with other autophagy-related proteins, such as ULK1, to form the ULK1 complex, which initiates autophagosome formation. Its activity is regulated by mTOR signaling, linking nutrient availability to autophagy induction.

4E-BP1 (eIF4E-binding protein 1) Is a key signaling protein involved in the regulation of protein synthesis.

AGC family of kinases Is a group of serine/threonine kinases that includes over 60 enzymes, named after three of its main members: PKA (protein kinase A), PKG (protein kinase G), and PKC (protein kinase C). These kinases play crucial roles in regulating a wide array of cellular processes such as cell growth, survival, metabolism, and differentiation.

AKT The term "AKT" doesn't stand as an abbreviation for a phrase but is rather a name derived historically from its association with the transforming retrovirus AKT8, where the AKT gene was first identified. It is also known as *Protein Kinase B (PKB)* and is a serine/threonine kinase that plays a critical role in regulating diverse cellular processes, including metabolism, growth, cell survival, and proliferation. AKT is activated by phosphoinositide-dependent kinase-1 (PDK1) in response to growth factors and insulin via the PI3K (phosphoinositide 3-kinase) signaling pathway. Once activated, AKT phosphorylates a variety of substrates involved in the regulation of cell survival, apoptosis, and glucose metabolism, making it a key player in cellular signaling.

Alpha helix A common structural motif in proteins, characterized by a right-handed coil, stabilized by hydrogen bonds.

AMPK (AMP-activated protein kinase) Is a critical energy sensor and regulator of cellular metabolism. It is activated by increases in the AMP/ATP ratio, indicating low energy in the cell, and it helps restore energy balance by stimulating catabolic pathways that generate ATP and inhibiting anabolic pathways that consume ATP.

Apoptosis Is a highly regulated process of programmed cell death that occurs naturally in the body as a means of maintaining homeostasis and removing damaged or unnecessary cells. It is characterized by distinct morphological changes such as cell shrinkage, chromatin condensation, nuclear fragmentation, and the formation of apoptotic bodies. The process is controlled by a variety of cell signals, which can trigger either the intrinsic (mitochondrial) or extrinsic (death receptor) apoptosis pathways. Caspases, a family of protease enzymes, play a crucial role in the execution phase of apoptosis, systematically dismantling the cell's structural components and signaling for its removal by phagocytes. This controlled cell death mechanism is essential for development, immune function, and disease prevention.

ARF (alternate reading frame) Is a tumor suppressor encoded by the CDKN2A locus. It stabilizes p53 by inhibiting MDM2, promoting cell cycle arrest and apoptosis in response to oncogenic stress.

ATG (autophagy-related genes) These genes encode a group of proteins essential for autophagy, the cellular degradation and recycling process. These proteins are involved in the formation of autophagosomes, the vesicles that capture and transport cellular components to the lysosome for degradation.

ATP/ADP Adenosine triphosphate (ATP) is the main energy carrier in cells. Adenosine diphosphate (ADP) is a product of ATP dephosphorylation and can be converted back to ATP.

Autophagy A cellular degradation process where cells recycle cytoplasmic components, often regulated by nutrient availability and stress.

BAD (Bcl-2-associated death promoter) BAD is a pro-apoptotic member of the Bcl-2 protein family, which is known for its role in regulating apoptosis. BAD promotes apoptosis by binding to and inhibiting the function of anti-apoptotic Bcl-2 family members, such as Bcl-2 and Bcl-xL. This inhibition frees the pro-apoptotic proteins Bax and Bak, allowing them to induce mitochondrial dysfunction and caspase activation, leading to cell death. BAD's activity is regulated by phosphorylation; when phosphorylated, BAD is sequestered by the 14-3-3 proteins and prevented from inducing apoptosis.

BAMBI (BMP and activin membrane-bound inhibitor) Is a transmembrane pseudoreceptor that structurally resembles type I receptors but lacks an intracellular kinase domain. It acts as a negative regulator of TGF-β and BMP signaling by sequestering ligands or receptors, thereby modulating processes such as development and fibrosis.

BAX (Bcl-2-associated X protein) Is a pro-apoptotic member of the Bcl-2 protein family. It plays a critical role in apoptosis by promoting the release of cytochrome c from mitochondria, a key step in the activation of caspases that execute cell death.

BECLIN1 (BECN1) Is a key protein in the regulation of autophagy, a cellular process for degrading and recycling cellular components. It is involved in the formation of autophagosomes and interacts with various other proteins to initiate and regulate autophagy. BECLIN1 also plays a role in tumor suppression, with its dysfunction linked to cancer development. Additionally, it is involved in various cellular processes, including development, immune response, and neurodegeneration.

Beta sheets They consist of beta strands connected laterally by at least two or three backbone hydrogen bonds, forming a pleated sheet.

BH3-only proteins Are a subfamily of the Bcl-2 protein family, which play a pivotal role in the regulation of apoptosis, or programmed cell death. These proteins are named for the presence of a single Bcl-2 Homology 3 (BH3) domain, which is critical for their pro-apoptotic activity. BH3-only proteins act as essential initiators of apoptosis by binding to and inhibiting the function of anti-apoptotic Bcl-2 family members, thereby promoting cell death in response to various stress signals. Key members include Bim, Bid, Bad, and Noxa, each with distinct regulatory mechanisms and roles in apoptosis.

BIM (Bcl-2-interacting mediator of cell death) BIM is another pro-apoptotic protein belonging to the BH3-only subgroup of the Bcl-2 family. It is essential for initiating apoptosis in response to various cell stress signals, including cytokine deprivation, toxin exposure, and other apoptotic stimuli. BIM binds to and neutralizes anti-apoptotic Bcl-2 family proteins, facilitating activation of BAX and BAK, thereby promoting apoptosis.

BMP signaling (bone morphogenetic protein signaling) Is a subset of the TGF-β superfamily, regulates eye morphogenesis, lens induction, retinal differentiation, and corneal development through Smad1/5/8 phosphorylation and non-Smad pathways. BMPs are categorized based on sequence homology and function:

Group 1: Prototypical BMPs (Involved in Bone, Cartilage, and Eye Development)

- BMP2, BMP4 → Optic vesicle, lens, and retinal development
- BMP5, BMP6, BMP7 → Corneal differentiation, lens fiber formation
- BMP8a, BMP8b → Less studied in ocular biology

Group 2: GDF Subfamily (Growth and Differentiation Factors)

- GDF5, GDF6, GDF7 → Retina, neural crest, and scleral development

Group 3: Divergent BMPs (Act in Morphogenesis and Neurogenesis)

- BMP9, BMP10 → Retinal vascularization and angiogenesis

Bnip3 (BCl2/adenovirus E1B 19 kDa protein-interacting protein) Bnip3 is a pro-apoptotic protein and a member of the Bcl-2 family. It regulates mitochondrial quality control and induces mitophagy by interacting with autophagy machinery, particularly under hypoxic or stress conditions.

c-Jun Is a protein belonging to the AP-1 (Activator Protein-1) transcription factor complex. It regulates gene expression in response to cellular stimuli, such as stress, growth factors, and cytokines.

C-Terminal Is the end of the protein and contains the carboxyl group (-COOH) of the last amino acid.

c-Myc Is a well-known transcription factor that enhances mTOR expression by binding to its promoter in response to growth signals.

Caspase Caspases are a family of cysteine proteases that play essential roles in programmed cell death (apoptosis) and inflammation. They are named for their ability to cleave proteins at specific cysteine residues adjacent to aspartic acid. Caspases are produced as inactive precursors (zymogens) that are activated through proteolytic cleavage in response to pro-apoptotic signals. Once activated, they execute apoptosis by cleaving key cellular proteins, leading to the orderly disassembly of the cell.

CASTOR (cytosolic arginine sensor for mTORC1) CASTOR1 and CASTOR2 are proteins that directly bind arginine and function as cytosolic sensors for arginine. They regulate mTORC1 activity in response to cellular arginine levels, with CASTOR1 inhibiting mTORC1 when arginine is scarce.

Demethylation Demethylation is the process of removing a methyl group (CH_3) from a molecule. In genetics, it commonly refers to the removal of methyl groups from DNA or histones, leading to changes in gene expression.

DEPTOR (DEP domain containing mTOR-interacting protein) DEPTOR is an endogenous inhibitor of the mTOR (mechanistic target of rapamycin) pathway. It interacts with mTOR complexes (mTORC1 and mTORC2) and regulates their activity. By inhibiting mTOR signaling, DEPTOR plays a crucial role in controlling cell growth, proliferation, and survival.

DNA (deoxyribonucleic acid) The molecule that carries genetic information in cells.

(DNA-PKcs) DNA-dependent protein kinase catalytic subunit Is a critical enzyme in the non-homologous end joining (NHEJ) pathway of DNA double-strand break repair. It forms a complex with the Ku protein (Ku70/Ku80) to recognize and bind DNA breaks. DNA-PKcs phosphorylates itself and other proteins to facilitate the repair process. It plays essential roles in maintaining genomic stability and is implicated in cancer and other diseases when its function is compromised.

Drosha-DGCR8 complex Also known as the Microprocessor complex, is a key component in the biogenesis of microRNAs (miRNAs). Drosha, an RNase III enzyme, works in partnership with DGCR8, a double-stranded RNA-binding protein, to cleave primary miRNAs (pri-miRNAs) into precursor miRNAs (pre-miRNAs) within the nucleus. This processing is essential for the maturation of miRNAs, which play crucial roles in post-transcriptional gene regulation.

EFTFs (eye field transcription factors) Regulates eye specification and development and including Pax6, Rx, Six3, Lhx2, and Otx2.

eIF4B (eukaryotic initiation factor 4B) Is a protein that plays a crucial role in the initiation of translation in eukaryotic cells. It facilitates the recruitment of ribosomes to mRNA by promoting the unwinding of secondary structures in the 5′ untranslated region of mRNAs. eIF4B works in conjunction with other initiation factors, such as eIF4A and eIF4F, to enhance the efficiency of translation initiation, which is essential for protein synthesis and cell growth.

Elk Is a member of the ETS-domain transcription factor family and is primarily involved in regulating gene expression in response to extracellular signals

FasL (Fas ligand) Is a transmembrane protein belonging to the tumor necrosis factor (TNF) family. It plays a crucial role in inducing apoptosis by binding to its receptor, Fas (CD95), triggering the death receptor pathway. FasL is vital for immune system regulation, particularly in maintaining immune privilege and eliminating harmful or unnecessary cells.

FcεRI (high-affinity IgE receptor) Is a key receptor on mast cells, basophils, and dendritic cells, responsible for initiating allergic responses. Upon binding IgE antibodies, FcεRI triggers mast cell degranulation, leading to the release of histamine, prostaglandins, and cytokines, which drive allergic inflammation.

FAT (FRAP, ATM, TRRAP domain) Is a protein interaction domain found in a family of kinases, including FRAP (mTOR), ATM (ataxia-telangiectasia mutated), and TRRAP (transformation/transcription domain-associated protein). This domain is involved in the regulation of these kinases and plays a key role in various cellular processes such as cell cycle control, DNA repair, and signal transduction.

FATC (FAT C-terminal domain) Is the highly conserved C-terminal domain of the PIKK family of protein kinases, which includes mTOR, ATM, and ATR. This domain is involved in the regulation of kinase activity and is essential for the function of these enzymes, often through interactions with regulatory proteins and other domains within the kinase.

FKBP12 (FK506 binding protein 12 kDa) Is a small 12 kDa protein that belongs to the immunophilin protein family, which plays a role in immunosuppression and neuronal signaling. It binds to immunosuppressant drugs like FK506 (tacrolimus) and rapamycin. In the context of mTOR signaling, FKBP12 binds to rapamycin and then to the FRB domain of mTOR, inhibiting its activity and affecting cell growth and proliferation.

FOXO (Forkhead box O) Which refers to a subgroup within the larger family of Forkhead transcription factors. These transcription factors are characterized by a distinct DNA-binding domain known as the Forkhead box. FOXO proteins play crucial roles in regulating gene expression involved in various cellular processes such as apoptosis, cell-cycle control, glucose metabolism, oxidative stress resistance, and longevity. The FOXO family includes several members, such as FOXO1, FOXO3, FOXO4, and FOXO6, which are involved in different signaling pathways, notably those mediated by insulin and growth factors.

FRB (FKBP12-rapamycin binding domain) Is part of mTOR and is the binding site for the immunosuppressant drug rapamycin when it forms a complex with FKBP12 (a peptidyl-prolyl isomerase). The binding of the FKBP12-rapamycin complex to the FRB domain inhibits mTOR function, particularly affecting the mTORC1 pathway involved in cell growth and proliferation.

GABARAPs (GABA type A receptor-associated proteins) Are a subfamily of Atg8 proteins crucial for autophagy. They assist in autophagosome formation, autophagy-lysosome fusion, and selective autophagy processes like mitophagy. Beyond autophagy, GABARAPs regulate intracellular trafficking of key receptors, such as the γ-GABAA and angiotensin II AT1 receptors. Their involvement in cellular homeostasis links them to various diseases, including cancer, cardiovascular disease, and neurodegenerative disorders, making them potential therapeutic targets and biomarkers for disease prognosis.

GAP (GTPase-activating protein) Proteins are a family of regulatory molecules that accelerate the hydrolysis of GTP bound to GTPases, which are molecular switches involved in cellular signaling. By enhancing the GTPase activity of these switches, GAPs convert them from their active GTP-bound state to their inactive GDP-bound state, effectively turning off the signal transduction pathways they control. This regulation is essential for controlling a wide range of cellular functions including growth, differentiation, and movement. GAPs play crucial roles in the regulation of various types of GTPases, including the Rho, Ras, and Rab families, each of which is involved in different cellular processes and signaling pathways.

GATORs (GAP activity towards Rags) Are multiprotein complexes that play a crucial role in regulating the mTORC1 (mechanistic target of rapamycin complex 1) pathway, which is vital for cell growth and nutrient response. GATORs are composed of two distinct complexes:

1. *GATOR1:* This complex functions as a negative regulator of mTORC1. It is composed of three subunits: DEPDC5, NPRL2, and NPRL3. GATOR1 acts as a GTPase-activating protein (GAP) for RagA and RagB, which are GTPases that regulate mGameTORC1 activity in response to amino acid levels. By inactivating RagA and RagB, GATOR1 inhibits mTORC1, reducing cell growth and proliferation under nutrient-poor conditions.
2. *GATOR2:* In contrast to GATOR1, GATOR2 acts to promote mTORC1 activity and consists of subunits such as Mios, WDR24, WDR59, SEH1L, and Sec13. GATOR2 inhibits the activity of GATOR1, thereby facilitating the activation of mTORC1 in the presence of sufficient nutrients.

The interplay between GATOR1 and GATOR2 complexes is critical for amino acid-sensitive regulation of mTORC1, linking cellular growth signals to nutrient availability and ensuring that cellular growth does not occur under nutrient-restricted conditions.

GATSL3 Is an arginine sensor that negatively regulates mTORC1, a pathway crucial for aging and lifespan regulation. Its varying expression levels across different age groups suggest it could be pivotal in age-related changes in mTORC1 activity. Targeting GATSL3 may offer therapeutic benefits for age-related conditions by modulating mTORC1 signaling.

Gli transcription factor GLI transcription factors (GLI1, GLI2, and GLI3) are key mediators of the Hedgehog (Hh) signaling pathway. They regulate gene expression involved in cell proliferation, differentiation, and tissue development. GLI1 acts as an activator, while GLI2 and GLI3 can function as both activators and repressors, depending on Hh signaling activity.

GPCRs (G-protein-coupled receptors) These are a large family of cell surface receptors that respond to various external signals, such as hormones, neurotransmitters, and light. Upon ligand binding, GPCRs activate intracellular G-proteins, which then trigger various signaling pathways, regulating physiological processes like vision, taste, immune response, and cell growth. GPCRs play a critical role in many biological functions and are important drug targets.

GRB 10 Is a protein that is activated by mTORC1 and acts to inhibit insulin and other growth factor signaling pathways, further reducing PI3K/AKT activity.

GSK3β (glycogen synthase kinase 3 beta) Is a serine/threonine kinase involved in various cellular processes, including metabolism, cell proliferation, and apoptosis. It is constitutively active and regulated by phosphorylation. GSK3β plays significant roles in the Wnt signaling pathway and is implicated in diseases such as diabetes, Alzheimer's disease, and cancer, making it a potential target for therapeutic intervention.

GTPase Is a family of enzymes that hydrolyze guanosine triphosphate (GTP) into guanosine diphosphate (GDP) and a phosphate molecule, a process that releases energy. GTPases function as molecular switches in many cellular processes, including signal transduction, protein synthesis, and cell division.

HEAT repeats Protein motifs consisting of tandemly repeated alpha-helical structures, involved in intracellular transport processes.

HIF-1α (hypoxia-inducible factor-1α) Under low oxygen conditions, HIF-1α can increase mTOR transcription, linking mTOR activity to hypoxic responses.

HSF1 (heat shock factor 1) Is a transcription factor that regulates the expression of heat shock proteins (HSPs), which are critical for maintaining protein homeostasis and protecting cells from stress-induced damage.

IGF (insulin-like growth factors) Which play a role in growth and development and are involved in the regulation of cell growth and survival.

Histones Histones are proteins that help package and organize DNA into structural units called nucleosomes. They play a crucial role in regulating gene expression by controlling the accessibility of DNA to transcription factors and other proteins.

HKII (hexokinase II) It can influence mTOR signaling by affecting cellular energy status. By catalyzing the first step of glycolysis, HKII promotes ATP production. High ATP levels support mTOR activation, promoting cell growth and proliferation. Additionally, HKII's interaction with mitochondria can integrate metabolic signals with mTOR pathways, linking glucose metabolism to mTOR-mediated anabolic processes.

IKK (IκB kinase) Is a critical enzyme complex involved in the NF-κB (nuclear factor kappa-light-chain-enhancer of activated B cells) signaling pathway. It consists of two kinase subunits, IKKα and IKKβ, and a regulatory subunit, IKKγ (also known as NEMO). IKK is activated in response to various stimuli, including inflammatory cytokines and microbial infections. Once activated, IKK phosphorylates IκB proteins, leading to their degradation and the subsequent release and nuclear translocation of NF-κB. This activation promotes the transcription of genes involved in inflammation, immune response, cell survival, and proliferation.

Immunophilins Immunophilins are a family of highly conserved proteins that have the ability to bind to immunosuppressive drugs such as cyclosporin, tacrolimus (FK506), and sirolimus (rapamycin). They are characterized by their peptidyl-prolyl cis-trans isomerase (PPIase) activity, which helps in protein folding by catalyzing the rotation of proline residues in polypeptide chains. Immunophilins are divided into two main classes based on their drug-binding properties:

1. *FK506-binding proteins (FKBPs):* These bind to FK506 (tacrolimus) and rapamycin. They play roles in protein folding, immune response regulation, and signal transduction pathways involving calcineurin and mTOR.
2. *Cyclophilins (Cyps):* These bind to cyclosporin A and are involved in similar cellular processes as FKBPs, including protein folding and modulation of the immune response through their role in the calcineurin signaling pathway.

Both types of immunophilins are involved in complex formation with their respective immunosuppressive drugs to inhibit specific phosphatases like calcineurin, thus preventing activation of T-cells and reducing immune responses. This makes them crucial targets for immunosuppressive therapy, particularly in organ transplantation and autoimmune diseases.

IRS Insulin receptor substrates, key adaptor proteins that transmit signals from the insulin and IGF-1 receptors to intracellular pathways.

Kinase An enzyme that catalyzes the transfer of phosphate groups, usually from ATP to specific substrates, a critical step in many signaling pathways.

LATS1/2 (large tumor suppressor 1 and 2) Are serine/threonine kinases in the Hippo signaling pathway. They phosphorylate and inhibit YAP/TAZ, preventing their nuclear translocation and suppressing cell proliferation and tumorigenesis, thus maintaining tissue homeostasis.

LC3 (microtubule-associated protein 1A/1B-light chain 3) Is a protein involved in autophagy, specifically in the formation of autophagosomes. It exists in two forms, LC3-I and LC3-II, with LC3-II being associated with the autophagosome membrane. LC3 is widely used as a marker for autophagy due to its role in autophagosome maturation and degradation.

Lhx2 (LIM homeobox 2) Is a key transcription factor essential for early eye development. It is required for optic vesicle formation, retinal progenitor maintenance, and eye field specification. It is controlled by FGF and other signaling pathways to ensure proper eye formation.

LKB1 (liver kinase B1) Is a tumor suppressor protein that acts as a serine/threonine kinase. It activates AMPK (AMP-activated protein kinase) and other related kinases, regulating cellular energy homeostasis. LKB1 plays a crucial role in controlling cell growth, metabolism, and polarity, and its dysfunction is linked to various cancers.

MDM2 (mouse double minute 2) Is an E3 ubiquitin ligase that regulates the tumor suppressor protein p53. MDM2 binds to p53, promoting its ubiquitination and subsequent degradation by the proteasome. This interaction controls p53 levels and activity, thereby modulating cell cycle progression, apoptosis, and DNA repair. Overexpression of MDM2 can lead to decreased p53 activity, contributing to tumorigenesis.

mEAK7 (mammalian EAK-7) Is a protein involved in cellular growth and proliferation. It functions as a regulator of the mTOR (mechanistic target of rapamycin) signaling pathway, particularly influencing mTORC1 activity. mEAK7 plays a role in processes like autophagy and metabolism, and its dysregulation is associated with cancer progression, making it a potential target for therapeutic research.

miR-29 Is a family of microRNAs (miR-29a, miR-29b, and miR-29c) involved in regulating gene expression at the post-transcriptional level. It plays critical roles in various biological processes, including fibrosis, apoptosis, and extracellular matrix remodeling.

mLST8 (mammalian lethal with SEC13 protein 8) Is a core component of mTORC1, mTORC2, and mTORC4 complexes. It stabilizes these complexes by binding to the kinase domain of mTOR, contributing to their activity in cellular growth, metabolism, and autophagy. Dysregulation of mLST8 and mTOR signaling is associated with diseases such as cancer, metabolic disorders, and neurodegenerative diseases.

MORG1 (mitogen-activated protein kinase organizer 1) Is a WD-repeat protein that interacts with the selective autophagy receptor SQSTM1/p62 and the regulator complex on the lysosomal surface. It inhibits mTORC1 activity to enable basal autophagy flux and controls the spatiotemporal localization of mTORC1, ensuring its proper activation in response to nutrient availability.

Myc transcription factor Is a transcription factor that regulates the expression of genes involved in cell growth, proliferation, metabolism, and apoptosis. It binds to specific DNA sequences to activate or repress target gene transcription, playing a critical role in normal cellular functions and cancer development when dysregulated.

mSIN1 (mammalian stress-activated protein kinase interacting protein 1) Is a crucial component of the mTORC2 complex, it interacts directly with mTOR and is essential for the activation of Akt, a key regulator of cell survival and growth. Through its interaction with mTORC2, mSIN1 influences various cellular processes including cytoskeletal organization and ion transport. Its function is pivotal in regulating the cellular response to environmental stresses and growth signals.

MSK (mitogen- and stress-activated kinase) These proteins are a group of serine/threonine kinases activated by the ERK and p38 MAPK pathways. They play a role in regulating gene expression in response to stress and mitogenic signals by phosphorylating transcription factors like CREB and histones, thereby modulating chromatin structure and transcriptional activity.

MST1/2 (mammalian STE20-like kinases 1 and 2) Are key serine/threonine kinases in the *Hippo signaling pathway*, regulating cell proliferation, apoptosis, and organ size. They activate downstream effectors like LATS1/2, leading to the inhibition of transcriptional co-activators YAP/TAZ, thereby suppressing uncontrolled growth and tumorigenesis.

N-terminal The N-terminal is the start of the protein and contains the amino group (-NH2) of the first amino acid.

NF-κB (nuclear factor kappa-light-chain-enhancer of activated B cells) Is a transcription factor involved in regulating immune response, inflammation, cell survival, and proliferation. It is activated by various stimuli, including cytokines, stress, and pathogens. Once activated, NF-κB translocates to the nucleus, where it promotes the expression of target genes involved in immune and inflammatory responses, cell growth, and survival. Dysregulation of NF-κB is associated with chronic inflammation, autoimmune diseases, and cancer.

NFAT (nuclear factor of activated T-cells) Is a family of transcription factors that play a central role in regulating gene expression in response to calcium signaling.

NOXA Stands for *"Damage"* in Latin and is a pro-apoptotic protein regulated by p53, belonging to the BCL-2 family. It promotes apoptosis by antagonizing anti-apoptotic proteins like MCL-1, facilitating mitochondrial outer membrane permeabilization and cytochrome c release.

OPTX2 (Six6) Is a homeobox transcription factor essential for eye and pituitary development. It regulates retinal progenitor cell proliferation and differentiation. Mutations are linked to microphthalmia and anophthalmia.

P21 (Waf1/Cip1) P21 (Waf1/Cip1) is a cyclin-dependent kinase inhibitor (CDKI) that regulates cell cycle progression by binding to and inhibiting cyclin-CDK complexes. It is a transcriptional target of p53 and plays a key role in cell cycle arrest, particularly in response to DNA damage, to allow for repair or initiate apoptosis if the damage is irreparable.

P27 (Kip1) P27 (Kip1) is a cyclin-dependent kinase inhibitor (CDKI) that regulates cell cycle progression by inhibiting cyclin-CDK complexes, particularly those involved in the G1 to S phase transition. It acts as a tumor suppressor and is critical for maintaining cell cycle control and cellular quiescence.

p53 Is a tumor suppressor protein that plays a crucial role in regulating the cell cycle, DNA repair, apoptosis, and genomic stability. It acts as a transcription factor, responding to cellular stress and damage by activating genes that halt cell proliferation, initiate DNA repair, or trigger programmed cell death (apoptosis). Mutations or inactivation of p53 is commonly associated with cancer development.

p70S6K (ribosomal protein S6 kinase beta-1) Is a serine/threonine kinase that plays a crucial role in the regulation of cell growth, proliferation, and survival. It is a downstream target of the mTOR (mammalian target of rapamycin) signaling pathway and is involved in protein synthesis and cell cycle progression.

p110 Is the catalytic subunit of PI3K (Phosphoinositide 3-kinase). It phosphorylates phosphatidylinositols to produce PIP3, activating downstream signaling pathways, including AKT, which regulate cell growth, survival, and metabolism. Different isoforms of p110 (e.g., p110α, p110β, p110δ) are involved in various cellular processes and have distinct roles in health and disease.

PAX6 (Paired Box 6) Is a key transcription factor crucial for eye, brain, and pancreatic development. It regulates genes involved in ocular morphogenesis, neurogenesis, and cell differentiation. Mutations in *PAX6* cause aniridia, microphthalmia, and other congenital eye disorders. It also influences corneal and retinal development, playing a role in ocular disease pathogenesis.

PDGF (platelet-derived growth factor) Is a mitogenic signaling molecule that plays crucial roles in cell proliferation, survival, migration, and differentiation, particularly in development, wound healing, and angiogenesis.

PDK1 (phosphoinositide-dependent kinase-1) Is a crucial signaling protein that plays a central role in cellular signaling pathways, particularly those regulating growth, survival, and metabolism. PDK1 is best known for its function in the phosphoinositide 3-kinase (PI3K)/Akt pathway, where it phosphorylates and activates Akt (also known as protein kinase B, PKB) at the threonine 308 position near its amino terminus. This activation is a critical step in the PI3K pathway, leading to a cascade of downstream effects that promote cell survival, growth, and proliferation. PDK1 itself is activated in response to signals from growth factors and other extracellular cues that stimulate PI3K to produce phosphatidylinositol (3,4,5)-trisphosphate (PIP3), a lipid molecule that anchors PDK1 to the plasma membrane where it can interact with its substrates. Beyond Akt, PDK1 also phosphorylates a range of other AGC kinases (a group of protein kinases including PKA, PKG, and PKC families), affecting various cellular processes. Its universal role in multiple signaling pathways underscores its importance in cellular regulation and has made it a target of interest for therapeutic intervention in diseases such as cancer and diabetes.

PGC-1α (peroxisome proliferator-activated receptor gamma coactivator 1-alpha) Is a transcriptional coactivator that plays a pivotal role in regulating cellular energy metabolism. Activation of PGC-1α enhances mitochondrial biogenesis, oxidative metabolism, and thermogenesis. It is activated by various physiological stimuli, including exercise, cold exposure, and fasting. PGC-1α promotes the expression of genes involved in energy production, fat oxidation, and glucose metabolism, thereby improving metabolic efficiency and endurance. Its activation is crucial for maintaining metabolic health and has therapeutic potential in metabolic disorders, neurodegenerative diseases, and muscle function.

PI3K (phosphoinositide 3-kinase) Is a family of enzymes involved in cellular functions such as growth, proliferation, differentiation, motility, survival, and intracellular trafficking. PI3Ks phosphorylate the 3′ position of the inositol ring of phosphatidylinositol, a critical step in the activation of the AKT signaling pathway. The activation of PI3K is often triggered by receptor tyrosine kinases and G-protein-coupled receptors. Dysregulation of PI3K activity is commonly associated with cancer, making it a target for therapeutic intervention.

PIKK (phosphatidylinositol 3-kinase-related kinase) Is a family of serine/threonine. These kinases are involved in a wide range of cellular processes including DNA damage response, cell cycle control, and growth regulation. They share a similar structure and mechanism, using phosphatidylinositol lipids as substrates to initiate various signaling pathways critical for cellular stress responses, development, and maintenance of genomic integrity.

PGC-1α (peroxisome proliferator-activated receptor gamma coactivator 1-alpha) Is a transcriptional coactivator that regulates genes involved in energy metabolism. It plays a crucial role in mitochondrial biogenesis, oxidative phosphorylation, and adaptive thermogenesis. PGC-1α is highly expressed in tissues with high energy demands, such as skeletal muscle, heart, and brown adipose tissue. It is also involved in the regulation of glucose and lipid metabolism and is associated with various metabolic disorders, including diabetes and obesity.

Phosphorylation The addition of a phosphate group to a protein or other organic molecules, a common mechanism for regulating protein activity.

PLCγ (phospholipase C gamma) pathway Is activated downstream of receptor tyrosine kinases, leading to hydrolysis of PIP2 into IP3 and DAG. This generates intracellular calcium release and activates protein kinase C (PKC), mediating diverse cellular processes like proliferation, differentiation, and migration.

PTEN-induced kinase 1 (PINK1) Is a mitochondrial serine/threonine-protein kinase that regulates mitochondrial quality control by activating mitophagy, and is the process that removes damaged mitochondria. It is essential for cellular energy homeostasis and is implicated in neurodegenerative diseases like Parkinson's disease.

PIP2 (phosphatidylinositol 4,5-bisphosphate) PIP2 is a minor component of the cell membrane lipids but plays a major role in cellular signaling pathways. It acts as a substrate for several key enzymes, including phospholipase C (PLC), which cleaves PIP2 to produce inositol triphosphate (IP3) and diacylglycerol (DAG), second messengers involved in calcium signaling and protein kinase C activation.

PIP3 (phosphatidylinositol 3,4,5-trisphosphate) PIP3 is generated from PIP2 by the action of phosphoinositide 3-kinase (PI3K). It serves as a crucial signaling molecule, particularly in the AKT signaling pathway. PIP3 recruits AKT and other signaling proteins to the cell membrane, where they are activated to regulate various cellular functions, including growth, survival, and metabolism. The activity of PIP3 is negatively regulated by PTEN, which dephosphorylates PIP3 back to PIP2, thus inhibiting the signaling pathway.

PKC (protein kinase C) Is a family of enzymes regulating cell signaling, activated by diacylglycerol (DAG) and sometimes calcium. It controls processes like growth, apoptosis, and migration, with dysfunction linked to diseases like cancer.

PRAS40 (proline-rich Akt substrate 40 kDa) Is a signaling protein that acts as an important regulator of the mTORC1 (mechanistic target of rapamycin complex 1) pathway. It binds directly to mTORC1 and inhibits its activity in an Akt-dependent manner. PRAS40 phosphorylation by Akt leads to its dissociation from mTORC1, thereby promoting mTORC1 activation and subsequent protein synthesis. PRAS40 is involved in cellular processes such as growth, survival, and metabolism, playing a key role in integrating signals from growth factors and nutrients.

Protein kinase C delta (PKCδ) Is a serine/threonine kinase involved in apoptosis, cell growth, and differentiation. It is activated by signals like diacylglycerol (DAG) and reactive oxygen species (ROS). PKCδ plays key roles in cancer, cardiovascular diseases, and neurodegenerative disorders, making it a potential therapeutic target.

PTEN (phosphatase and tensin homolog) Is a tumor suppressor gene that negatively regulates the PI3K/AKT signaling pathway. PTEN is a critical tumor suppressor gene that encodes a protein phosphatase involved in regulating the PI3K/Akt signaling pathway. This protein acts by dephosphorylating phosphatidylinositol (3,4,5)-trisphosphate (PIP3), thereby acting as an antagonist to PI3K and inhibiting downstream signaling that promotes cell growth and survival. Mutations or deletions in the PTEN gene are common in a variety of cancers, emphasizing its key role in cell cycle regulation and preventing tumorigenesis.

RAG (recombination activating gene) Has two variations as RAG1 and RAG2 and are essential proteins that mediate V(D)J recombination, a process necessary for the development of diverse antigen receptors in B and T lymphocytes. This diversity allows the adaptive immune system to recognize a vast array of pathogens: Rag GTPases function as heterodimers, with each dimer consisting of either RAGA or RAGB paired with RAGC or RAGD. These proteins play a critical role in activating mTORC1 by sensing amino acid availability in the cellular environment.

RAPTOR (regulatory-associated protein of mTOR) It is a critical component of the mTOR complex 1 (mTORC1), serving as an adaptor protein that recruits mTORC1's substrates for phosphorylation. RAPTOR facilitates the assembly of the mTORC1 complex and helps determine its substrate specificity and localization within the cell. It plays a pivotal role in regulating cell growth and metabolism in response to nutrient availability and other environmental signals.

RAS (rat sarcoma) It originates from the discovery of the RAS gene in rats, where it was identified as an oncogene capable of inducing sarcoma, a type of cancer. RAS proteins are small GTPases that play critical roles in signal transduction pathways, regulating cellular processes such as growth, differentiation, and survival. RAS mutations are notably prevalent in many types of human cancers, emphasizing their importance in medical research and cancer biology. They are the family of GTPases involved in transmitting signals from cell surface receptors to intracellular signaling pathways, and affect cell growth, differentiation, and survival. RAS proteins act as binary molecular switches, cycling between an active and inactive state. They are a focal point in various signaling pathways, primarily the MAPK/ERK pathway, which influences cell division and survival. Dysregulation and mutations in RAS genes are common in cancer, making them significant targets in oncology research.

Rax (retina and anterior neural fold homeobox) Is a crucial transcription factor involved in early eye development. It plays a key role in the specification and maintenance of the eye field during embryogenesis.

REDD1 (regulated in development and DNA damage responses 1) Is a stress-responsive protein that plays a significant role in the regulation of the mTOR signaling pathway. It is involved primarily in the cellular response to hypoxia, as well as other stress conditions such as DNA damage, energy stress, and nutrient deprivation.

Rheb (Ras homolog enriched in brain) Is a small GTPase protein that plays a crucial role in cell growth and metabolism. It is a key regulator of the mechanistic target of rapamycin complex 1 (mTORC1). Rheb activates mTORC1 by binding to it directly when in its GTP-bound state. This activation promotes anabolic processes, including protein and lipid synthesis. Rheb's activity is tightly controlled by the TSC1/TSC2 complex, which functions as a GTPase-activating protein (GAP) to convert Rheb-GTP to its inactive GDP-bound form, thereby inhibiting mTORC1 signaling.

Rho family Small GTPases are signaling proteins that regulate cytoskeletal dynamics, cell migration, division, and adhesion. Key members, including RhoA, Rac1, and Cdc42, act as molecular switches, cycling between active (GTP-bound) and inactive (GDP-bound) states, influencing processes like cell shape and motility.

RICTOR (rapamycin-insensitive companion of mTOR) Is a key component of the mTOR Complex 2 (mTORC2). Unlike RAPTOR, RICTOR is involved in forming mTORC2, which is insensitive to the drug rapamycin in most contexts. RICTOR contributes to the regulation of the actin cytoskeleton, cell survival, and lipid metabolism. It is particularly important for the activation of AKT by phosphorylating it at Ser473, a crucial step required for full AKT activation and its subsequent downstream signaling effects.

RNA (ribonucleic acid) A molecule essential for coding, decoding, regulation, and expression of genes.

RTKs (receptor tyrosine kinases) They are a class of cell surface receptors that, upon binding to ligands such as growth factors, dimerize and auto-phosphorylate on tyrosine residues. This activation triggers downstream signaling pathways, including the MAPK, PI3K-AKT, and JAK-STAT pathways, regulating cell proliferation, differentiation, survival, and metabolism. RTKs are crucial in development and tissue homeostasis, and their dysregulation is associated with various cancers and other diseases.

Rx (Rax) Is a homeobox gene essential for retinal development. It regulates progenitor cell proliferation and eye formation. Mutations cause anophthalmia and microphthalmia.

S6K (ribosomal protein S6 kinase) Refers to a family of protein kinases, including S6K1 and S6K2, which are downstream effectors of mTORC1. These kinases phosphorylate the S6 ribosomal protein, leading to an increase in protein synthesis and cell growth. S6K is a critical component of the signaling pathways that regulate cell size and metabolism.

SAMTOR (S-adenosylmethionine sensor upstream of mTORC1) Is a protein that senses levels of S-adenosylmethionine (SAM), a critical methyl donor in the cell. It interacts with GATOR1, a component of the amino acid sensing pathway upstream of mTORC1, linking methionine metabolism and mTORC1 signaling.

SGK1 (serum- and glucocorticoid-inducible kinase 1) Is a serine/threonine kinase that is part of the AGC family of kinases. It plays significant roles in regulating ion transport, cell survival, and cell proliferation. It shares functional similarities with Akt, influencing several cellular pathways by phosphorylating a range of substrates involved in apoptosis, transcription, and other metabolic processes.

Signaling cascades Sequential processes where a signal is transmitted through a series of molecular events, often involving phosphorylation, to elicit a cellular response.

Six3 Is a homeobox transcription factor critical for forebrain and eye development. It regulates progenitor cell proliferation and lens formation. Mutations cause holoprosencephaly and eye malformations.

Six6 (sine oculis homeobox 6) Is a transcription factor crucial for eye development. Regulates retinal progenitor proliferation and differentiation. Influenced by FGF and other signaling pathways.

SLC (solute carrier family) The SLC family includes numerous membrane-bound transporters that facilitate the transport of a wide variety of solutes across cellular membranes. These transporters are crucial for many physiological processes, including nutrient uptake, ion transport, and waste removal.

SMAD proteins "SMAD" does not stand for an acronym; rather, it is a name derived from the fusion of two words from the names of the first two proteins of this type to be discovered: "Sma" from the *Caenorhabditis elegans* gene Sma, and "Mad" from the *Drosophila* gene Mothers against decapentaplegic. Together, these form the term "SMAD." SMAD proteins are intracellular signal transducers and transcriptional modulators that mediate the effects of the TGF-β (transforming growth factor beta) superfamily of cytokines on cell processes such as proliferation, differentiation, and apoptosis. They are critical components of pathways essential for developmental biology and cellular homeostasis. They are crucial for translating extracellular signals from TGF-beta ligands into specific transcriptional responses that regulate cell proliferation, differentiation, and death. Upon activation, SMAD proteins translocate to the nucleus where they influence gene expression.

SMO (smoothened) protein Is a G-protein-coupled receptor-like protein that transduces Hedgehog (Hh) signaling by activating GLI transcription factors, regulating cell growth and development.

Smurf2 Is an E3 ubiquitin ligase that targets TGF-β signaling proteins, including receptor-regulated Smads, for degradation, thereby modulating cellular processes like proliferation, differentiation, and fibrosis.

SQSTM1/p62 Also known as sequestosome 1, is a multifunctional adaptor protein involved in various cellular processes, including autophagy, cell signaling, and the degradation of ubiquitinated proteins. It acts as a link between ubiquitinated proteins and the autophagy machinery, facilitating their degradation. p62 also plays a role in regulating inflammation and oxidative stress, making it significant in the context of diseases such as cancer and neurodegeneration.

SREBP pathway (sterol regulatory element-binding protein) Is a transcription factor that regulates lipid homeostasis by controlling the expression of genes involved in cholesterol, fatty acid, and triglyceride biosynthesis. It is activated in response to low cellular lipid levels.

STAT proteins (signal transducers and activators of transcription) These proteins are key components of the JAK-STAT signaling pathway. They are activated in response to cytokines and growth factors. Upon activation, STAT proteins are phosphorylated, dimerize, and then translocate to the nucleus where they act as transcription factors to regulate the expression of genes involved in development, immune function, and cell survival.

TEAD1-4 Are transcription factors in the TEAD (TEA Domain) family, crucial mediators of the Hippo signaling pathway. They regulate gene expression related to cell proliferation, differentiation, and survival by interacting with co-activators like YAP and TAZ. Dysregulation of TEAD proteins is linked to cancer and organ size abnormalities.

TERT (telomerase reverse transcriptase) Is the catalytic subunit of the enzyme telomerase. It maintains telomere length by adding repetitive nucleotide sequences to the ends of chromosomes, preventing cellular aging and allowing cells to divide indefinitely. TERT is crucial for the immortality of cancer cells and plays a significant role in cellular aging and stem cell function.

TFEB (transcription factor EB) Is a master regulator of lysosomal biogenesis and autophagy. It belongs to the MiT/TFE subfamily of basic helix-loop-helix leucine zipper transcription factors. TFEB controls the expression of genes involved in the autophagy-lysosome pathway, enhancing the clearance of cellular debris and damaged organelles. Its activity is regulated by nutrient availability and cellular stress, primarily through phosphorylation that controls its localization between the cytoplasm and nucleus.

TGF-β (transforming growth factor beta) TGF-β is a multifunctional cytokine that regulates ocular development, immune homeostasis, and fibrosis. It signals via Smad-dependent and Smad-independent pathways to control cell proliferation, differentiation, and extracellular matrix (ECM) remodeling.

TRIM (tripartite motif) family of proteins They comprise a large group of E3 ubiquitin ligases characterized by a conserved tripartite structure: a RING finger, one or two B-boxes, and a coiled-coil domain. They regulate diverse cellular processes, including protein degradation, immune response, and cell proliferation.

TSC1 (tuberous sclerosis complex 1) TSC1, also known as Hamartin, is a protein that plays a key role in cellular growth and proliferation regulation. TSC1 forms a complex with TSC2, acting as a tumor suppressor. This complex inhibits the mTORC1 pathway, which is involved in cell growth and division. Mutations in the TSC1 gene are associated with the genetic disorder tuberous sclerosis, which causes non-malignant tumors to grow in the brain and other vital organs.

TSC2 (tuberous sclerosis complex 2) TSC2, also known as Tuberin, partners with TSC1 to form the tuberous sclerosis complex, functioning as a GTPase-activating protein (GAP) for the small G protein Rheb, a direct activator of mTORC1. By inhibiting Rheb, the TSC1-TSC2 complex effectively suppresses mTORC1 activity, thereby regulating cell growth and proliferation. Like TSC1, mutations in TSC2 are linked to tuberous sclerosis, highlighting its critical role in controlling cell growth and preventing tumor formation.

TSP1 (thrombospondin-1) Is a glycoprotein that regulates cell adhesion, angiogenesis, and immune responses. It inhibits angiogenesis by activating TGF-β and interacting with CD36, suppressing endothelial cell proliferation. TSP1 also modulates extracellular matrix remodeling and promotes immune cell recruitment, playing roles in cancer, wound healing, and vascular diseases.

ULK (Unc-51 like autophagy activating kinase) ULK1 and ULK2 are serine/threonine kinases that play a pivotal role in the initiation of autophagy. They form a complex with several other proteins to initiate autophagy in response to nutrient depletion or other stress signals.

WD-repeat protein Is characterized by the presence of WD repeats, which are minimally conserved regions of approximately 40 amino acids that typically end with a tryptophan-aspartic acid (WD) dipeptide. These repeats facilitate protein-protein interactions, enabling the formation of multiprotein complexes. WD-repeat proteins play key roles in various cellular processes, including signal transduction, cell cycle control, and apoptosis, by providing a stable scaffold for the assembly of protein complexes.

Wnt pathway (wingless-integration) Is a cell signaling system essential for embryonic development, cell proliferation, and tissue homeostasis. It involves Wnt proteins binding to Frizzled receptors and LRP5/6 co-receptors, leading to the inhibition of a destruction complex. This inhibition allows β-catenin to accumulate and move into the nucleus, where it activates gene transcription. Dysregulation of the Wnt pathway is linked to cancers and other diseases.

Wortmannin Is a potent and specific inhibitor of phosphoinositide 3-kinases (PI3Ks). It is a steroidal metabolite originally isolated from the fungus *Talaromyces wortmannii*. Wortmannin works by binding irreversibly to the catalytic subunit of PI3K, thereby inhibiting its activity. This inhibition affects various cellular processes that PI3K regulates, including cell growth, survival, metabolism, and migration.

XPC (xeroderma pigmentosum, complementation group C) Is a DNA damage recognition protein critical for nucleotide excision repair (NER), identifying and initiating repair of helix-distorting lesions caused by UV radiation and chemical damage.

YAP/TAZ (yes-associated protein and WWTR1 transcription co-activator) YAP and TAZ are transcriptional co-activators regulated by the Hippo signaling pathway. They play crucial roles in cell proliferation, survival, and differentiation by modulating gene expression. Dysregulation of YAP/TAZ is associated with cancer, fibrosis, and regenerative processes.

Acknowledgments

I acknowledge the use of controlled AI-assisted tools in the preparation, drafting, and refinement of this book. These technologies were employed to enhance clarity, structure, and accuracy while ensuring adherence to scientific rigor and integrity. All interpretations, conclusions, and insights presented remain my own, guided by established literature, professional references, and expertise.

No grants, financial assistance, or compensation were received from any organizations, universities, or companies for the preparation of this book.

The author declares that there are no financial interests or personal relationships that could be considered potential competing interests.

All expenses related to the preparation of this book were personally financed by the author.

I extend my gratitude to my graphic designer, *David Folender*, for his collaboration in creating all the images featured in this book.

A special thanks to my brother, *Hamid R. Moazed*, for his invaluable assistance in the preparation and editing of this book

Contents

Chapter 1
Molecular Biology of mTOR

Contents

Abstract Molecular biology of mTOR (mechanistic target of rapamycin) introduces the structure, function, and regulation of the mTOR complexes, which are essential in integrating both intracellular and extracellular signals in a cell. In this chapter, we explore the structure of the mechanistic target of rapamycin (mTOR) molecule, delving into its role across various functions, and brief signaling pathways as we discuss the more detailed mTOR signaling pathways in the next chapter. While the molecular intricacies of mTOR and its pathways might seem daunting, our goal is to demystify these complexities by explaining the basic key players involved in these molecular interactions, for a better understanding the essentials of mTOR complexes. We hope that this chapter would be more accessible and relevant to a broader audience beyond molecular biologists.

K. T. Moazed, *mTOR Signaling in Ophthalmology*,
https://doi.org/10.1007/978-3-032-05044-1_1

Discussions

In biology, mTOR regulates and orchestrates critical cellular functions such as growth, metabolism, and autophagy (cellular recycling), ensuring that cells respond appropriately to environmental cues. However, when dysregulated, mTOR signaling contributes to the pathogenesis of numerous diseases, including cancer, neurodegenerative disorders, cardiovascular and metabolic syndromes. By modulating key pathways, mTOR balances the delicate equilibrium between cellular growth and stress responses, making it a pivotal node in the network of cellular homeostasis (Figs. 1.1 and 1.2).

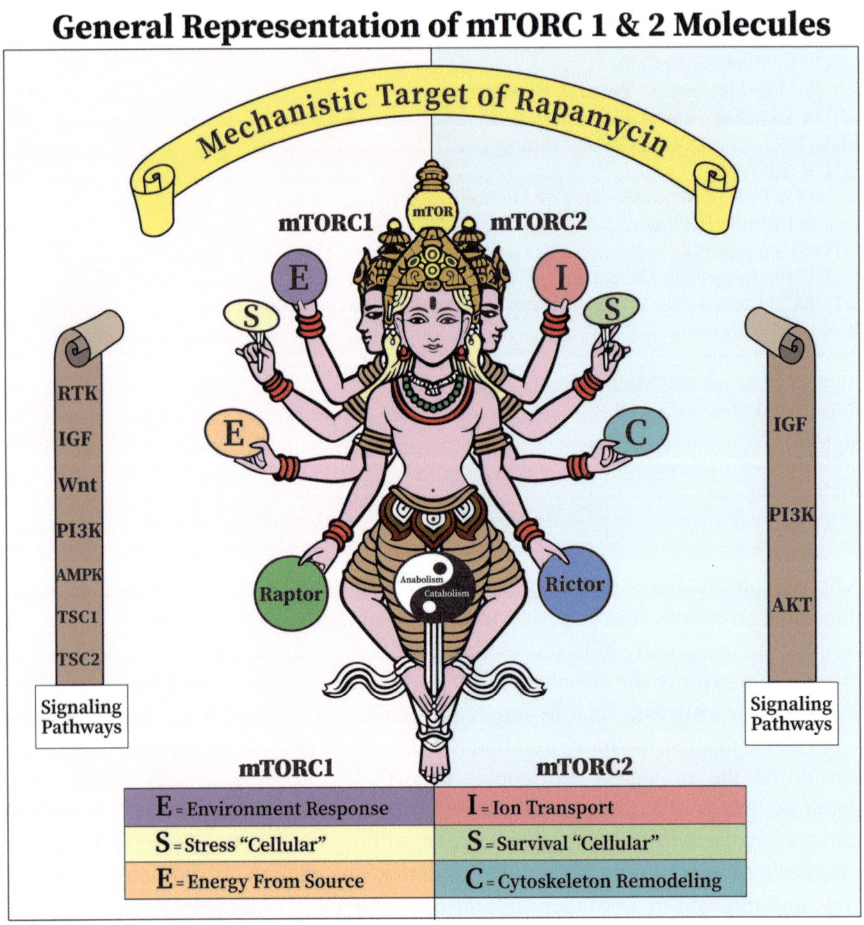

Fig. 1.1 The image represents the complex molecules of mTOR which at present is consistent with four complexes; the first two mTORC1 and mTORC2 are represented above. Each complex has its own signaling pathways and cellular functions as shown

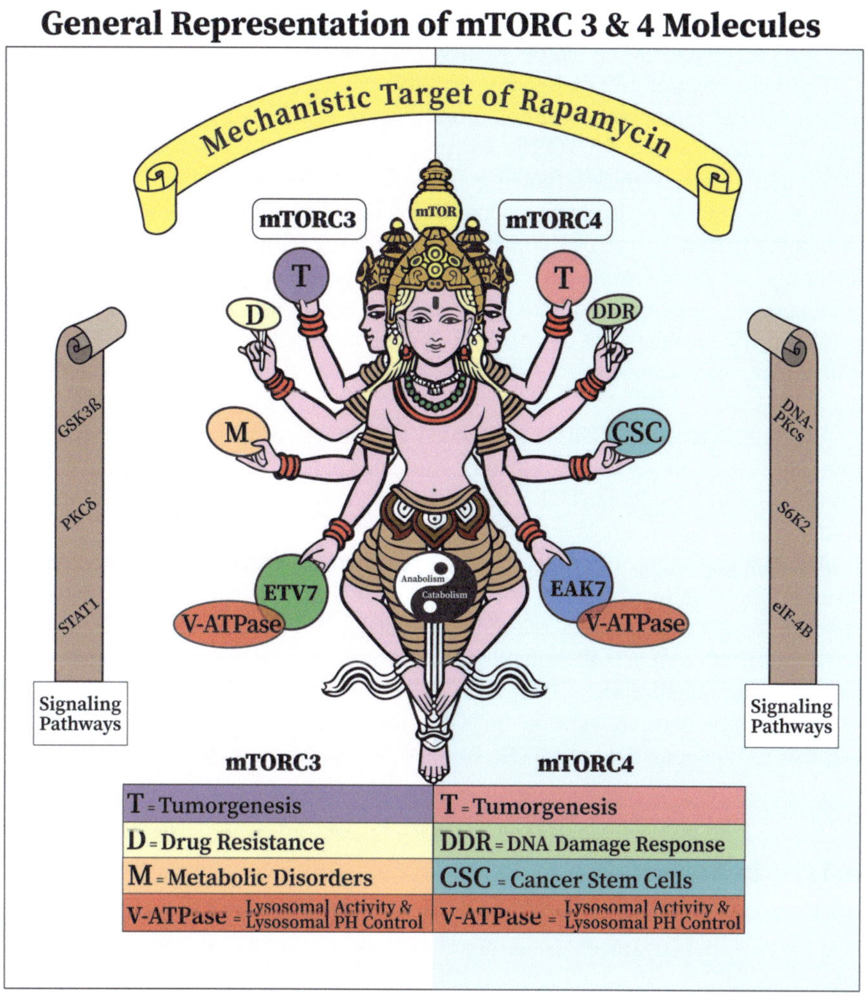

Fig. 1.2 The image represents the complex molecules of mTOR which at present is consistent with four complexes; of which, mTORC3 and mTORC4 are represented above. Each complex has its own signaling pathways and cellular functions as shown

The dual role of mTOR in regulating autophagy underscores the complexity of its involvement in cellular homeostasis and disease, particularly in cancer. The dynamic nature of mTOR's control over autophagy, where it can both inhibit and promote this process depending on cellular conditions, highlights its critical role in balancing cellular survival and stress responses.

The fact that mTOR suppresses autophagy in nutrient-rich conditions to favor growth and anabolism, while autophagy is promoted when mTOR activity is inhibited, reflects the adaptability of cells to fluctuating environmental and internal signals. This adaptability is especially pertinent in cancer, where the modulation of autophagy by mTOR can have paradoxical effects—either supporting tumor growth and survival or sensitizing tumors to therapeutic interventions.

The many roles of mTOR signaling are also critical in the central nervous system (CNS) and has implications for both normal brain function and neurological disorders. The involvement of mTOR in key processes such as neuronal survival, synaptic plasticity, and cognitive functions underscores its importance in maintaining brain health. The tight mechanistic connection between mTOR and the TSC1/TSC2 complexes (tuberous sclerosis complexes), especially in the context, illustrates how disruptions in this pathway can lead to a wide range of neurological manifestations, from epilepsy to neuropsychiatric disorders and brain tumors. The upregulation of mTOR in TSC patients and its potential as a therapeutic target for epilepsy is a significant area of research, particularly given the challenges in managing epilepsy in these patients.

The link between mTORC1-associated autophagy and neurodegenerative diseases like Alzheimer's and Parkinson's further expands the relevance of mTOR in the CNS, suggesting that mTOR's regulatory functions extend beyond developmental disorders to age-related neurodegeneration.

Another important role of mTOR is in cardiac physiology and cardiovascular diseases, highlighting the broad impact of this signaling pathway. The regulation of conditions such as pulmonary arterial hypertension, myocardial infarction, and atherosclerosis through mTOR signaling adds another dimension to its significance in human health and disease.

This comprehensive view of mTOR's roles across different organ systems emphasizes the potential for mTOR-targeted therapies in a wide range of diseases.

mTOR in Mammalian Cells

The study of mTOR (mechanistic target of rapamycin) has its roots in the 1960s, when researchers embarked on an expedition to Easter Island, known by its inhabitants as Rapa Nui. This expedition aimed to identify natural products from plants and soil that might have therapeutic potential [28]. In 1972, Suren Sehgal and his colleagues made a significant discovery: they identified a small molecule produced by the soil bacterium *Streptomyces hygroscopicus* which initially garnered attention for its potent antifungal properties [46].

Streptomyces hygroscopicus is a species of soil-dwelling bacterium known for its production of several important bioactive compounds. Most notably, it is the source of rapamycin (also known as sirolimus), a potent inhibitor of the mTOR (mechanistic Target of Rapamycin) pathway. The compound was named rapamycin after the indigenous name of the island, Rapa Nui. Later on, some other effects of this molecule were discovered which are briefly summarized below:

- *Antifungal Activity:* Rapamycin was initially studied for its ability to inhibit the growth of fungi, making it a candidate for antifungal treatments.

- *Immunosuppressive Properties:* Further research revealed that rapamycin had powerful immunosuppressive effects, making it useful for preventing organ transplant rejection. This led to its development as a drug, known as sirolimus.
- *Cancer Research*: mTOR inhibitors are now being explored and used as treatments for various cancers, as mTOR signaling is often dysregulated in cancer cells.
- *Metabolic Diseases*: Understanding mTOR's role in metabolism has led to insights into diseases such as diabetes and obesity.
- *Neurodegenerative Diseases*: mTOR plays a critical role in the pathogenesis of neurodegenerative diseases through its regulation of autophagy, protein synthesis, and cellular metabolism.
- *Cardiovascular Diseases:* Dysregulation of mTOR is linked to a variety of cardiovascular diseases, including atherosclerosis, hypertension, heart failure, and cardiac hypertrophy. Inhibition of mTOR, particularly mTORC1, has been explored as a therapeutic strategy to reduce vascular inflammation, prevent arterial plaque formation, and improve heart function.
- *Aging and Longevity*: mTOR is also implicated in the regulation of lifespan and aging, with studies suggesting that modulating mTOR activity can influence aging processes.
- *Viral diseases*: mTOR plays a dual role in viral infections, supporting viral replication while also impacting the host immune response.

Before discussing the function of the mTOR molecule, it's essential to understand the basic molecular structure of proteins and become familiar with their molecular biology. Proteins are intricate molecules that play critical roles in almost all biological processes.

The human body uses about 20 amino acids to build proteins, but only nine of them are considered essential because they cannot be synthesized by the body and must be obtained from the diet. The 20 amino acids can be categorized as essential, conditionally essential and non-essential (Fig. 1.3).

Essential Amino Acids

1. *Histidine*: Important for growth and tissue repair
2. *Isoleucine*: Involved in muscle metabolism and immune function
3. *Leucine*: Key for protein synthesis and muscle repair
4. *Lysine*: Necessary for protein synthesis, hormone, and enzyme production
5. *Methionine*: A precursor to other amino acids and essential for metabolism and detoxification
6. *Phenylalanine*: Precursor for neurotransmitters like dopamine
7. *Threonine*: Crucial for collagen and elastin production
8. *Tryptophan*: Precursor for serotonin, a neurotransmitter that regulates mood and sleep
9. *Valine*: Important for muscle growth and tissue repair

Fig. 1.3 The table above contains approximately 20 consequential amino acids in 3 groups; essential amino acids, conditionally essential amino acids and non-essential amino acids

Amino Acids

Essential Amino Acids	3 Letter	1 Letter
Histidine	His	H
Isoleucine	Ile	I
Leucine	Leu	L
Lysine	Lys	K
Methionine	Met	M
Phenylalanine	Phe	F
Threonine	Thr	T
Tryptophan	Trp	W
Valine	Val	V
Conditionally Essential Amino Acids		
Arginine	Arg	R
Cysteine	Cys	C
Glycine	Gly	G
Glutamine	Gln	Q
Proline	Pro	P
Tyrosine	Tyr	Y
Non-Essential Amino Acids		
Alanine	Ala	A
Aspartic Acid	Asp	D
Asparagine	Asn	N
Glutamic Acid	Glu	E
Serine	Ser	S

Conditionally Essential

10. *Arginine*: Important for immune function and hormone secretion
11. *Cysteine*: Important for protein structure and detoxification
12. *Glycine*: Important for collagen formation and central nervous system function
13. *Glutamine*: Involved in immune function and intestinal health
14. *Proline*: Crucial for collagen stability
15. *Tyrosine*: Precursor for neurotransmitters and hormones like dopamine and thyroid hormones

Non-essential Amino Acids

16. *Alanine*: Plays a role in glucose metabolism
17. *Aspartic Acid*: Plays a role in the citric acid cycle
18. *Asparagine*: Involved in metabolic control of cell functions
19. *Glutamic Acid*: A key neurotransmitter
20. *Serine*: Involved in metabolism and immune function

These amino acids work together to support various physiological processes, including protein synthesis, enzyme function, and cellular communication.

There is a specific set of vocabulary and abbreviations in molecular biology, for the molecular interaction between the signaling proteins and enzymes, which is described in "Pretext" part of this book, making it crucial for understanding these processes.

Since all biological events occur at a molecular and an atomic level, the foundation of biology and the medical science is based on these interactions, which are critical for understanding how proteins like mTOR functions within the cell.

Basic Protein Structure

The structure of a protein is intricately linked to its function. From the linear sequence of amino acids forming the primary structure to the complex interactions that define the higher levels of structure, each aspect of a protein's architecture is essential for its role in life processes. Proteins are fundamental molecules within biological systems, playing a myriad of roles from structural support to catalyzing biochemical reactions. Understanding the basic structure of a protein molecule is essential for grasping how these versatile molecules function in various biological processes, as these structures are essential not only in biochemistry and molecular biology, but also in developing new therapies and treatments in medicine.

Here is a simplified structure of a basic protein molecule (Fig. 1.4).

Levels of Protein Structure

Proteins have four levels of structure: primary, secondary, tertiary, and quaternary. Each level of structure plays a critical role in defining the final shape and function of the protein.

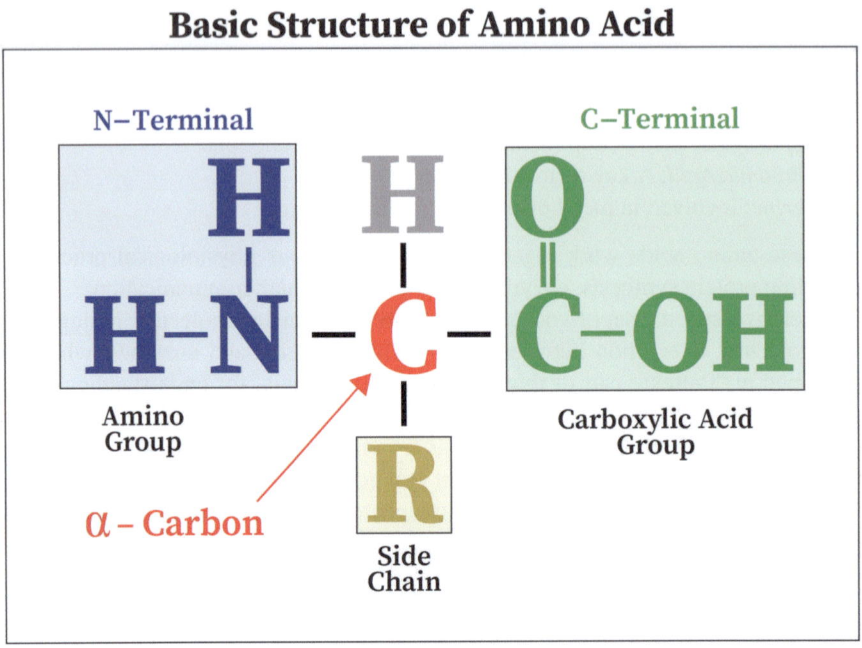

Fig. 1.4 The basic structure of amino acids consists of central alpha carbon, which is attached to side chain residue. One end contains amino group (n-terminal), and the other end contains carboxylic acid group (c-terminal)

Primary Structure

- The primary structure of a protein is its unique sequence of amino acids.
- Proteins are made up of around 20 different amino acids, each with a unique side chain (R group) that affects the protein's properties and function.
- The amino acids are linked by peptide bonds, which are formed between the carboxyl group of one amino acid and the amino group of another.
- The sequence of a protein might be written as Ala-Gly-Ser-His, where each name represents an amino acid.

Secondary Structure

The secondary structure refers to the regular, repeating patterns in regions of a protein, primarily due to hydrogen bonding between backbone atoms (Fig. 1.5).

- *Alpha Helix:* This is a right-handed coiled structure, where each turn of the coil involves 3.6 amino acids, and the backbone is stabilized by hydrogen bonds between nearby residues. For example, the helical structure of the protein keratin, found in hair and nails, is an alpha helix.

Fig. 1.5 Illustration of secondary structure of proteins. On the top is the alpha helix structure and on the bottom is the beta sheets

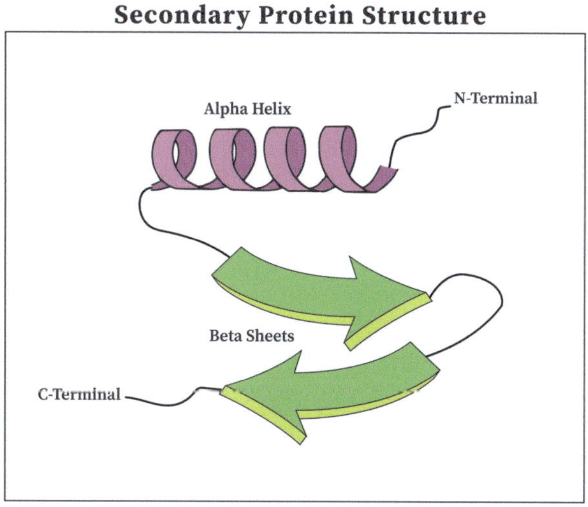

- *Beta Sheet:* This structure can be parallel or anti-parallel, formed by hydrogen bonding between different protein strands (or segments of the same strand), resulting in a flat, pleated sheet appearance. Immunoglobulins contain beta-sheets in their variable and constant regions, providing structural stability necessary for antigen binding.

Tertiary Structure

- The tertiary structure is the overall three-dimensional shape of a single protein molecule.
- The structure is stabilized by a number of interactions, including:
  - *Hydrophobic Interactions:* Non-polar side chains tend to cluster away from water, contributing to the folding of the protein.
  - *Hydrogen Bonds:* Polar side chains can form hydrogen bonds with each other or with surrounding water molecules.
  - *Ionic Bonds:* Also known as salt bridges, these are electrostatic interactions between positively and negatively charged side chains.
  - *Disulfide Bonds:* Covalent bonds that form between cysteine residues, stabilizing the protein's structure.
  - *Van der Waals Forces:* These weak interactions also play a role in stabilizing the protein's shape.

Quaternary Structure

- The quaternary structure is the arrangement and interaction of multiple protein subunits (polypeptide chains) in a multi-subunit complex.
- Similar to those stabilizing the tertiary structure, including hydrophobic interactions, hydrogen bonds, ionic bonds, and sometimes covalent disulfide bonds.
- *For example,* hemoglobin, the oxygen-carrying protein in blood, consists of four subunits (two alpha and two beta chains) that form its quaternary structure.

Protein Function and Importance

The function of proteins can be summarized as follows.

- *Enzymatic Activity:* Many proteins are enzymes that catalyze biochemical reactions, which are crucial for metabolism and other cellular processes.
- *Structural Role:* Proteins like collagen provide structural support in tissues and are key components of connective tissues.
- *Transport and Storage:* Proteins like hemoglobin transport oxygen in the blood, while others store essential nutrients.
- *Signaling:* Proteins are involved in transmitting signals within and between cells to regulate biological processes.
- *Immune Response:* Antibodies are proteins that bind to specific foreign particles, such as viruses and bacteria, to help protect the body.

Basic and Simplified Cellular Process of Protein Synthesis in a Cell

The process of protein synthesis in a cell, particularly in response to external signals, involves a complex series of steps, beginning from the interaction at the cell surface and culminating in the production of a specific protein. Here's a streamlined overview of this process (Fig. 1.6):

Initiation by Ligand Binding: The process starts when a ligand, such as a hormone or growth factor, binds to a specific cell surface receptor. This binding changes the conformation of the receptor and activates it.

Receptor Conformation Change: The activated receptor undergoes a conformational change which often exposes or activates its intrinsic enzymatic activity, such as kinase activity.

Activation of Signal Transduction via Phosphorylation: The conformational change typically activates the receptor's kinase domain, allowing it to phosphorylate itself and/or other target proteins on specific tyrosine, serine, or threonine residues. This phosphorylation serves as a signal to recruit and activate various intracellular signaling proteins.

Domino Effect of Signaling Proteins: These phosphorylated residues create docking sites for signaling molecules containing SH2 (Src Homology 2) or other phospho-

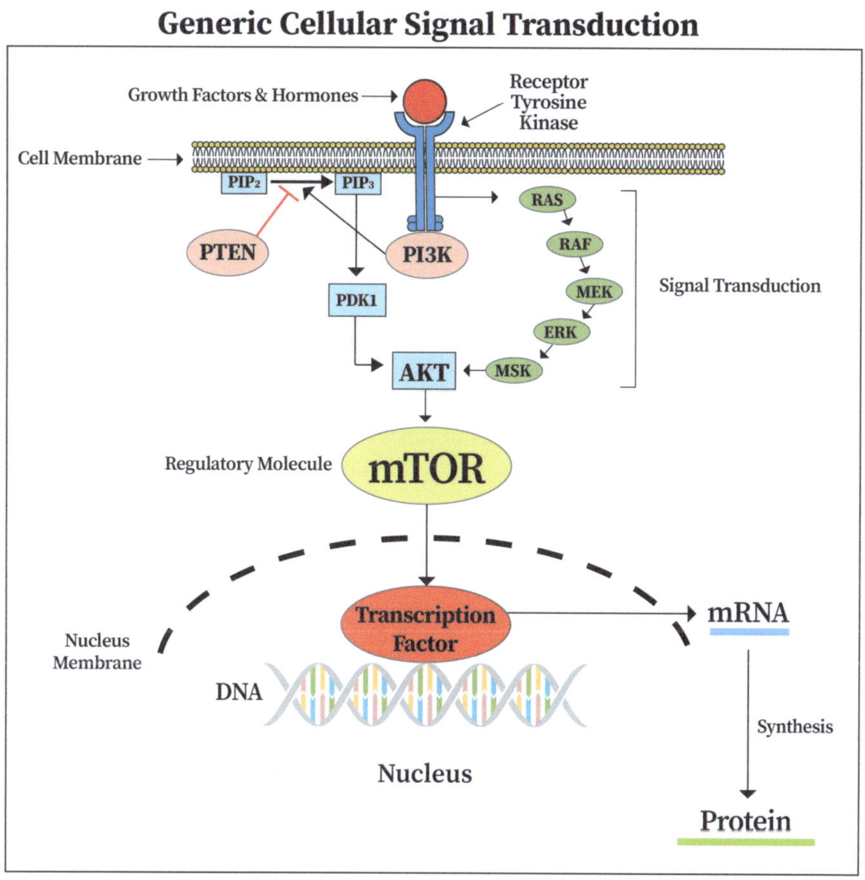

Fig. 1.6 Typical cellular signal transduction begins with attachment of a ligand to the cell membrane receptors which causes confirmation of the receptor and activation of signal transduction proteins. This will activate the regulatory molecule of mTOR which in turn activates the transcription factors in the nucleus producing mRNA for synthesis of necessary proteins

recognizing domains. This triggers a cascade of further phosphorylation, leading to the activation of multiple downstream signaling pathways. Key proteins like SOS (Son of Sevenless) can be activated, which in turn activate small GTPases like Ras.

Activation of mTOR Pathway: Among the pathways activated, the PI3K (phosphoinositide 3-kinase) pathway leads to the production of PIP3 (phosphatidylinositol (3,4,5)-trisphosphate), which recruits and activates protein kinase B (AKT). Activated AKT can then activate mTOR (mechanistic target of rapamycin). mTOR, as part of the mTORC complexes, regulates various cellular functions including cell growth and protein synthesis.

Transcription Factor Activation: mTORC1, for example, can lead to the activation of transcription factors such as SREBP (sterol regulatory element-binding protein) or "ican" indirectly leads to the activation of transcription factors like TFEB (transcription factor EB) by inhibiting their sequestration. These transcription factors then move into the nucleus.

DNA Binding and mRNA Production: Once inside the nucleus, these transcription factors bind to specific DNA sequences near the genes they regulate. The binding initiates or enhances the transcription of these genes into messenger RNA (mRNA).

mRNA Processing and Translation: The newly formed mRNA is processed (capping, tailing, and splicing) and then exported from the nucleus to the cytoplasm. In the cytoplasm, ribosomes read the mRNA sequences and translate them into polypeptides.

Protein Synthesis: These polypeptides fold into functional proteins, sometimes with the aid of chaperones, completing the process of protein synthesis. These proteins can then perform their specific functions in the cell, including acting as enzymes, structural components, or signaling molecules.

Each step in this pathway is tightly regulated and critical for ensuring that cells respond appropriately to their external and internal environments. Disruptions in any part of this chain can lead to diseases such as cancer, metabolic disorders, and inflammatory conditions.

mTOR (The Mechanistic Target of Rapamycin)

The mechanistic target of rapamycin (mTOR) is a central component of the cellular signaling network, regulating growth, proliferation, and survival in response to nutrients, growth factors, and cellular energy status. The mTOR molecule is characterized by multiple structural domains that mediate its function, each playing a critical role in the protein's activity and its interaction with other cellular components mTOR [24].

mTOR is also a central player in cellular regulation, particularly in processes such as autophagy (recycling), growth, and survival. It integrates signals from nutrients, growth factors, and cellular energy status to modulate various cellular processes. mTOR's ability to integrate various signals makes it a central regulator of cellular physiology. Its role is important in maintaining cellular homeostasis and responding to environmental changes. Understanding mTOR's mechanisms and interactions is crucial for developing therapeutic strategies for diseases related to dysregulated mTOR signaling, such as cancer, metabolic disorders, neurodegenerative diseases and viral infections such as HIV. Understanding the intricate regulatory networks involving mTOR and its complexes is essential for developing effective therapies.

mTOR gene is located on the "p" arm of chromosome 1, at location 1p36.22, as seen in Fig. 1.7.

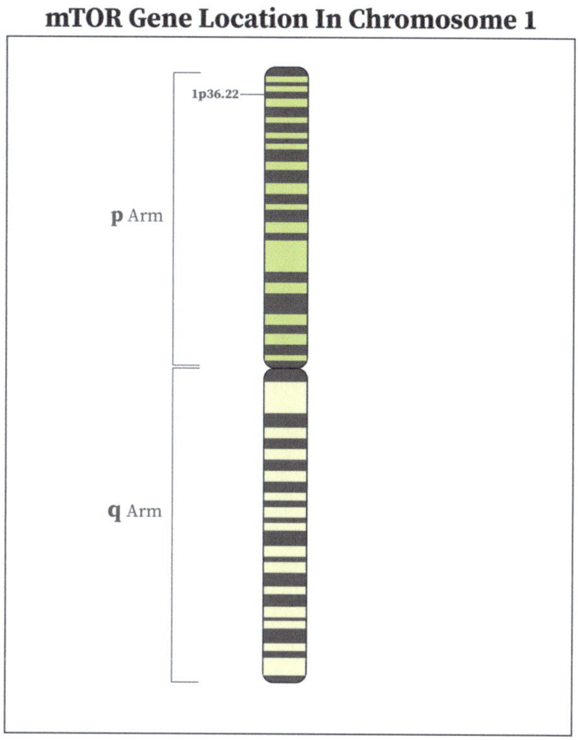

Fig. 1.7 The mTOR gene is located on the short arm (p arm) of chromosome 1 at position 1p36.22, as shown above

The Molecular Structure of mTOR

The mechanistic target of rapamycin (mTOR) is a conserved serine/threonine kinase and a member of the PI3K-related kinase (PIKK) family. It contains several conserved domains.

mTOR was initially discovered in the budding yeast *Saccharomyces cerevisiae* through the screening of rapamycin-resistant mutants. Remarkably, all studied organisms possess a single mTOR kinase, underscoring its evolutionary conservation and fundamental role in cellular biology.

The mechanistic target of rapamycin (mTOR) protein contains several important structural domains that contribute to its function as a key regulator of cell growth and metabolism. In summary, these main structural domains are (Fig. 1.8):

- Heat domains (N-Heat and M-Heat) (Huntingtin, elongation factor 3, A subunit of protein phosphatase 2A, and TOR1)
- FAT (FRAP, ATM, and TRRAP) domain
- FRP domain (FATC-rapamycin binding)
- Kinase domain
- Serine- and threonine-rich negative regulatory domain (NRD)
- FATC domain (FAT C-terminal)

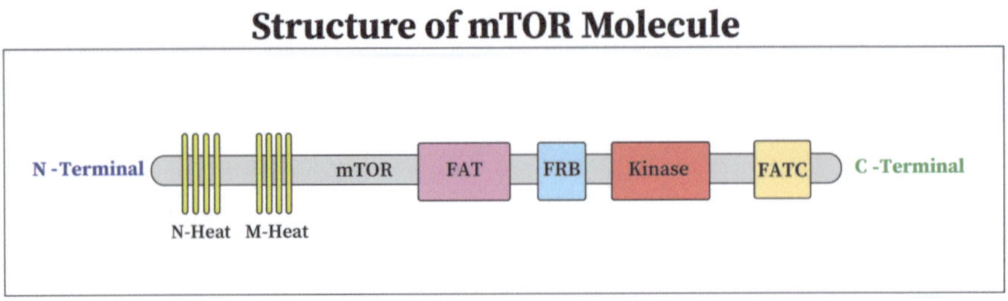

Fig. 1.8 Structural domains of mTOR molecule composed of N-Heat & M-Heat domains, FAT domain, FRB domain, Kinase domain and FATC domain

Here is a structured overview of the domains of the mTOR molecule:

1. HEAT Repeats in mTOR (N-HEAT and M-HEAT Domains)

   HEAT repeats contribute to the overall structural stability of mTOR, ensuring that it maintains its functional conformation and plays a crucial role in the structural organization and function of mTOR. HEAT repeats are named after four proteins: Huntingtin, elongation factor 3, the A subunit of protein phosphatase 2A, and TOR1. These repeats are involved in protein-protein interactions and are found in multiple copies within the mTOR protein.

   - *The N-HEAT domain*: It is located at the N-terminal region of the mTOR protein. This domain is thought to be involved in the regulation of mTOR's interaction with other proteins, including regulatory components of the mTORC1 and mTORC2 complexes. It provides a scaffold that helps stabilize the structure of mTOR and facilitates its interactions with other proteins and complexes.
   - *The M-HEAT Domain*: It is located in the middle region of the mTOR protein. Similar to the N-HEAT domain, the M-HEAT domain contributes to the structural integrity of mTOR. It also plays a role in the binding of mTOR to various regulatory proteins and complexes, influencing the assembly and function of mTORC1 and mTORC2.

   HEAT repeat is a structural motif found in many proteins and are crucial for understanding protein function and interaction networks within the cell, making them a significant focus in molecular biology and structural biochemistry research. They are located at the N-terminus, and in the middle of mTOR, there are more than 20 HEAT repeats, typically consisting of two alpha-helices connected by a short loop, and these repeats often stack together to form elongated solenoid structures. These repeats create a hydrophobic surface that is crucial for protein-protein interactions. The structure of these repeats facilitates the localization of mTOR to the cell membrane, where many of its upstream signaling interactions occur.

   HEAT repeats in mTOR provide a scaffold for the binding of various regulatory proteins and complexes, which enable mTOR to interact with and be regulated by proteins such as Raptor, Rictor, and other components of mTOR complexes. This localization is essential for the protein to receive and process signals that dictate cellular growth and survival. HEAT repeats are involved in various cellular processes, such as intracellular transport, signaling, and the structural organization of protein complexes. They are known for providing a flexible scaffold that can adapt to different functional needs, making them integral to protein-protein interactions and the dynamic aspects of cellular machinery. HEAT repeats play a crucial role in the activation and inhibition of mTOR. This regulation is essential for the proper functioning of mTOR in response to cellular signals such as nutrient availability and growth factors.

2. *Focal Adhesion Targeting (FAT) Domain*: This domain, composed of approximately 568 amino acids, is essential for the specific interactions that mTOR mediates within the cell. The FAT domain interacts with another FAT domain located at the C-terminus (FATC). This interaction is vital for exposing the kinase domain (KIN), allowing it to become active or accessible to other regulatory proteins and substrates.
3. *FKBP12-Rapamycin Binding (FRB) Domain*: The FRB domain of mTOR is a crucial mediator of its interaction with external inhibitory molecules. When rapamycin binds to the FK506-binding protein of 12 kD (FKBP12), this complex then interacts with the FRB domain of mTOR. This interaction leads to allosteric conformational changes in the KIN domain, inhibiting its kinase activity. This inhibition is a key therapeutic mechanism exploited by rapamycin and similar compounds to modulate mTOR activity in various diseases, including certain cancers and cardiac hypertrophy.
4. *Kinase Domain (KIN)*: The kinase domain of mTOR is where ATP binds, facilitating the transfer of a phosphate group from ATP to specific serine and threonine residues on substrate proteins. This domain is also where ATP-competitive inhibitors bind, providing another mechanism for regulating mTOR activity. The kinase activity of this domain is central to the function of mTOR, as it phosphorylates a variety of substrates that govern cellular processes such as protein synthesis, autophagy, and metabolism.
5. *Serine-Threonine-Rich Negative Regulatory Domain (NRD)*: Located between the KIN and FATC domains, the NRD is rich in serine and threonine residues. This region acts as a negative regulatory domain; phosphorylation of residues in this region can inhibit mTOR activity. The NRD serves as a critical modulator of mTOR function, ensuring that the kinase activity is precisely controlled in response to cellular conditions.
6. *Focal Adhesion Targeting C-terminus (FATC) Domain*: At the very C-terminus of the mTOR protein, the FATC domain interacts with the FAT domain near the N-terminus. This interaction is critical for the structural integrity of mTOR and for the proper exposure and function of the kinase domain. The FATC domain contributes to the overall conformational stability of mTOR and its ability to respond to regulatory signals.

mTOR Signaling Pathways

The mTOR signaling pathway is crucial for regulating cell growth, survival, and proliferation. The phosphorylation of mTOR substrates and the binding of regulatory components significantly influence these downstream processes. These substrates and regulatory components can be subdivided into categories of recognition and regulation, affecting the outputs of signaling cascades associated with the mTOR complexes [24]. The regulation of the balance between cell recycling process (autophagy) and cell death (apoptosis) is one of the fundamental responsibilities of mTOR complexes.

In mammalian cells, mTOR forms the core of several distinct complexes, each with specific components and functions. At present there are four mTOR complexes that have been explored and are discussed here, and also there is a possibility of more complexes to be discovered in the future. mTORC1 and mTORC2 have been studied well in recent years, and ongoing research into the newly discovered functions and interactions of mTORC3 and mTORC4 holds promise for uncovering new mechanisms of disease and identifying novel therapeutic targets.

The signaling pathways affecting mTOR is very complex and will be discussed in the next chapter in more details. Basically, there are "upstream" and "downstream" signals that ae involved in mTOR function. In intracellular signal transduction, the terms "upstream" and "downstream" refer to the direction and sequence of signaling events within a cell. These pathways are crucial for cells to respond appropriately to various stimuli, such as hormones, growth factors, and environmental changes.

Signal Transduction Pathways in mTOR in a nutshell

1. *Upstream Signals*:
   - Nutrients, growth factors, and energy status activate upstream sensors, for example, kinases like PI3K and Akt, which in turn regulate mTOR activity.
2. *mTOR Activation*:
   - mTOR complex integrates these signals to control cellular processes.
3. *Downstream Effects*:
   - mTOR regulates many proteins' synthesis by phosphorylating key targets such as S6K1 and 4E-BP1.
   - They also influence many other functions such as lipid synthesis, autophagy, and metabolism.

Understanding these upstream and downstream pathways is crucial for elucidating how cells process external and internal signals to maintain homeostasis and respond to environmental changes.

Many Roles of mTOR in Cellular Biology

mTOR (mechanistic target of rapamycin) is a key regulator in cellular biology, orchestrating numerous processes related to growth, metabolism, and survival. It controls cell growth by regulating protein synthesis, lipid biosynthesis, and nutrient uptake, responding to signals like nutrients, growth factors, and energy status. mTOR also plays a critical role in autophagy, where it inhibits the degradation of cellular components in nutrient-rich conditions. Furthermore, it regulates immune responses, cell cycle progression, and mitochondrial function, impacting aging, cancer, neurodegeneration, and metabolic diseases.

Some of the many important roles of mTOR are briefly mentioned here, with more detailed descriptions provided later in the text:

mTOR and Autophagy

Autophagy is a cellular degradation process that recycles damaged organelles and proteins to maintain cellular homeostasis [74]. mTOR acts as a key negative regulator of autophagy [12]:

- *Nutrient Sensing*: When nutrients are abundant, mTOR is active and inhibits autophagy by phosphorylating key components of the autophagic machinery, such as ULK1 (Unc-51 like autophagy activating kinase 1).
- *Energy Status*: High energy levels (e.g., ATP) also activate mTOR, further suppressing autophagy. Conversely, low energy levels (high AMP/ATP ratio) inhibit mTOR activity, thereby promoting autophagy to provide an alternative energy source.

Autophagy consists of three primary mechanisms [78] (Fig. 1.9):

1. *Microautophagy*: In this process, the lysosome directly engulfs small portions of the cytoplasm by invagination of the lysosomal membrane. It is a non-selective form of autophagy and plays a role in general cellular maintenance.
2. *Macroautophagy*: Often referred to simply as "autophagy," this is the most well-studied mechanism. It involves the formation of a double-membrane vesicle called an autophagosome, which engulfs larger cellular components (such as damaged organelles or protein aggregates). The autophagosome then fuses with the lysosome to degrade and recycle the contents. Macroautophagy can be selective or non-selective.
3. *Chaperone-Mediated Autophagy (CMA)*: This selective process involves chaperone proteins that recognize specific target proteins containing a KFERQ-like motif. These proteins are transported directly to the lysosome, where they are unfolded and translocated across the lysosomal membrane for degradation.

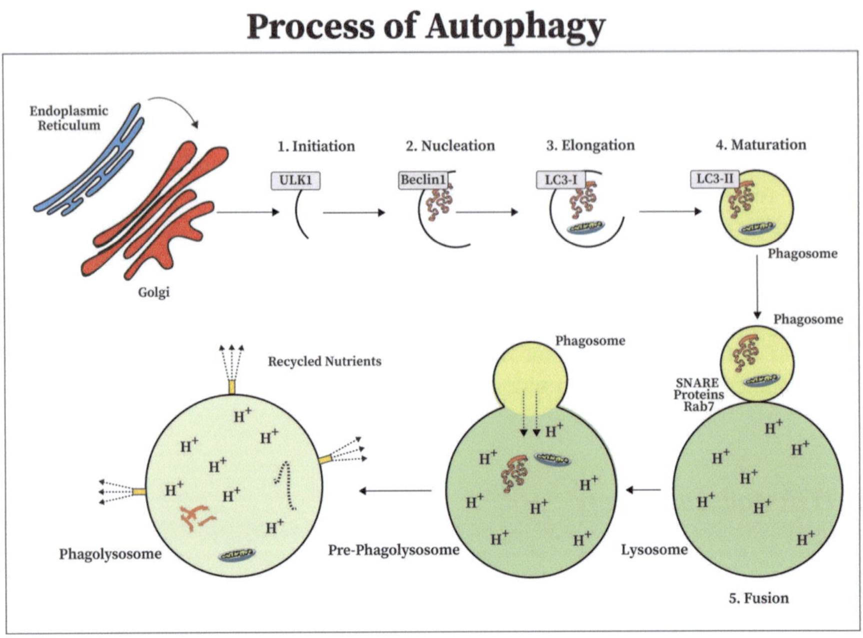

Fig. 1.9 The schematic above represents the process of autophagy (recycling) in the cell. In this process the cellular byproducts are being engulfed by phagosomes which then fuse with lysosomes and form phagolysosomes which further produces recycled nutrients used in the cells for production of new proteins

mTOR and Cellular Growth

mTOR promotes cellular growth and proliferation by stimulating anabolic processes and inhibiting catabolic processes[15]:

- *Protein Synthesis*: mTOR enhances protein synthesis through the phosphorylation of downstream targets like S6K1 (ribosomal protein S6 kinase beta-1) and 4E-BP1 (eukaryotic translation initiation factor 4E-binding protein 1).
- *Lipid Synthesis*: mTOR activation leads to increased lipid synthesis by upregulating key enzymes involved in fatty acid and cholesterol biosynthesis.
- *Nucleotide Biosynthesis*: mTOR promotes the synthesis of nucleotides, which are essential for DNA and RNA production.

mTOR and Cell Survival

mTOR signaling is crucial for cell survival, particularly under stress conditions [24]:

- *Response to Stress*: mTOR helps cells survive by modulating the response to various stresses, including hypoxia and oxidative stress. It does this by regulating pathways involved in mitochondrial function and antioxidant defense.
- *DNA Damage Response*: mTOR influences the DNA damage response and repair mechanisms, contributing to the maintenance of genomic stability.

mTOR and Immune Response

The mechanistic target of rapamycin (mTOR) is a key regulator in cellular immune response. mTOR influences both innate and adaptive immune responses through its effects on various immune cells, including T cells, B cells, dendritic cells, and macrophages. Here's an overview of how mTOR is involved in the immune response [44]:

1. *T Cells:*
   - *Activation and Differentiation:* mTOR is crucial in T-cell activation and differentiation. When T cells are activated by antigen-presenting cells, mTOR signaling promotes the differentiation of naïve T cells into different subsets of T helper (Th) cells, such as Th1, Th2, Th17, and regulatory T cells (Tregs).
   - *Effector T Cells:* mTORC1 (one of the complexes mTOR forms) drives the differentiation of effector T cells, which are necessary for responding to infections and eliminating pathogens.
   - *Regulatory T Cells:* On the other hand, mTORC2 signaling is essential for the development and function of regulatory T cells, which help maintain immune tolerance and prevent autoimmune responses.
2. *B Cells:*
   - mTOR signaling is involved in B-cell development, activation, and differentiation. It influences the generation of plasma cells and memory B cells, which are crucial for long-term immunity.
   - mTORC1, in particular, promotes B cell proliferation and antibody production in response to antigens.
3. *Dendritic Cells:*
   - mTOR affects dendritic cell metabolism and function. It regulates the maturation of dendritic cells and their ability to present antigens to T cells, thereby influencing the initiation of adaptive immune responses.
   - mTOR signaling modulates the production of cytokines by dendritic cells, which in turn affects the polarization of T-cell responses.

4. *Macrophages:*

   - In macrophages, mTOR controls the balance between pro-inflammatory (M1) and anti-inflammatory (M2) phenotypes. mTORC1 promotes the M1 phenotype, which is associated with a strong inflammatory response, while mTORC2 is linked to the M2 phenotype, which is involved in tissue repair and anti-inflammatory functions [54].
   - This balance is crucial in controlling infection, inflammation, and tissue homeostasis.

5. *Autophagy:*

   - mTOR is a major inhibitor of autophagy, a cellular process that is important for degrading and recycling cellular components. Autophagy plays a role in regulating immune responses by controlling the degradation of pathogens, the presentation of antigens, and the survival of immune cells under stress conditions.
   - The inhibition of mTOR can enhance autophagy, which may influence immune cell survival and function, particularly in the context of infections and inflammation.

6. *Immune Diseases and Cancer:*

   - Dysregulation of mTOR signaling is associated with various immune-related diseases, including autoimmune disorders, chronic inflammation, and cancer. Targeting mTOR with specific inhibitors (such as rapamycin) has therapeutic potential in these conditions by modulating the immune response.

Overall, mTOR is a central player in coordinating the immune response, influencing both the activation and suppression of various immune cells. Understanding the precise mechanisms by which mTOR regulates immunity is crucial for developing targeted therapies for immune-related diseases such as HIV.

mTOR and Viral Infections

The mechanistic target of rapamycin (mTOR) plays a significant role in viral infections, influencing both the host's immune response and the replication of viruses. Its involvement can be summarized in two primary aspects:

1. Viral Replication

   - Positive regulation of viral replication: Many viruses exploit the mTOR pathway to promote their replication. mTOR enhances protein synthesis, lipid biosynthesis, and energy production, all of which are essential for the efficient replication of viral particles.
   - Examples: Viruses like HIV[34], human papillomavirus[69], and herpes simplex virus [71] are known to manipulate mTOR signaling to create favorable conditions for their replication.

2. Host Immune Response

   - Immune activation and response: mTOR regulates immune cells, including T cells, dendritic cells, and macrophages, all crucial for mounting antiviral responses. Through mTORC1 and mTORC2, it modulates:

     – T-cell activation: mTOR promotes the differentiation and proliferation of T cells, enhancing the immune system's ability to fight off viral infections.
     – Autophagy regulation: mTOR inhibits autophagy, a process that can either help or hinder viral survival. Some viruses are destroyed via autophagy, while others evade immune detection through its inhibition.

Dual mTOR Role in Viral Infections:

- mTOR as a target for viral therapy: In some cases, inhibiting mTOR with drugs like rapamycin can block viral replication and enhance antiviral autophagy.
- Conversely, inhibiting mTOR might suppress immune functions, potentially worsening viral infections in certain contexts, such as HIV.
- The complexity of mTOR role in HIV infection and its effect on viral reservoir is an example of many functions of mTOR in the cell. One such example is explained in a nutshell: The activation of AKT leads to the inhibition of TSC1, which in turn activates Rheb by converting it to its active GTP-bound state. This activation of Rheb is crucial for mTORC1 signaling, which also depends on an amino acid-sensing branch. DEPDC5, part of the GATOR1 complex, acts as a GTPase-activating protein (GAP) that inhibits the amino acid-sensing branch of mTORC1. Once activated, mTORC1 phosphorylates S6K1 and inhibits the phosphorylation of 4EBP1, thereby promoting mRNA translation. TSC1 and DEPDC5 may help maintain HIV-1 latency by suppressing the AKT-mTORC1 pathway, as shown by evidence where TSC1- or DEPDC5-knockout enhances AKT-mTORC1 signaling and reactivates latent HIV-1, an effect that can be blocked by the mTORC1 inhibitor rapamycin.

mTOR and Cancer

mTOR plays a critical role in cancer by promoting cell growth, survival, and metabolic reprogramming. The dysregulation of mTOR signaling is a hallmark of many cancers, making it a key target for therapeutic intervention. While mTOR inhibitors have shown promise in treating certain cancers, challenges such as drug resistance and the identification of predictive biomarkers remain. Continued research into the role of mTOR in cancer and the development of novel inhibitors and combination therapies holds the potential to improve cancer treatment outcomes [28, 35].

Cancer Cells and Dormancy Cancer cells can also exploit mTOR inhibition to enter a dormant state. By shutting down mTOR signaling, cancer cells may evade therapeutic interventions that target rapidly proliferating cells. This dormancy contributes to cancer recurrence, as dormant cells can survive chemotherapy or radiotherapy and later reactivate under favorable conditions [35].

1. *mTORC1 and Cancer:*
    - *Cell Growth and Proliferation:* mTORC1 promotes cell growth and proliferation by enhancing protein synthesis, lipid biosynthesis, and nucleotide synthesis. This contributes to the rapid growth and division of cancer cells.
    - *Metabolic Reprogramming:* Cancer cells often exhibit altered metabolism, known as the Warburg effect, where they rely on aerobic glycolysis for energy production. mTORC1 supports this metabolic shift by promoting glycolysis and inhibiting oxidative phosphorylation.
    - *Inhibition of Autophagy:* mTORC1 inhibits autophagy, a cellular process that degrades damaged organelles and proteins. In cancer, reduced autophagy can lead to the accumulation of damaged components, promoting genomic instability and tumor progression.
2. *mTORC2 and Cancer:*
    - *Survival and Proliferation:* mTORC2 activates AKT, which promotes cell survival and proliferation. AKT activation leads to the inhibition of pro-apoptotic factors and enhances the activity of proteins involved in cell cycle progression.
    - *Cytoskeleton Organization:* mTORC2 regulates the actin cytoskeleton, which is essential for cell migration and invasion. This regulation supports cancer cell metastasis and the spread of tumors.
3. *mTORC3 and cancer:* mTORC3 appears to play a distinct role in cancer biology, particularly in promoting tumor growth and resistance to certain therapies, such as rapamycin. mTORC3 has been implicated in enhancing the oncogenic potential of cells, as seen in experimental models like rhabdomyosarcoma, where its activation accelerates tumorigenesis.
4. *mTORC4 and cancer:* mTORC4 is a newly proposed complex within the mTOR signaling pathway, potentially involved in regulating cell proliferation and migration through mEAK-7, S6K2, and 4E-BP1. It may also play a role in tumorigenesis and drug resistance by influencing the DNA damage response and cancer stem cell (CSC) maintenance, suggesting its importance in cancer progression and therapy resistance.

Signaling pathways and oncogenesis:

1. *Mutations and Amplifications*
    - *PI3K/AKT Pathway:* Mutations or amplifications in the PI3K/AKT pathway can lead to constitutive activation of mTOR signaling, promoting oncogenesis. For example, activating mutations in PIK3CA (encoding the p110α subunit of PI3K) or loss of function mutations in PTEN (a tumor suppressor that inhibits PI3K) are common in various cancers.

- *mTOR Itself:* Mutations in the mTOR gene can lead to its hyperactivation. These mutations often result in increased mTORC1 and mTORC2 signaling, contributing to tumor growth and survival.

2. *Growth Factors and Nutrients*

   - Cancer cells often have increased sensitivity to growth factors, leading to enhanced mTOR signaling. Additionally, cancer cells can adapt to nutrient availability by altering mTOR activity, ensuring continued growth and survival even under nutrient-deprived conditions.

Clinical Implications

1. *Therapeutic Targeting of mTOR:*

   - *mTOR Inhibitors:* Drugs like rapamycin (sirolimus) and its analogs (rapalogs, e.g., everolimus, temsirolimus) inhibit mTORC1 and have been used in cancer therapy. These inhibitors can reduce tumor growth and enhance the efficacy of other treatments.
   - *Dual mTORC1/mTORC2 Inhibitors:* Second-generation inhibitors target both mTORC1 and mTORC2, potentially providing more effective suppression of mTOR signaling and overcoming resistance to Rapalogs.
   - *Combination Therapies:* mTOR inhibitors are often used in combination with other treatments, such as chemotherapy, targeted therapies, and immunotherapy, to enhance their efficacy and reduce resistance.

2. *Biomarkers for mTOR Inhibition:*

   - Identifying biomarkers that predict response to mTOR inhibitors can help personalize cancer treatment. For example, patients with mutations in the PI3K/AKT/mTOR pathway may benefit more from mTOR-targeted therapies.

3. *Resistance Mechanisms:*

   - Resistance to mTOR inhibitors is a significant challenge in cancer therapy. Mechanisms of resistance include activation of compensatory pathways (e.g., MAPK/ERK), mutations in mTOR pathway components, and feedback activation of upstream signaling pathways.

Few Examples of mTOR in Specific Cancers

1. *Breast Cancer:*

   - mTOR signaling is often dysregulated in breast cancer, particularly in hormone receptor-positive and HER2-positive subtypes. mTOR inhibitors, like everolimus, are approved for the treatment of hormone receptor-positive, HER2-negative advanced breast cancer [40].

2. *Renal Cell Carcinoma:*

   - mTOR inhibitors, such as temsirolimus and everolimus, are used in the treatment of advanced renal cell carcinoma . These inhibitors have shown efficacy in delaying disease progression [63].

3. *Glioblastoma:*

   - Glioblastoma, an aggressive brain tumor, often exhibits hyperactivation of the PI3K/AKT/mTOR pathway. Clinical trials are ongoing to evaluate the efficacy of mTOR inhibitors in this cancer [14].

mTOR and Aging

mTOR Pathway and Cellular Aging

- *Cellular Senescence:* mTOR signaling is associated with cellular senescence, a state where cells cease to divide but remain metabolically active. Senescent cells accumulate with age and contribute to tissue dysfunction and chronic inflammation. mTOR promotes the growth and maintenance of these senescent cells, thereby contributing to the aging process.
- *Protein Synthesis and Quality Control:* mTOR enhances protein synthesis, which is essential for growth and cellular function. However, excessive mTOR activity can lead to the accumulation of damaged or misfolded proteins, overwhelming the cellular protein quality control systems, such as autophagy and the ubiquitin-proteasome system, which are vital for cellular homeostasis and longevity.
- *Inhibition of Autophagy:* mTOR is a major inhibitor of autophagy, a cellular process that degrades and recycles damaged organelles and proteins. Autophagy is known to be critical for longevity and cellular health. By inhibiting autophagy, mTOR can contribute to the accumulation of cellular damage, which is a hallmark of aging.
- *Enhancing Autophagy for Longevity:* Inhibition of mTOR (e.g., using rapamycin) can activate autophagy, which has been shown to extend lifespan in various organisms, including yeast, worms, flies, and mice. This suggests that modulating mTOR activity to enhance autophagy could be a potential strategy for promoting healthy aging.

Mechanisms by Which mTOR Influences Aging

mTOR is a central regulator of aging, influencing key processes such as protein synthesis, autophagy, metabolism, stem cell function, and inflammation. Inhibition of mTOR signaling has been shown to extend lifespan and improve health span in various model organisms by enhancing cellular maintenance mechanisms and reducing the burden of age-related damage. These findings have significant implications for the development of interventions targeting mTOR to promote healthy aging and treat age-related diseases. Continued research into mTOR signaling and its modulation holds promise for improving longevity and quality of life in humans [41].

- *Protein Synthesis:*
  - *Anabolic Processes:* mTORC1 promotes protein synthesis, lipid biosynthesis, and nucleotide synthesis, which are essential for cell growth and proliferation. While these anabolic processes are crucial during development and growth, excessive mTOR activity in later life can contribute to the accumulation of damaged proteins and cellular senescence.
  - *Proteostasis:* High mTORC1 activity can impair proteostasis (the balance of protein synthesis, folding, and degradation), leading to the accumulation of misfolded proteins and aggregates that are associated with age-related diseases such as Alzheimer's and Parkinson's.
- *Autophagy:*
  - *Cellular Cleanup:* mTORC1 inhibits autophagy, a process that degrades and recycles damaged organelles and proteins. Reduced autophagy with age leads to the accumulation of cellular debris, contributing to cellular dysfunction and aging.
  - *Lifespan Extension:* Inhibition of mTORC1, which activates autophagy, has been shown to extend lifespan and improve health span in various organisms. Enhanced autophagy helps maintain cellular homeostasis and reduce the accumulation of damaged components.
- *Metabolism:*
  - *Nutrient Sensing:* mTORC1 integrates signals from nutrients (especially amino acids), growth factors, and energy status to regulate cellular metabolism. Dysregulation of mTOR signaling can lead to metabolic disorders, which are often associated with aging.
  - *Caloric Restriction:* Caloric restriction, which reduces mTORC1 activity, is one of the most robust interventions known to extend lifespan and delay age-

related diseases. This suggests that mTORC1 inhibition mimics some of the beneficial effects of caloric restriction.

- *Stem Cell Function:*
  - *Stem Cell Maintenance:* mTOR signaling plays a role in the maintenance and function of stem cells. Dysregulation of mTOR can lead to stem cell exhaustion, reducing the regenerative capacity of tissues and contributing to aging.
  - *Tissue Regeneration:* Inhibition of mTOR has been shown to enhance stem cell function and tissue regeneration in aged organisms, thereby improving health span.
- *Inflammation and Immune Function:*
  - *Inflammation:* Chronic inflammation, often termed "inflammaging," is a hallmark of aging. mTOR signaling is involved in the regulation of immune responses and inflammation. Inhibition of mTOR can reduce chronic inflammation, which is associated with various age-related diseases.
  - *Immune Senescence:* Aging is associated with a decline in immune function, known as immune senescence. mTOR inhibition has been shown to rejuvenate immune function in aged organisms, enhancing their ability to respond to infections and vaccines.

mTOR Inhibition, Aging, and Longevity

mTOR is a critical regulator of aging processes. Inhibition of mTOR has been shown to extend lifespan in several organisms by modulating cellular maintenance and stress responses. The mechanistic target of rapamycin (mTOR) is a key regulator of cellular growth, metabolism, and survival, and it plays a significant role in the aging process and longevity. The relationship between mTOR and longevity has been a major focus of aging research, with evidence suggesting that modulation of mTOR activity can influence lifespan and health span across various organisms [57].

The inhibition of the mTOR kinase is indeed a critical event that facilitates the entry of cells (including stem cells and certain cancer cells) into a state of quiescence or "cellular hibernation." This state allows cells to conserve energy, reduce metabolic activity, and resist stressful conditions, such as nutrient deprivation or hypoxia.

Ongoing research continues to explore how mTOR signaling can be optimized to promote healthy aging and longevity. Inhibition of mTOR signaling has been shown to extend lifespan and improve health and aging [52]. Life span varies in different organisms, including yeast, worms, flies, mice, primates, and humans [19].

Because mTOR plays a central role in regulating the aging process and longevity, its inhibition, particularly of mTORC1, has been shown to extend lifespan and improve health span in various organisms by promoting autophagy, reducing protein synthesis, and mitigating metabolic stress. However, the effects of mTOR inhibition are complex and context-dependent, requiring careful modulation to balance the benefits of extended lifespan with potential side effects. Ongoing research continues to explore how mTOR signaling can be optimized to promote healthy aging and longevity. The key processes of modulation of cellular aging are as follows:

- *Rapamycin and Lifespan Extension*: Rapamycin, a well-known mTOR inhibitor, has been shown to extend lifespan in various model organisms, including yeast, worms, flies, and mice. The longevity effects of rapamycin are primarily attributed to its inhibition of mTORC1, which leads to enhanced autophagy, reduced protein synthesis, and altered metabolism, all of which are associated with delayed aging and increased lifespan.
- *Autophagy and Cellular Maintenance:* One of the key mechanisms by which mTOR inhibition promotes longevity is through the activation of autophagy. Autophagy is a cellular process that degrades and recycles damaged proteins and organelles, maintaining cellular homeostasis. Enhanced autophagy helps to clear out cellular debris and mitigate the accumulation of damaged macromolecules, which are hallmarks of aging. This process is thought to contribute to the anti-aging effects of mTOR inhibition.
- *Reduced Protein Synthesis and Metabolic Stress:* mTORC1 promotes protein synthesis, which is necessary for growth and maintenance of cellular functions. However, excessive protein synthesis, particularly in aging cells, can lead to metabolic stress and accumulation of misfolded proteins, contributing to cellular dysfunction. mTOR inhibition reduces protein synthesis, thereby decreasing the burden on the protein quality control systems and potentially reducing the rate of age-related cellular damage.

mTOR and Age-Related Diseases

Many age-related diseases have been associated with dysregulation of mTOR molecule and its role in autophagy [78].

- Cancer*:* As was mentioned earlier, mTOR activity is often upregulated in cancer cells, driving their growth and proliferation. By inhibiting mTOR, rapamycin and other mTOR inhibitors can suppress tumor growth, which may contribute to their longevity-promoting effects by reducing the incidence of age-related cancers.
- Metabolic Disorders*:* mTOR is a key regulator of metabolism, and its dysregulation is linked to metabolic diseases such as obesity, type 2 diabetes, and cardiovascular diseases. By modulating mTOR activity, it is possible to improve metabolic health and potentially extend lifespan by delaying the onset of these age-related diseases.
- Neurodegenerative Diseases*:* mTOR signaling is also involved in the regulation of neuronal function and maintenance. Dysregulation of mTOR has been impli-

cated in neurodegenerative diseases such as Alzheimer's and Parkinson's. mTOR inhibition may offer neuroprotective effects by enhancing autophagy and reducing the accumulation of toxic protein aggregates, which are characteristic of these conditions.

- Muscle disorders are associated with the aging process, and mTOR signaling is crucial for muscle growth and repair. Dysregulation can lead to muscle wasting diseases and conditions such as sarcopenia. Sarcopenia, the age-related loss of muscle mass and strength, is a significant health issue, particularly in older adults. The mechanistic target of rapamycin (mTOR) pathway plays a crucial role in the regulation of muscle growth and maintenance, making it a key player in the development and potential treatment of sarcopenia [62].

mTOR and Muscle Protein Synthesis

1. Muscle Growth and Maintenance: mTOR is a central regulator of muscle protein synthesis. It responds to various stimuli, including nutrients (particularly amino acids like leucine), insulin, and mechanical stress (such as exercise). When activated, mTOR promotes the synthesis of muscle proteins by initiating the translation of specific mRNAs involved in muscle growth. This process is vital for maintaining muscle mass and function.
2. Aging and mTOR Signaling: In younger individuals, mTOR activity is robust, supporting muscle protein synthesis and growth. However, with aging, mTOR signaling becomes dysregulated. This dysregulation can lead to impaired protein synthesis, contributing to the progressive loss of muscle mass seen in sarcopenia.

mTOR and Muscle Autophagy

Role of Autophagy in Muscle Health: Autophagy, a cellular process that degrades and recycles damaged proteins and organelles, is essential for maintaining muscle health. mTOR negatively regulates autophagy; when mTOR is highly active, autophagy is suppressed. While mTOR-mediated suppression of autophagy is beneficial for muscle growth in the short term, chronic suppression can lead to the accumulation of damaged proteins and organelles, contributing to muscle dysfunction and sarcopenia over time.

mTOR Inhibition and Sarcopenia

1. Rapamycin and Muscle Health: Rapamycin, an mTOR inhibitor, has been shown to extend lifespan in various model organisms, partly by enhancing autophagy. However, in the context of muscle health, mTOR inhibition can have mixed

effects. While rapamycin may promote autophagy and reduce the accumulation of cellular damage, its inhibition of mTOR can also impair muscle protein synthesis, potentially exacerbating sarcopenia.
2. Balancing mTOR Activity: The key to managing sarcopenia may lie in finding the right balance of mTOR activity. On the one hand, sufficient mTOR activity is needed to support muscle protein synthesis and maintain muscle mass. On the other hand, too much mTOR activity, particularly when combined with reduced autophagy, can contribute to the aging-related decline in muscle function. Therapeutic strategies that selectively modulate mTOR activity to support muscle maintenance while enhancing autophagy could be beneficial in combating sarcopenia.

Exercise and Nutritional Interventions

mTOR is a critical regulator of muscle mass and function, making it highly relevant to the development and potential treatment of sarcopenia. While mTOR promotes muscle protein synthesis and growth, its dysregulation with age contributes to the decline in muscle mass and strength. Therapeutic strategies that balance mTOR activity—supporting protein synthesis while maintaining autophagy—alongside exercise and nutritional interventions, hold promise for mitigating the effects of sarcopenia and improving muscle health in aging populations [70].

1. Exercise*:* Resistance training is one of the most effective ways to stimulate mTOR signaling in muscles, promoting muscle protein synthesis and countering sarcopenia. Regular exercise helps maintain mTOR activity at levels that support muscle growth and function.
2. Nutrition*:* Adequate protein intake, especially of essential amino acids like leucine, is crucial for maintaining mTOR activity and muscle health in older adults. Nutritional strategies that optimize mTOR signaling can help mitigate the effects of sarcopenia [3].

Balancing mTOR Activity for Longevity

While mTOR inhibition has been shown to extend lifespan in various models, the effects are context-dependent. Chronic inhibition of mTOR can lead to side effects such as impaired wound healing, immunosuppression, and metabolic disturbances. Therefore, the timing, dosage, and duration of mTOR inhibition are critical factors that need to be carefully considered to maximize the benefits while minimizing potential harms.

1. *Intermittent Fasting and Dietary Restriction:* Caloric restriction and intermittent fasting are known to extend lifespan in many organisms, and these effects are

mediated in part through the downregulation of mTOR activity. These dietary interventions mimic some of the effects of mTOR inhibitors by reducing nutrient signaling and promoting autophagy, thereby contributing to increased longevity [22].

2. *Exercise:* mTOR is a key regulator that integrates growth signals and nutritional status to control protein synthesis. Given that skeletal muscle is the largest protein reservoir in the human body, it is unsurprising that mTOR plays a pivotal role in determining skeletal muscle phenotype. Through its regulation of protein synthesis and muscle growth, mTOR influences muscle mass, function, and adaptation in response to stimuli like exercise and nutrient availability, making it central to muscle health and development [55, 80].
3. *Metformin:* This common diabetes drug is known to indirectly inhibit mTOR by activating AMPK, a cellular energy sensor. This inhibition reduces cell growth and proliferation, which has potential benefits in conditions like cancer, aging, and metabolic disorders, where mTOR activity is dysregulated [6].

   Metformin is a widely used oral medication for type 2 diabetes. Metformin's activation of AMPK can inhibit mTORC1, making it a potential therapeutic strategy for conditions related to overactive mTOR signaling, such as certain cancers and metabolic disorders. It primarily works by:

   - *Decreasing hepatic glucose production:* Reduces gluconeogenesis in the liver
   - *Increasing insulin sensitivity*: Enhances glucose uptake by peripheral tissues
   - *mTOR Pathway*: Indirectly affects the mTOR pathway by activating AMP-activated protein kinase (AMPK), which can inhibit mTORC1 activity, thus influencing cellular metabolism and growth

4. *Resveratrol:* Resveratrol is a natural polyphenolic compound found in grapes, berries, and peanuts. It is known for its antioxidant and anti-inflammatory properties. It inhibits mTOR by activating AMPK and promoting autophagy. Resveratrol through SIRT1 and AMPK activation can modulate mTOR activity, contributing to its potential health benefits, including lifespan extension and disease prevention. This mTOR inhibition is linked to its potential anti-aging, anticancer, and cardioprotective effects . Its mechanisms include:

   - *Sirtuin Activation:* Activates sirtuin 1 (SIRT1), which is involved in cellular stress responses and longevity.
   - *AMPK Activation:* Similar to metformin, it can activate AMPK, indirectly affecting the mTOR pathway and promoting autophagy and metabolic regulation.
   - *Cardioprotective and Neuroprotective Effects:* Studies suggest benefits in cardiovascular health and neuroprotection, potentially linked to its effects on mTOR and related pathways.

5. *Rapamycin:* Rapamycin directly inhibits mTOR, specifically mTORC1, reducing cell growth and promoting autophagy. It has therapeutic uses in cancer, organ transplantation, and age-related diseases due to its ability to modulate cellular processes controlled by mTOR .

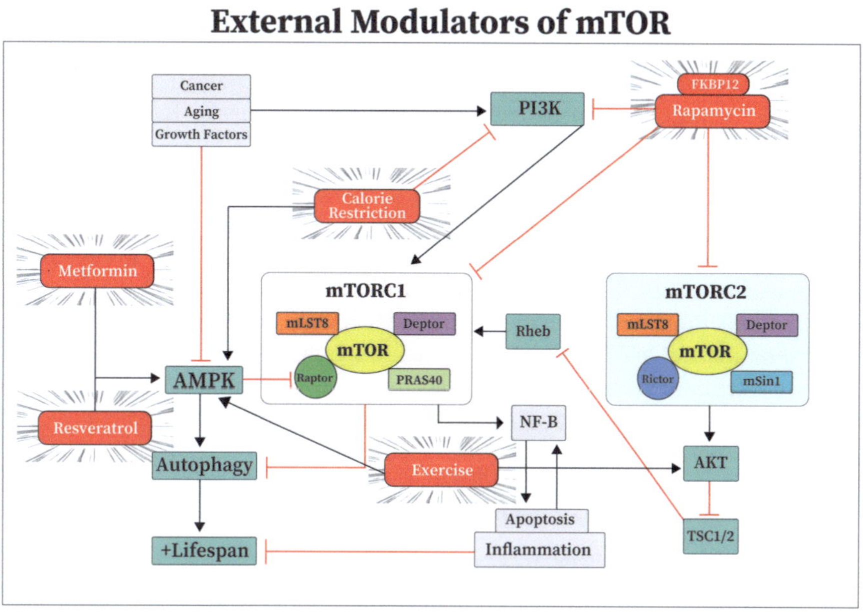

Fig. 1.10 The five most influential modulators of mTOR complexes are shown above. Each modulator (rapamycin, calorie restriction, metformin, resveratrol & exercise) is highlighted in red, and the site of its action are shown by black arrows as an activator and red t-bars as inhibitors

Rapamycin (Sirolimus) is an immunosuppressant and mTOR inhibitor, primarily affecting mTORC1. Direct inhibition of mTORC1 by rapamycin has therapeutic applications in organ transplantation, cancer therapy, and possibly anti-aging interventions. Its effects include:

- *Inhibition of mTORC1:* Suppresses protein synthesis and cell proliferation.
- *Autophagy induction:* Promotes the breakdown of damaged cells and components.
- *Anti-aging and longevity:* Has been studied for its potential to extend lifespan by modulating mTOR activity.
- *Potential Side Effects*: While mTOR inhibition has therapeutic potential, it also has side effects, including impaired wound healing, hyperlipidemia, and glucose intolerance, which must be carefully managed in patients with cardiovascular disease (Fig. 1.10).

Clinical Implications

1. *Rapamycin and Rapalogs:*

- *Lifespan Extension:* Rapamycin, an mTOR inhibitor, has been shown to extend lifespan in various animal models. Studies in mice have demonstrated that rapamycin treatment can improve healthspan, reducing the incidence of age-related diseases and enhancing overall health.

- *Human Studies:* Clinical trials are investigating the potential of rapamycin and rapalogs to treat age-related conditions in humans. Early results are promising, suggesting benefits in terms of immune function and disease markers.

Benefits of Rapamycin:

- *Immunosuppression*: Used to prevent organ transplant rejection by inhibiting immune responses.
- *Anti-aging*: Promotes longevity in animal models by reducing cellular senescence.
- *Cancer*: Inhibits mTOR, which is implicated in tumor growth, offering potential as a cancer therapeutic.
- *Neuroprotection*: Shows promise in protecting against neurodegenerative diseases like Alzheimer's.
- *Autophagy promotion*: Enhances cellular autophagy, which can support cellular maintenance and stress resilience.

Side Effects of Rapamycin:

- *Immunosuppression*: Increases the risk of infections and delayed wound healing.
- *Metabolic issues*: May cause hyperlipidemia, hyperglycemia, and insulin resistance.
- *Hematologic effects*: Can lead to anemia, thrombocytopenia, and leukopenia.
- *Mouth sores*: Common side effect in many users.
- *Pulmonary toxicity*: In rare cases, it causes lung-related issues, including pneumonitis (Figs. 1.11 and 1.12).

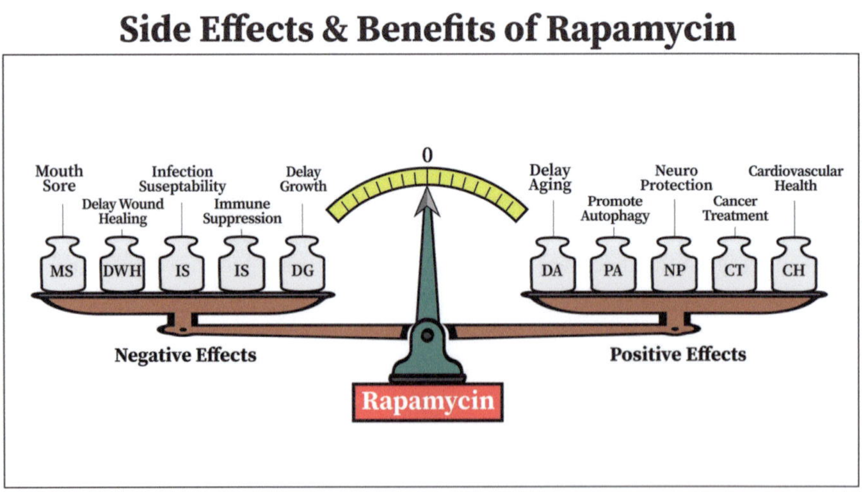

Fig. 1.11 Schematic representation of rapamycin treatment with its side effects on the left side of the scale and the benefits on the right

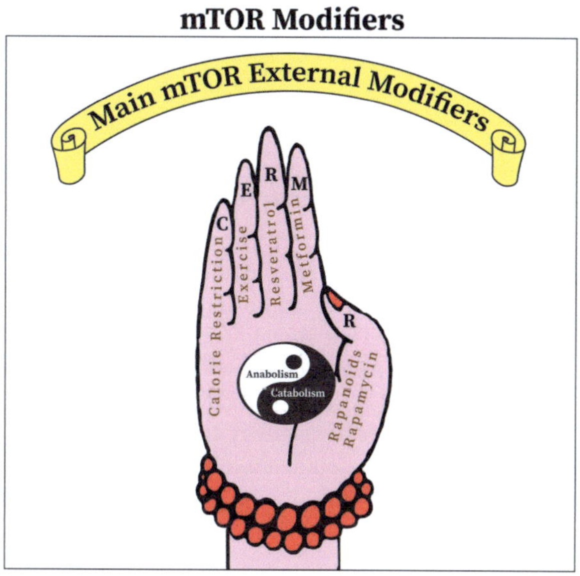

Fig. 1.12 Another representation emphasizing the mTOR's five external modifiers signifying the five most influential activators and inhibitors

2. *Age-Related Diseases:*

- *Neurodegenerative Diseases:* mTOR inhibition has potential therapeutic benefits for neurodegenerative diseases, as enhanced autophagy can help clear protein aggregates associated with conditions like Alzheimer's and Parkinson's.
- *Cardiovascular Health:* mTOR inhibitors may improve cardiovascular health by reducing inflammation and enhancing the repair and maintenance of vascular tissues.
- *Metabolic Health:* Modulation of mTOR signaling can improve metabolic health, potentially reducing the risk of type 2 diabetes, obesity, and other metabolic disorders.
- *Sarcopenia:* The mTOR pathway is crucial in regulating muscle homeostasis, and its dysregulation in aging leads to muscle wasting and functional decline characteristic of sarcopenia.
- *Menopause:* During menopause, decline in estrogen levels affects the mTOR pathway, influencing various cellular processes.
- *Delayed Wound Healing:* mTOR plays a crucial role in wound healing by regulating cell growth, protein synthesis, and tissue repair.

Role of mTOR in Neurodegenerative Diseases

mTOR (mechanistic target of rapamycin) plays a significant role in neurodegenerative diseases, primarily through its regulation of autophagy, protein synthesis, and cellular metabolism. Dysregulation of mTOR signaling has been implicated in the pathogenesis of various neurodegenerative disorders, including Alzheimer's disease, Parkinson's disease, Huntington's disease, and amyotrophic lateral sclerosis (ALS) .

mTOR and Neurodegenerative Diseases

mTOR plays a critical role in the pathogenesis of neurodegenerative diseases through its regulation of autophagy, protein synthesis, and cellular metabolism. Dysregulation of mTOR signaling contributes to the accumulation of toxic protein aggregates, impaired mitochondrial function, and metabolic dysfunction. Modulating mTOR activity, particularly through the inhibition of mTORC1, holds promise as a therapeutic strategy to enhance autophagy, clear protein aggregates, and protect neurons. Continued research into the role of mTOR in neurodegeneration and the development of targeted therapies offers hope for improving the treatment and outcomes of neurodegenerative diseases.

1. *Autophagy and Protein Aggregation:*
    - *Autophagy Regulation:* mTORC1 is a key inhibitor of autophagy. In neurodegenerative diseases, the accumulation of misfolded and aggregated proteins is a common pathological feature. Impaired autophagy, due to hyperactive mTORC1 signaling, contributes to the buildup of these toxic protein aggregates .
    - *Therapeutic Potential:* Inhibition of mTORC1 can enhance autophagy, promoting the clearance of protein aggregates and potentially ameliorating disease symptoms. For example, rapamycin and other mTOR inhibitors have shown promise in preclinical models of neurodegenerative diseases by reducing the accumulation of pathogenic proteins.
2. *Alzheimer's Disease:*
    - Amyloid Beta and Tau Pathology: Alzheimer's disease is characterized by the accumulation of amyloid-beta plaques and tau tangles. mTOR signaling is implicated in both the production of amyloid-beta and the phosphorylation of tau. Hyperactive mTORC1 can exacerbate these pathological processes .
    - Cognitive Function: mTOR inhibition has been shown to improve cognitive function in animal models of Alzheimer's disease, likely through enhanced autophagy and reduced amyloid-beta and tau pathology.
3. *Parkinson's Disease:*
    - Alpha-Synuclein Aggregation: Parkinson's disease is marked by the accumulation of alpha-synuclein in Lewy bodies. Dysregulated mTOR signaling can impair the autophagic degradation of alpha-synuclein, contributing to its accumulation .

- Neuroprotection: mTOR inhibitors have demonstrated neuroprotective effects in models of Parkinson's disease by promoting autophagy and reducing alpha-synuclein levels.

4. *Huntington's Disease:*

   - Huntingtin Protein Aggregation: Huntington's disease involves the accumulation of mutant huntingtin protein. mTORC1 inhibition has been shown to enhance the clearance of mutant huntingtin aggregates through autophagy, improving disease outcomes in animal models.

5. *Amyotrophic Lateral Sclerosis (ALS):*

   - Motor Neuron Degeneration: *This is characterized by the degeneration of motor neurons. mTOR* signaling affects protein homeostasis and cellular metabolism, which are critical in ALS pathology. Enhancing autophagy through mTOR inhibition may help in the clearance of misfolded proteins and support motor neuron survival .

Mechanisms and Interactions

1. *Autophagy:*

   - *Activation of Autophagy:* Inhibiting mTORC1 activates autophagy, a crucial process for the degradation and recycling of damaged cellular components and protein aggregates.
   - *Neuroprotective Autophagy:* Enhanced autophagy can reduce the toxic burden of protein aggregates in neurons, providing neuroprotection and improving cellular health.

2. *Protein Synthesis and Homeostasis:*

   - Control of Protein Synthesis: mTORC1 promotes protein synthesis, but excessive protein synthesis can contribute to the accumulation of misfolded proteins. Modulating mTOR activity can help balance protein synthesis and degradation.
   - Onaka 2024Dysregulated protein synthesis can lead to endoplasmic reticulum (ER) stress and the activation of the unfolded protein response (UPR), which are implicated in neurodegenerative diseases. mTOR inhibition can mitigate ER stress and support protein homeostasis.

3. *Mitochondrial Function and Metabolism:*

   - Mitochondrial Health: mTOR signaling influences mitochondrial function and biogenesis. Dysregulated mTOR activity can impair mitochondrial dynamics and function, contributing to neurodegeneration. Modulating

mTOR activity can improve mitochondrial health and cellular energy metabolism .
- Metabolic Reprogramming: Neurodegenerative diseases often involve metabolic dysfunction. mTOR regulation of cellular metabolism can impact neuronal survival and function, with potential therapeutic benefits from mTOR modulation.

4. *Lysosomal Influence*: mTOR regulates lysosomal function by controlling the lysosomal biogenesis and activity through the TFEB transcription factor. When nutrients are abundant, active mTOR inhibits TFEB, reducing lysosomal activity. Under nutrient-deprived conditions, mTOR activity decreases, allowing TFEB to translocate into the nucleus and promote the expression of lysosomal and autophagy-related genes, enhancing lysosomal degradation and recycling processes. This regulation is critical for maintaining cellular homeostasis and metabolism .
5. *Microtubule Organization*: mTOR plays a role in microtubule organization by regulating microtubule dynamics and stability. Through its downstream effectors, mTOR influences the phosphorylation of microtubule-associated proteins, such as stathmin, which in turn modulates microtubule polymerization and depolymerization. This regulation is crucial for various cellular processes, including cell division, migration, and intracellular transport .

Clinical Implications

1. *Therapeutic Interventions:*
   - *mTOR Inhibitors:* Drugs like rapamycin and its analogs are being explored for their potential to treat neurodegenerative diseases. These drugs can enhance autophagy, reduce protein aggregates, and improve neuronal survival.
   - *Combination Therapies:* Combining mTOR inhibitors with other therapeutic agents, such as proteostasis modulators or mitochondrial protectors, may provide synergistic benefits in treating neurodegenerative diseases.
2. *Biomarkers and Personalized Medicine:*
   - *Identifying Biomarkers:* Biomarkers for mTOR pathway activity and autophagy function can help identify patients who may benefit from mTOR-targeted therapies. Personalized approaches based on these biomarkers can optimize treatment outcomes.
3. *Challenges and Considerations:*

Selective Targeting While mTOR inhibition has potential benefits, long-term systemic inhibition of mTOR can have adverse effects, including immune suppression and metabolic disturbances. Strategies to selectively target mTOR signaling in neurons or specific brain regions are being investigated to minimize side effects [31].

mTOR and Cardiovascular Diseases

mTOR plays a role in cardiac hypertrophy, atherosclerosis, and other cardiovascular conditions by affecting cellular growth and metabolism in heart tissues. The mechanistic target of rapamycin (mTOR) plays a significant role in cardiovascular health and disease. mTOR is a serine/threonine kinase that integrates various signals, including nutrients, growth factors, and energy status, to regulate cellular growth, proliferation, metabolism, and survival. Given its central role in these processes, mTOR is implicated in various cardiovascular diseases (CVDs). mTOR plays a complex and multifaceted role in cardiovascular diseases, influencing processes like inflammation, lipid metabolism, cell growth, and autophagy. Therapeutic modulation of mTOR, particularly its inhibition, holds promise for treating various cardiovascular conditions, but it requires careful consideration of potential side effects and the specific context of the disease. Ongoing research continues to explore the nuanced roles of mTOR in cardiovascular health and disease [30].

Here's an overview of how mTOR influences cardiovascular diseases:

1. Atherosclerosis
   - mTOR and Lipid Metabolism*:* mTOR regulates lipid metabolism, which is crucial in the development of atherosclerosis. Dysregulation of mTOR signaling can lead to increased lipid accumulation in the arterial walls, promoting atherosclerosis.
   - Inflammation*:* mTOR influences inflammatory responses, which are central to atherosclerosis. Inhibition of mTOR can reduce the inflammatory processes involved in the progression of atherosclerotic plaques.
2. Cardiac Hypertrophy
   - mTOR in Cardiac Growth*:* mTOR is a key regulator of cardiac hypertrophy, which is the enlargement of the heart muscle cells in response to increased workload or stress. While physiological hypertrophy (e.g., from exercise) is generally beneficial, pathological hypertrophy (e.g., from hypertension) can lead to heart failure. mTOR signaling is often upregulated in pathological hypertrophy, and its inhibition has been shown to reduce or prevent the development of this condition.
3. Heart Failure
   - mTOR and Autophagy*:* mTOR inhibits autophagy, a cellular process involved in the degradation and recycling of cellular components. In heart failure, impaired autophagy can contribute to cellular damage and dysfunction. Inhibition of mTOR with agents like rapamycin can enhance autophagy and potentially protect against heart failure.
   - Metabolic Regulation*:* mTOR is also involved in the regulation of cardiac metabolism. Dysregulation of mTOR can lead to metabolic disturbances that exacerbate heart failure.

4. Ischemia-Reperfusion Injury
   - *mTOR and Cell Survival:* During ischemia-reperfusion injury, which occurs when blood supply returns to the heart after a period of ischemia (lack of blood flow), mTOR signaling is critical in determining cell survival. mTOR can contribute to both protective and harmful effects depending on the context. Modulation of mTOR activity has been explored as a potential therapeutic strategy to reduce tissue damage during reperfusion.
5. Vascular Diseases
   - mTOR and Endothelial Function*:* mTOR signaling plays a role in endothelial cell function, which is crucial for maintaining vascular health. Dysregulation of mTOR can lead to endothelial dysfunction, a precursor to various vascular diseases, including hypertension and atherosclerosis.
   - Vascular Smooth Muscle Cells (VSMCs)*:* mTOR regulates the proliferation and migration of VSMCs, which are critical in the development of neointimal hyperplasia and restenosis following vascular injury or intervention.

mTOR in Metabolic Disorders and Obesity

mTORC1 hyperactivation plays a pivotal role in the pathogenesis of obesity and its related metabolic disorders. It promotes lipid accumulation, impairs insulin sensitivity, and disrupts energy balance, contributing to the metabolic derangements seen in obesity, insulin resistance, and type 2 diabetes. Therapeutic strategies targeting mTOR must balance its anabolic and metabolic functions while minimizing side effects. Dysregulation of mTOR signaling is implicated in various metabolic disorders, including obesity, type 2 diabetes, and other related conditions.

Here is an overview of mTOR's role in metabolic disorders and obesity:

mTOR signaling metabolic pathways are more related to mTORC1 and mTORC2

- *mTORC1 (mTOR Complex 1):* This complex is primarily involved in promoting cell growth, protein synthesis, and lipid metabolism. It is highly responsive to nutrients (especially amino acids like leucine), growth factors (e.g., insulin), and energy levels.
- *mTORC2 (mTOR Complex 2):* This complex is more involved in cytoskeletal organization, cell survival, and insulin signaling.

mTORC1 and Obesity

mTORC1 plays a crucial role in regulating lipid and glucose metabolism, and its hyperactivation is closely linked to obesity and metabolic dysfunction:

- *Lipid Metabolism:* mTORC1 promotes lipogenesis (the synthesis of fatty acids) by upregulating the activity of key enzymes involved in this process, such as SREBP-1 (sterol regulatory element-binding protein 1). Overactive mTORC1 increases fat accumulation, contributing to obesity.
- *Energy Balance:* mTORC1 is sensitive to nutrient availability and energy status. When energy levels are high, mTORC1 is activated, which promotes anabolic processes, including fat storage. Chronic overnutrition (as seen in obesity) leads to sustained mTORC1 activation, exacerbating fat deposition.
- *Appetite Regulation:* mTORC1 signaling in the hypothalamus also plays a role in controlling appetite and energy expenditure. Dysregulation of hypothalamic mTORC1 can lead to hyperphagia (overeating) and reduced energy expenditure, further contributing to obesity.

mTORC1 and Insulin Resistance

One of the key metabolic abnormalities in obesity is insulin resistance, which can progress to type 2 diabetes. mTORC1 is intricately linked to insulin signaling:

- *Insulin Sensitivity:* mTORC1 is activated by insulin through the PI3K-Akt pathway. However, chronic overactivation of mTORC1 leads to a negative feedback loop that dampens insulin signaling by inhibiting IRS-1 (insulin receptor substrate 1), a key component of insulin signaling. This results in reduced insulin sensitivity, contributing to insulin resistance.
- *Glucose Homeostasis:* By promoting insulin resistance, mTORC1 dysregulation affects glucose uptake and metabolism, worsening hyperglycemia and increasing the risk of developing type 2 diabetes.

mTORC2 and Insulin Resistance

- *Insulin Signaling and Akt Activation:* mTORC2 is crucial for full activation of Akt, a key kinase in the insulin signaling pathway. Impaired mTORC2 activity can reduce Akt-mediated glucose uptake, worsening insulin resistance. In obesity and metabolic disorders, mTORC2 dysfunction is also implicated in impaired insulin sensitivity.

mTOR and Adipose Tissue

- *Adipogenesis:* mTORC1 signaling regulates the differentiation of pre-adipocytes into mature adipocytes (fat cells). This process is essential for fat storage, and hyperactivation of mTORC1 can enhance adipogenesis, leading to excessive fat accumulation in obese individuals.

- *Brown Adipose Tissue (BAT):* mTORC1 and mTORC2 have also been implicated in regulating the function of brown adipose tissue, which is involved in thermogenesis (heat production) and energy expenditure. Dysfunctional mTOR signaling in BAT may contribute to reduced energy expenditure in obesity.

Therapeutic Implications

Given the central role of mTOR in metabolism and obesity, it is a potential target for therapeutic interventions:

- *Rapamycin (mTOR Inhibitors):* Rapamycin inhibits mTORC1, and studies suggest that it could improve insulin sensitivity and reduce fat mass in some models. However, its clinical use is limited due to side effects, including impaired glucose tolerance and disruption of immune function.
- *mTOR Modulators:* There is ongoing research into developing more selective modulators of mTORC1 and mTORC2, which could target the metabolic dysregulation seen in obesity without the adverse effects of broad mTOR inhibition.

mTOR, Obesity, and Other Related Metabolic Disorders

- *Non-alcoholic Fatty Liver Disease (NAFLD):* Chronic mTORC1 activation contributes to lipid accumulation in the liver, promoting NAFLD, which is commonly associated with obesity.

mTOR and Sarcopenia

mTOR pathway is crucial in regulating muscle homeostasis, and its dysregulation in aging leads to muscle wasting and functional decline characteristic of sarcopenia (loss of muscle mass). The mTOR pathway plays a central role in the regulation of muscle mass and is critically involved in the pathogenesis of sarcopenia. In skeletal muscle, the mTOR pathway, particularly through the mTORC1 complex, mediates muscle protein synthesis and growth in response to anabolic signals like nutrients (especially amino acids), insulin, and mechanical stimuli (e.g., exercise). However, in the context of aging and sarcopenia, the mTOR pathway becomes dysregulated [62].

Key points about the mTOR pathway in sarcopenia:

1. *Diminished Activation*: In sarcopenia, there is often reduced responsiveness of the mTORC1 pathway to anabolic stimuli like nutrition and exercise. This leads to decreased protein synthesis, which is a critical factor in the loss of muscle mass.

2. *Impaired Muscle Regeneration*: mTORC1 signaling is essential for the activation of satellite cells, which are responsible for muscle repair and regeneration. Aging results in a decline in the efficiency of this process, leading to impaired muscle regeneration and contributing to sarcopenia.
3. *Inhibition of Autophagy*: Chronic activation of mTORC1 in aging muscle inhibits autophagy, the process by which damaged proteins and organelles are degraded and recycled. This leads to the accumulation of dysfunctional cellular components, which exacerbates muscle degradation.
4. *Nutrient and Hormonal Sensitivity*: With aging, the muscle's sensitivity to anabolic signals like insulin and amino acids decreases. This reduced sensitivity leads to lower mTORC1 activation and impaired protein synthesis, a phenomenon known as "anabolic resistance." This contributes significantly to the muscle wasting seen in sarcopenia.
5. *Inflammation and Oxidative Stress*: Chronic low-grade inflammation and increased oxidative stress, common in aging, can further impair mTOR signaling. Inflammation activates pathways that antagonize mTORC1, while oxidative damage may disrupt mTOR regulation, both of which contribute to muscle atrophy.

Sarcopenia is indeed a complex condition driven by multiple molecular, cellular, and environmental factors, and aging serves as a primary hallmark in its development.

The more detailed and specific highlights of several key mechanisms involved in the progression of sarcopenia are as follows:

1. *Genomic Instability and Telomere Attrition*: As cells age, they experience increased genomic instability and telomere shortening, which leads to cellular senescence and a decline in regenerative capacity. This instability contributes to muscle degeneration.
2. *Proteostasis and Epigenetic Alterations*: Aging disrupts proteostasis, which is the balance of protein synthesis, folding, and degradation. Inefficient proteostasis causes an accumulation of misfolded or damaged proteins, further accelerating muscle wasting. Additionally, epigenetic modifications in aging muscles affect gene expression, contributing to sarcopenia.
3. *Smad and Akt Signaling Pathways*: Smad and Akt are essential in muscle signaling and atrophy. Akt is involved in the IGF-1 pathway, promoting muscle growth through protein synthesis, while Smad signaling is activated by transforming growth factor-β (TGF-β), which promotes muscle atrophy. Increased Smad4 activity in aging inhibits muscle regeneration by preventing satellite cell differentiation.
4. *Hormonal Influence*: Hormonal changes during aging, particularly the rise of glucocorticoids, promote muscle atrophy. These hormones interfere with anabolic pathways, including IGF-1 and insulin signaling, both of which are crucial for maintaining muscle mass.
5. *Oxidative Stress and Free Radicals*: Aging muscles accumulate oxidative stress due to the excessive production of free radicals, which damage proteins, lipids,

and DNA in muscle cells. This oxidative damage disrupts normal cellular signaling and contributes to the decline in muscle function.
6. *Satellite Cell Depletion*: The decrease in satellite cells, which are essential for muscle regeneration, is another key factor in sarcopenia. Elevated Smad4 levels impair satellite cell differentiation, reducing their ability to repair and regenerate muscle tissue.
7. *Role of Nrf2 and Redox Homeostasis*: The loss of redox-dependent transcription factors like Nrf2, which regulates antioxidant defenses, leads to apoptosis and a reduction in the stem cell population. This diminishes the muscle's ability to counteract oxidative stress, further weakening muscle regeneration capacity.

These interconnected molecular and cellular mechanisms underscore the complexity of sarcopenia and highlight potential therapeutic targets, such as modulating signaling pathways (Akt/Smad), reducing oxidative stress, and enhancing satellite cell function, to slow or reverse muscle degeneration.

Therapeutic Implications Interventions targeting the mTOR pathway, such as resistance exercise, protein supplementation (particularly leucine), and potential pharmacological approaches (e.g., rapamycin or mTOR modulators), are being explored to mitigate the effects of sarcopenia. However, these approaches must balance promoting muscle growth without causing excessive mTORC1 activation, which can have negative consequences.

mTOR and Menopause

As mentioned previously, the mechanistic target of rapamycin (mTOR) plays a significant role in cellular metabolism, growth, and aging, and its dysregulation has been implicated in various aging-related processes, including menopause. Menopause, which marks the end of a woman's reproductive years, is characterized by a decline in ovarian function, reduced estrogen levels, and various metabolic and physiological changes. The mTOR pathway interacts with these processes in several ways .

1. mTOR and Ovarian Aging

   Menopause is strongly associated with ovarian aging, as the number of oocytes and the quality of follicles in the ovaries decline with age. mTOR signaling plays a critical role in regulating the function of ovarian cells, particularly granulosa cells, which are important for follicular development and estrogen production.

   - *Follicular Development:* mTORC1 activity in ovarian follicles is crucial for follicle growth and the survival of oocytes. As women age, mTOR signaling in the ovaries tends to decline, leading to reduced follicle numbers and impaired oocyte quality. This process is linked to the onset of menopause.

- *Oocyte Quality:* mTOR also affects the quality of oocytes by regulating autophagy, a cellular process involved in maintaining cell health by clearing damaged organelles. Impaired autophagy, often due to age-related mTOR dysregulation, may contribute to the reduction in oocyte quality seen in older women, which accelerates the onset of menopause.

2. mTOR and Estrogen Production

   Estrogen production primarily occurs in the ovaries, and mTOR is involved in regulating the synthesis of estrogen:

- *mTORC1 and Granulosa Cells:* mTORC1 activity in granulosa cells enhances estrogen synthesis by promoting the activity of steroidogenic enzymes. As mTOR signaling decreases with age, the ovaries produce less estrogen, contributing to the hormonal changes characteristic of menopause.
- *Hormonal Regulation of mTOR:* Estrogen can also regulate mTOR activity. In postmenopausal women, lower estrogen levels are associated with a decline in mTOR signaling, which affects various tissues and metabolic processes, including bone health, fat distribution, and cardiovascular function.

3. Metabolic Changes in Menopause

   Menopause is associated with a variety of metabolic changes, such as increased fat mass, insulin resistance, and changes in lipid metabolism. mTORC1 plays a significant role in these processes:

- *Weight Gain and Fat Distribution:* Estrogen depletion after menopause is linked to increased mTORC1 activity in adipose tissue, contributing to weight gain and the accumulation of visceral fat. This shift in fat distribution increases the risk of metabolic disorders, such as obesity and type 2 diabetes, which are common in postmenopausal women.
- *Insulin Resistance:* mTORC1 overactivation can impair insulin signaling, leading to insulin resistance, a condition that is more prevalent in postmenopausal women due to the combined effects of aging and hormonal changes. Estrogen normally helps to modulate insulin sensitivity, and its decline can exacerbate metabolic dysfunction through altered mTOR signaling.

4. *mTOR and Bone Health*

   Postmenopausal women are at increased risk for osteoporosis due to the loss of estrogen, which plays a critical role in bone homeostasis. mTOR signaling is important in regulating bone turnover:

- *Osteoblast and Osteoclast Function:* mTOR regulates the activity of both osteoblasts (cells that build bone) and osteoclasts (cells that break down bone). In postmenopausal women, mTOR signaling may become imbalanced, favoring bone resorption over bone formation, contributing to the development of osteoporosis.
- *Estrogen-mTOR Interplay in Bone:* Estrogen deficiency after menopause can lead to dysregulation of mTORC1 in bone cells, accelerating bone loss.

5. mTOR and Cardiovascular Health

   Menopause is also associated with an increased risk of cardiovascular diseases (CVD), partly due to changes in lipid metabolism and vascular health. mTOR is involved in:

   - *iVascular Aging:* mTORC1 regulates endothelial cell function and vascular smooth muscle cells. In postmenopausal women, reduced estrogen levels may lead to impaired mTOR signaling in vascular tissues, contributing to endothelial dysfunction and increased arterial stiffness, both of which are risk factors for CVD.
   - *Lipid Metabolism:* Menopause is linked to adverse changes in lipid profiles, such as increased LDL cholesterol and decreased HDL cholesterol. Dysregulated mTORC1 activity can exacerbate these lipid imbalances, further increasing cardiovascular risk.

6. Potential Therapeutic Interventions

   Given the role of mTOR in aging, ovarian function, and menopause-related metabolic changes, it is being explored as a therapeutic target:

   - *mTOR Inhibitors:* Rapamycin and other mTOR inhibitors have been studied for their potential to delay ovarian aging and extend reproductive lifespan in animal models. However, their application in humans is complex due to potential side effects.
   - *Hormone Replacement Therapy (HRT):* HRT, which provides estrogen, may help modulate mTOR activity and alleviate some menopause-related symptoms, including metabolic dysfunction and bone loss.
   - *Caloric Restriction and mTOR:* Caloric restriction is known to inhibit mTOR activity and has been shown to extend lifespan and improve metabolic health in some models. It may also have potential benefits in reducing menopause-related metabolic dysfunction by modulating mTOR activity.

Delayed Wound Healing

Rapamycin can delay wound healing. Rapamycin is an immunosuppressive drug that inhibits mTOR (mechanistic target of rapamycin), which plays a key role in cell growth, proliferation, and survival. While this inhibition has beneficial effects in terms of longevity and protection against certain age-related diseases, it can also negatively impact processes that require rapid cell proliferation and growth, such as wound healing. While rapamycin has valuable therapeutic uses, particularly in extending lifespan and treating certain diseases, its role in delaying wound healing underscores the need for careful management of patients who may require rapid tissue repair .

Mechanisms by Which Rapamycin Delays Wound Healing

1. *Inhibition of Cell Proliferation*:
   - mTOR signaling promotes the proliferation of various cell types, including fibroblasts, keratinocytes, and endothelial cells, which are essential for wound healing. Inhibiting mTOR with rapamycin reduces the proliferation of these cells, slowing the repair process.
2. *Reduced Angiogenesis*:
   - mTOR is involved in the formation of new blood vessels (angiogenesis) by endothelial cells. Angiogenesis is crucial for supplying nutrients and oxygen to the wound site. Rapamycin-induced inhibition of mTOR can impair angiogenesis, thereby delaying wound healing.
3. *Decreased Collagen Production*:
   - Fibroblasts produce collagen, a major component of the extracellular matrix that provides structural support to healing tissues. mTOR promotes collagen synthesis, and its inhibition by rapamycin can result in decreased collagen production, affecting tissue repair and strength.
4. *Impaired Immune Response*:
   - An effective immune response is necessary for clearing debris and pathogens from the wound site. Rapamycin suppresses immune function, which can delay the initial inflammatory phase of wound healing and prolong the overall healing process.

Clinical Implications

- *Post-surgical Healing*: Patients receiving rapamycin or other mTOR inhibitors, particularly those undergoing organ transplantation or cancer treatment, may experience delayed wound healing. This is an important consideration for post-surgical care and management.
- *Chronic Wounds*: In conditions where rapid wound healing is crucial, such as in diabetic ulcers or other chronic wounds, the use of rapamycin may need to be carefully evaluated against its benefits.

mTOR Complexes

mTOR is a crucial protein kinase that regulates cell growth, proliferation, motility, survival, protein synthesis, and transcription. mTOR molecule functions within distinct multiprotein complexes: mTORC1, mTORC2, and newly discovered mTORC3 and mTORC4, each with unique functions. The mTOR signaling pathway is a crucial regulator of the cell, and its activity is compartmentalized within the cell to optimize its function. The pathway leverages two distinct cellular membrane locations: the lysosomal membrane and the plasma membrane. Specific adapter proteins play a vital role in directing mTOR kinase to these locations, where it forms at least four distinct complexes—mTORC1, mTORC2, mTORC3, and mTORC4.

- *mTORC1*: Sensitive to rapamycin, controls protein synthesis, autophagy, and metabolism
- *mTORC2*: Insensitive to rapamycin, involved in cell survival, cytoskeletal organization, and metabolism
- *mTORC3*: Tumor genesis, drug resistance
- *mTORC4*: Protein synthesis, mobility, tumor genesis, drug resistance

Categories of Recognition and Regulation

The mTOR pathway's ability to phosphorylate specific substrates and integrate various regulatory components is fundamental to its role in controlling cell growth, survival, and proliferation. By subdividing substrates into categories of recognition and regulation, mTOR complexes effectively coordinate diverse signaling cascades, ensuring appropriate cellular responses to environmental cues.

Very brief highlights of these complexes are presented, and more detailed descriptions are to follow.

1. *mTORC1 (mTOR Complex 1)*:
   - *Components*: mTOR, mLST8 (mammalian lethal with Sec13 protein 8), PRAS40 (proline-rich AKT substrate 40 kDa), Deptor (DEP domain-containing mTOR-interacting protein), and Raptor (regulatory-associated protein of mTOR).
   - *Functions*: mTORC1 is involved in regulating protein synthesis, autophagy, ribosome biogenesis, stress-induced transcription, and cell cycle transition. It integrates signals related to nutrients, energy status, oxygen levels, and stress to control these processes.
2. *mTORC2 (mTOR Complex 2)*:
   - *Components*: mTOR, mLST8, Rictor (rapamycin-insensitive companion of mTOR), Deptor, hSin1 (stress-activated protein kinase-interacting protein 1), and Protor (protein observed with Rictor).

- *Functions*: mTORC2 phosphorylates and activates AGC family kinases, including AKT, PKC (protein kinase C), and SGK1 (serum- and glucocorticoid-induced protein kinase 1). It regulates cell survival, proliferation, mobility, invasion, and angiogenesis. Full activation of AKT by mTORC2 involves phosphorylation at Ser308 by PDK1 and Thr473 by mTORC2, enhancing PI3K-AKT-mTORC1 signaling and forming a positive feedback loop.

3. *mTORC3 (mTOR Complex 3)*:
   - *Components*: mTOR, mLST8, and ETS transcription factor ETV7.
   - *Functions*: This newly identified complex is rapamycin insensitive and formed independently of ETV7's transcriptional activity. The specific physiological roles and regulatory mechanisms of mTORC3 are still under investigation.
4. *mTORC4 (mTOR Complex 4)*:
   - *Components*: mTOR, mLST8, DNA-PKcs (DNA-dependent protein kinase catalytic subunit), and mEAK7 (mammalian elongation factor-associated kinase 7).
   - *Functions*: mTORC4 has been implicated in tumorigenesis and anticancer drug resistance by controlling DNA damage response (DDR) and the physiology of cancer stem cells (CSCs). It plays a role in maintaining genomic stability and regulating CSC functions, contributing to cancer progression and therapy resistance.

mTOR Complexes and Their Specific Regulatory Mechanisms

The mTOR pathways integrate signals from nutrient and growth factor inputs to make binary decisions that regulate cell growth and metabolism. For example, cytosolic sensors like Sestrin2 and CASTOR1 detect specific amino acids and modulate the activity of the GATOR2-Rag GTPase axis, ensuring mTORC1 activation only under nutrient-replete conditions. This precise regulation allows cells to adapt to their nutritional environment, promoting growth and metabolic efficiency.

mTOR Complexes and Their Key Regulatory Components

Recognition

Substrate Recognition:

- *Specificity of Phosphorylation Sites*: The substrates for mTORC1 and mTORC2 have specific amino acid sequences recognized by the complexes. For instance, the TOR signaling (TOS) motif in S6K1 and 4E-BP1 is crucial for their recognition by mTORC1.

- *Adapter Proteins*: Proteins like Raptor in mTORC1 and Rictor in mTORC2 play critical roles in recognizing and binding specific substrates for phosphorylation.

Regulation

Regulatory Effects:
- *Feedback Loops*: Phosphorylation of certain substrates creates feedback loops that can either enhance or inhibit further mTOR activity. For example, activated S6K1 can phosphorylate and inhibit IRS1, reducing PI3K signaling and indirectly decreasing mTORC1 activity.
- *Cross-Talk Between Pathways*: mTOR complexes integrate signals from various upstream pathways, such as PI3K/Akt for mTORC2 and amino acid sensing pathways for mTORC1. This integration ensures that cell growth and metabolism are coordinated with nutrient availability and growth signals.

Functional Outcomes

Cell Growth:
- *Protein Synthesis*: Through substrates like S6K1 and 4E-BP1, mTORC1 significantly enhances protein synthesis, promoting cell growth.
- *Lipid Biosynthesis*: mTORC1 also regulates lipid biosynthesis, crucial for membrane formation and energy storage.

Survival:
- *Anti-Apoptotic Signaling*: mTORC2-mediated activation of Akt leads to the phosphorylation and inhibition of pro-apoptotic proteins, enhancing cell survival.
- *Stress Response*: mTORC2 helps cells adapt to stress by regulating cytoskeletal dynamics and ion transport.

Proliferation:
- *Cell Cycle Progression*: mTORC1 influences cell cycle regulators, promoting progression from G1 to S phase.
- *Metabolic Adaptation*: Both mTORC1 and mTORC2 adjust cellular metabolism to meet the demands of proliferation, ensuring sufficient energy and biosynthetic precursors are available.

Activation

- *Regulated Cell Growth*:
  - *Protein Synthesis*: Activation of mTORC1 leads to the phosphorylation of downstream targets such as S6K1 and 4E-BP1, enhancing protein synthesis.
  - *Lipid Biosynthesis*: mTORC1 promotes lipid biosynthesis, necessary for membrane formation and energy storage.

- *Inhibition of Autophagy*: mTORC1 inhibits autophagy by phosphorylating and inhibiting ULK1, ensuring resources are directed toward growth rather than degradation.

- *Metabolic Control*:
  - *Glucose Metabolism*: mTORC1 influences glucose uptake and utilization, ensuring cells have sufficient energy for growth.
  - *Amino Acid Metabolism*: By sensing amino acid levels, mTORC1 adjusts metabolic pathways to balance synthesis and degradation of proteins.

Crosstalk with AMPK (AMP-Activated Protein Kinase)

There is a crosstalk between mTORC1 and AMPK to control cell survival, growth, and proliferation [64]. Inhibition of mTORC1 signaling networks by AMPK is executed by at least four distinct mechanisms: phosphorylation of TSC2 and Raptor to induce a growth arrest and cell survival, phosphorylation of FNIP1 to inhibit FLCN that leads to preferential activation of TFEB, and phosphorylation and destabilization of GATOR2 when cellular glucose supply is limited. AMPK inhibits mTORC1 through:

1. *Phosphorylation of TSC2*: Enhances TSC2 activity to inhibit Rheb and mTORC1.
2. *Phosphorylation of Raptor*: Disrupts mTORC1 assembly and activity.
3. *Phosphorylation of FNIP1*: Inhibits FLCN, activating TFEB and promoting autophagy.
4. *Phosphorylation and Destabilization of GATOR2*: Limits mTORC1 activation under low glucose conditions.

These mechanisms collectively ensure that cells can arrest growth and survive during periods of energy stress by downregulating mTORC1 activity and promoting catabolic processes.

- *mTORC1 Inhibits AMPK via Phosphorylation*:
  - *α2-S345*: Prevents lysosomal targeting and activation by LKB1, reducing AMPK activity.
  - *α1-S347 and α2-S377*: Control AMPK activity through unresolved mechanisms, likely contributing to the regulation of AMPK's response to metabolic cues.

This reciprocal regulation ensures a balanced cellular response to nutrient availability, coordinating anabolic and catabolic processes to maintain metabolic homeostasis.

mTORC: References for Comprehensive Overview of Its Complexes and Functions

The diverse roles of mTOR complexes in regulating key cellular processes make them critical targets for therapeutic intervention, particularly in cancer. Dysregulation of mTOR signaling is a common feature in various cancers, often leading to uncontrolled cell growth, proliferation, and survival. Targeting specific mTOR complexes with selective inhibitors could provide new avenues for cancer treatment, potentially overcoming drug resistance and improving patient outcomes.

Each mTOR complexes will be discusses in more detail with reference to:

1. How mTOR complex receive signals and receptors (upstream signal transduction)
2. Molecular components
3. The resulting effects as the function of mTOR complexes (downstream signal transduction) .

Although mTOR (mechanistic target of rapamycin) is a central regulator of cell growth, proliferation, metabolism, and survival, beyond its well-known roles in these processes, emerging evidence suggests that mTOR also plays a significant role in epigenetic control. Here's how mTOR influences epigenetic regulation:

mTOR and Epigenetic Mechanisms

mTOR is an essential regulator of cellular processes and also exerts significant control over the epigenetic landscape. Through its influence on histone modifications, DNA methylation, and non-coding RNAs, mTOR integrates signals from the cellular environment to modulate gene expression. This epigenetic regulation by mTOR has profound implications for understanding development, disease, and aging and offers potential avenues for therapeutic interventions [11]

1. *Histone Modifications:*
   - *Histone Acetylation:* mTOR signaling can influence histone acetylation by regulating the activity of histone acetyltransferases (HATs) and histone deacetylases (HDACs). For example, mTORC1 (a complex of mTOR) activation has been linked to increased acetylation of histones, promoting a more open chromatin structure and active transcription.
   - *Histone Methylation:* mTOR can modulate histone methylation by affecting the expression and activity of histone methyltransferases (HMTs) and demethylases. This regulation impacts gene expression patterns essential for cell growth and differentiation.

2. *DNA Methylation:*
   - mTOR signaling may affect DNA methylation indirectly by altering the availability and activity of enzymes like DNA methyltransferases (DNMTs). Changes in DNA methylation patterns can lead to long-term changes in gene expression.
3. *Non-coding RNAs:*
   - mTOR can regulate the biogenesis and function of non-coding RNAs, including microRNAs (miRNAs) and long non-coding RNAs (lncRNAs), which play roles in modulating gene expression epigenetically. For instance, certain miRNAs regulated by mTOR can target mRNAs of epigenetic regulators, thus influencing their expression.

Pathways and Interactions:

1. *Nutrient Sensing and Epigenetics:*
   - mTOR is a key sensor of cellular nutrient and energy status. Through its signaling pathways, it can modulate the activity of epigenetic modifiers in response to nutrient availability. For instance, nutrient deprivation can lead to changes in mTOR activity, subsequently altering the epigenetic landscape and affecting gene expression relevant to metabolic adaptation.
2. *Cell Cycle and Epigenetics:*
   - mTOR activity is tightly linked to cell cycle progression. It can regulate the expression of genes involved in cell cycle control through epigenetic mechanisms. This regulation ensures that epigenetic modifications are synchronized with the cell cycle, facilitating proper cell division and growth.
3. *Aging and Epigenetics:*
   - mTOR signaling has been implicated in the aging process and age-related diseases. Epigenetic changes are a hallmark of aging, and mTOR can influence these changes. For example, inhibition of mTOR has been shown to delay aging and improve lifespan, possibly through its effects on the epigenome.

mTOR Complexes and References to their Clinical Implications

The discoveries of mTOR complexes underscore the centrality of mTOR in various human diseases and highlight the therapeutic potential of targeting this pathway across a broad spectrum of health issues. The following is just a small example of growing fields of knowledge on variety of diseases associated with the dysregulation of mTOR complexes.

Cancer mTOR pathways are often hyperactivated in various cancers, promoting tumor growth and survival. Inhibitors targeting mTOR are being explored as cancer therapies. Aberrant mTOR signaling is common in many cancers, and it can lead to epigenetic alterations that promote oncogenesis. Targeting mTOR pathways with inhibitors (like rapamycin and its analogs) can potentially reverse some of these epigenetic changes, offering a therapeutic strategy for cancer treatment.

- mTOR in breast cancer [40]
- mTOR in colorectal cancer [38]
- mTOR in head and neck carcinoma [29]
- mTOR in gastric cancer [73]
- mTOR in pancreatic cancer [84]
- mTOR in malignant melanoma [85]
- mTOR in multiple myeloma [76]
- mTOR in lung cancer [49]
- mTOR in glioblastoma [14]
- Cancer and mTOR [86]

Metabolic Disorders mTOR dysregulation is linked to obesity, type 2 diabetes, and metabolic syndrome. It affects insulin signaling and glucose homeostasis. Given mTOR's role in metabolism, its influence on epigenetic regulation is also relevant in metabolic diseases such as diabetes and obesity. Modulating mTOR activity could help restore normal epigenetic patterns and improve metabolic function.

- mTOR in diabetic retinopathy [17]
- mTOR and obesity [13]

Neurodegenerative Diseases: Abnormal mTOR activity is associated with conditions such as Alzheimer's and Parkinson's diseases, influencing protein aggregation and neuronal survival. Epigenetic dysregulation is a feature of neurodegenerative diseases, and mTOR signaling has been implicated in the pathology of these conditions. Understanding the interplay between mTOR and epigenetic mechanisms could lead to novel therapeutic approaches for diseases such as:

- mTOR and neurodegenerative diseases [37]
- Alzheimer's and Parkinson's [11]
- mTOR and brain injury [68]
- mTOR and stroke [7]

- mTOR in autism [10, 77]
- mTOR and epilepsy [60]

Autoimmune disorders Dysregulation of mTOR signaling has been implicated in various autoimmune diseases, such as systemic lupus erythematosus (SLE), rheumatoid arthritis (RA), and multiple sclerosis (MS). In these conditions, abnormal mTOR activity contributes to immune system imbalances, leading to increased inflammation and autoimmunity.

- mTOR and RA [83]
- mTOR and autoimmune thyroid disease[27]

Other associated implications The mechanistic target of rapamycin (mTOR) is increasingly recognized for its role in a wide range of physiological disturbances in humans. Beyond its established connection to autoimmune diseases, ongoing research has identified its involvement in:

- mTOR and intervertebral disc degeneration [65]
- mTOR and inflammation [50]
- mTOR and endometriosis [8]
- mTOR in infertility (sperm motility) [39]
- mTOR and acupuncture

Viral Infections

mTOR plays a crucial role in viral infections by regulating the host cell's metabolic and immune responses. Many viruses exploit the mTOR pathway to enhance their replication and survival by manipulating cellular growth, protein synthesis, and autophagy. Inhibiting mTOR can reduce viral replication and boost antiviral immunity, making it a potential therapeutic target in managing viral infections [51]. The pathways of viruses hijacking the cellular molecular machinery are discussed in the next chapter.

mTORC1: Central Role in Signal Transduction and Cell Regulation

The compartmentalization of mTOR signaling via distinct membrane localizations and adapter proteins ensures precise regulation of its activity in response to varying cellular signals. The lysosomal membrane is central to nutrient-sensing and its activation. mTORC1 (mechanistic target of rapamycin complex 1) serves as a central hub in intracellular and extracellular signal transduction networks by integrating and processing multiple signals. It plays a crucial role in dictating the rates of macromolecule synthesis, thereby influencing cell growth, proliferation, and survival. The ability of mTORC1 to sense intracellular alterations, such as changes in amino acids, energy levels, oxygen, and various stresses, enables it to control a range of cellular processes [1] and includes:

1. *Protein Translation*: mTORC1 regulates the machinery responsible for protein synthesis, ensuring that cells produce the necessary proteins for growth and function.
2. *Autophagy*: mTORC1 modulates autophagy, a process where cells degrade and recycle their components, balancing cellular metabolism and responding to nutrient availability.
3. *Ribosome Biogenesis*: By controlling the production of ribosomes, mTORC1 influences the cell's capacity for protein synthesis.
4. *Stress-Induced Transcription*: mTORC1 coordinates the cellular response to stress by regulating transcriptional programs that help the cell cope with adverse conditions.
5. *Cell Cycle Transition*: Through its downstream pathways, mTORC1 manages the progression of cells through the cell cycle, promoting or inhibiting cell division as needed

Components of mTORC1

1. *mTOR*: The core kinase of the complex, responsible for phosphorylating downstream substrates that regulate cell growth and metabolism.
2. *RAPTOR (regulatory-associated protein of mTOR)*: Essential for mTORC1 localization and substrate recruitment. It helps mTORC1 interact with the lysosomal surface and recognize substrates.
3. *mLST8 (mammalian lethal with Sec13 protein 8)*: Important for mTOR stabilization and structural integrity of the complex.
4. *DEPTOR (DEP domain-containing mTOR-interacting protein)*: A negative regulator of mTOR that inhibits mTORC1 activity.
5. *PRAS40 (Proline-rich AKT substrate of 40 kDa)*: An insulin-responsive inhibitor that regulates mTORC1 activity through its interactions directly with *Raptor* (Regulatory-associated protein of mTOR) (Fig. 1.13).

Substrates and Outputs:

- *S6 Kinase (S6K1)*: Phosphorylation by mTORC1 activates S6K1, leading to increased protein synthesis through the ribosomal protein S6.
- *4E-BP1*: The phosphorylation of 4E-BP1 relieves its inhibition of eIF4E, thereby enhancing cap-dependent translation initiation and promoting protein synthesis.
- *ULK1*: Inhibition of ULK1 by mTORC1 suppresses autophagy (Fig. 1.14).

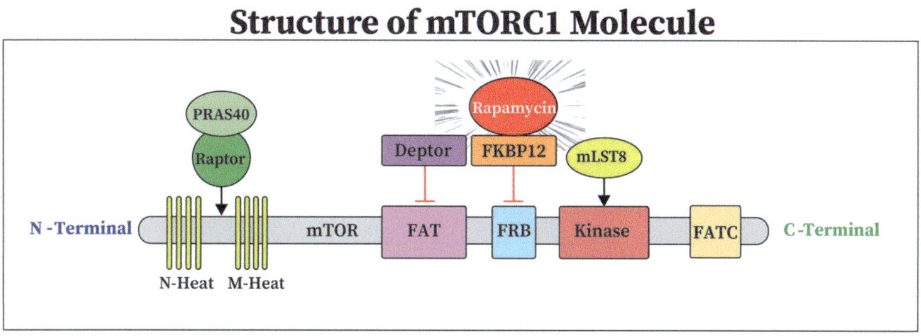

Fig. 1.13 This image represents the basic mTORC1 molecule, and the sites for attachment of both activator (black arrows) & inhibitor (red t-bars) molecules, each having their own specific function on the mTOR molecule as presented above

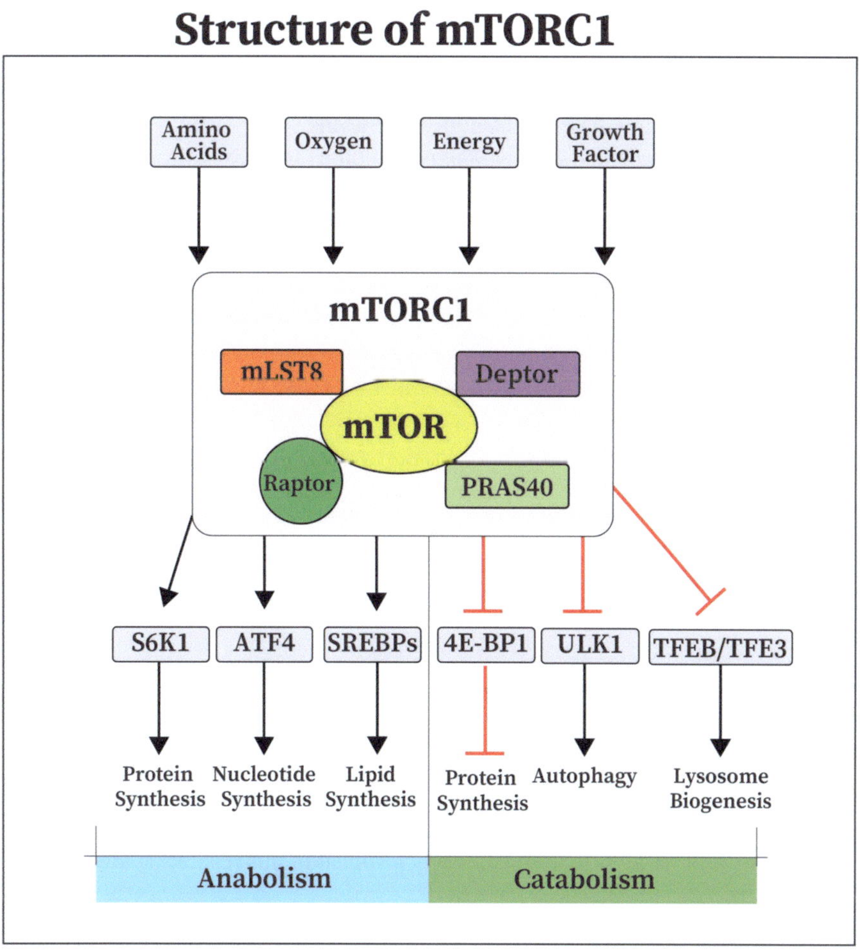

Fig. 1.14 The mTORC1 molecule's upstream pathways are shown above the image, while its downstream pathways are shown below. These end products are categorized as anabolic and catabolic

mTORC1 Activators

1. *Amino Acids*: Leucine, arginine
2. *Growth Factors*: Insulin, IGF-1 (insulin-like growth factor 1)
3. *Energy Status*: High ATP levels
4. *Lipids*: Lysophosphatidic acid (LPA)
5. *Glucose*: Via glycolysis, leading to increased ATP production.
6. *Rheb*: A small GTPase that directly activates mTORC1
7. *Rag GTPases*: Recruit mTORC1 to lysosomal surface in response to amino acids
8. *Nutrient Sensors*: Sestrins (in response to leucine)
9. *Hormones*: Estrogen
10. *Oxygen Levels*: Normoxia (normal oxygen levels)

mTORC1 Inhibitors

1. *Energy Status*: Low ATP levels, high AMP levels
2. *AMPK (AMP-Activated Protein Kinase)*: Inhibits mTORC1 through phosphorylation of TSC2 and Raptor
3. *TSC1/2 Complex*: Acts as a GTPase-activating protein (GAP) for Rheb, inhibiting mTORC1
4. *REDD1*: Induced by hypoxia, activates TSC1/2 complex
5. *PTEN (Phosphatase and Tensin Homolog)*: Dephosphorylates PIP3, reducing AKT signaling
6. *PP2A (Protein Phosphatase 2A)*: Dephosphorylates and inactivates mTORC1 components
7. *Stress Signals*: DNA damage (activates p53, which induces REDD1 and activates TSC1/2)
8. *Pharmacological Inhibitors*: Rapamycin, Torin1
9. *Cytokines*: IFN-γ (interferon-gamma)
10. *Nutrient Deprivation*: Low amino acids, glucose, or lipid levels (Fig. 1.15)

mTORC1 Upstream Pathways

Cell growth and proliferation are dependent not only on the availability of nutrients but also on extracellular growth factors. Growth factor signaling is crucial in determining the position and number of specific cell types within a tissue. The predominant growth-promoting signaling pathways involved in this regulation are:

- *PI3K-AKT Pathway*: The PI3K-AKT pathway is a key regulator of mTOR. When growth factors bind to their receptors, PI3K (phosphoinositide 3-kinase) is activated, producing PIP3, which recruits and activates AKT (protein kinase B).

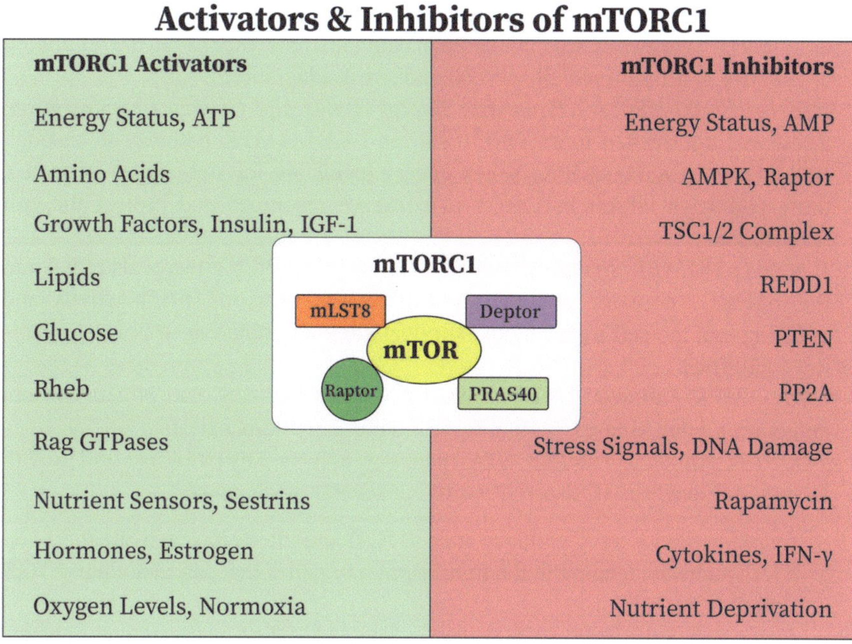

Fig. 1.15 The activators and inhibitors of mTORC1 molecule is categorized and presented in the table above

AKT phosphorylates and inhibits the TSC1/2 complex, leading to the activation of mTORC1. This pathway promotes cell growth, proliferation, and survival. This pathway activates mTORC1 and is frequently upregulated in cancers, driving cell growth and survival.

- *RAS-MAPK Pathway*: Similar to the PI3K-AKT pathway, the RAS-MAPK pathway activates mTORC1. The RAS-MAPK pathway regulates mTOR in response to growth signals. When activated, RAS initiates a cascade involving RAF, MEK, and ERK (MAPKs). ERK can phosphorylate and inhibit the TSC1/2 complex, leading to mTORC1 activation. This pathway promotes cell growth, differentiation, and proliferation by integrating external growth signals with mTORC1 activity.
- *Gator-Rag Pathway:* It regulates mTORC1 in response to amino acid availability. The Rag GTPases, regulated by the GATOR1 and GATOR2 complexes, sense amino acid levels. When amino acids are abundant, Rag GTPases are activated, facilitating the recruitment of mTORC1 to the lysosomal membrane where it becomes active. This activation promotes cell growth and metabolism. Conversely, in low amino acid conditions, GATOR1 inhibits Rag GTPases, leading to mTORC1 inactivation.
- *P53-Sestrin 1&2 Pathway:* The p53 tumor suppressor protein, along with the stress-inducible proteins Sestrin 1 and Sestrin 2, plays a critical role in cellular stress responses. p53 activates the transcription of Sestrin 1&2 and then activates

the TSC1/2 complex, which inhibits mTORC1 reducing cell growth and proliferation. Both pathways link p53's role in cellular stress response to the regulation of mTORC1, promoting cell survival and stress adaptation.
- *HIF-1–REDD1-TSC 1/2 Pathways: Energy Status and Oxygen Concentration*: These are transmitted to mTORC1 via the LKB1-AMPK pathway or through Reddl/2 and LKB1-AMPK. When energy levels are low or oxygen is scarce, these pathways inhibit mTORC1 to conserve resources and protect the cell from stress.
- *Wnt and p38MAPK Signaling*: Both Wnt and p38MAPK pathways also feed into the mTORC1 network, adding layers of regulation to mTORC1 activity and ensuring that the cell's growth and survival are finely tuned in response to varying conditions.
- *LKB1-AMPK Pathway:* LKB1activates AMPK (AMP-activated protein kinase) and other related kinases, regulating cellular energy homeostasis.
- *JAK-STAT pathway:* The JAK-STAT pathway, activated by cytokines and growth factors, influences mTOR activity through several mechanisms:
  - *Cytokine Signaling*: Cytokines such as IL-6 and interferons activate the JAK-STAT pathway, leading to the transcription of genes that can modulate mTOR signaling.
  - *Cross-Talk with PI3K-AKT Pathway*: The JAK-STAT pathway can enhance the PI3K-AKT pathway, which directly activates mTORC1 by inhibiting the TSC1/2 complex.
  - *Regulation of Cell Growth and Metabolism*: STAT proteins can regulate the expression of genes involved in cell growth, metabolism, and survival, thereby indirectly affecting mTOR activity.

This integration helps coordinate immune responses with cellular growth and metabolic regulation.

Role of Mitochondria

Mitochondria and mTOR signaling are intimately connected, with mitochondria providing the energy and metabolic intermediates necessary for mTORC1 activation. In turn, mTORC1 regulates mitochondrial biogenesis, dynamics, and function, integrating energy status with cellular growth and metabolic regulation. This interplay ensures that cells adapt to changing environmental conditions, maintaining energy homeostasis and cellular health. Mitochondria play a crucial role in the regulation of mTOR (mechanistic target of rapamycin) signaling, particularly through their involvement in energy production, metabolic processes, and cellular homeostasis [79].

Here's an elaboration on the interplay between mitochondria and mTOR:

1. Energy Production and mTOR Activation

Mitochondria are the primary source of cellular ATP through oxidative phosphorylation. mTORC1, a key component of the mTOR pathway, senses the energy status of the cell:

- *ATP Levels*: High ATP levels, indicating sufficient energy, promote mTORC1 activation. Active mTORC1 then enhances anabolic processes such as protein synthesis, lipid biosynthesis, and cell growth.
- *AMPK Activation*: Low ATP levels activate AMPK (AMP-activated protein kinase), which inhibits mTORC1. AMPK phosphorylates TSC2 (tuberous sclerosis complex 2) and Raptor, components of the mTORC1 complex, leading to mTORC1 inhibition. This conserves energy by reducing anabolic processes and promoting catabolic processes such as autophagy.

2. Mitochondrial Biogenesis

   5mTORC1 regulates mitochondrial biogenesis, the process by which new mitochondria are formed:

   - *PGC-1α Activation*: mTORC1 influences the expression of PGC-1α (peroxisome proliferator-activated receptor gamma coactivator 1-alpha), a master regulator of mitochondrial biogenesis. PGC-1α promotes the transcription of genes involved in mitochondrial replication and function.
   - *S6K1 Pathway*: mTORC1 activates S6K1 (ribosomal protein S6 kinase beta-1), which in turn can influence mitochondrial biogenesis and function.

3. Mitochondrial Dynamics and Function

   Mitochondria undergo continuous cycles of fusion and fission processes regulated by mTOR signaling:

   - *Mitochondrial Fusion*: mTORC1 activity is associated with enhanced mitochondrial fusion, leading to interconnected mitochondrial networks that optimize ATP production and reduce oxidative stress.
   - *Mitochondrial Fission*: Inhibition of mTORC1 can promote mitochondrial fission, resulting in fragmented mitochondria that are often targeted for mitophagy, a selective form of autophagy that degrades damaged mitochondria.

4. Metabolic Regulation

   mTOR signaling integrates mitochondrial metabolism with cellular growth and metabolic pathways:

   - *Glycolysis and Oxidative Phosphorylation*: mTORC1 promotes glycolysis by upregulating the expression of glycolytic enzymes and glucose transporters. Additionally, it supports oxidative phosphorylation by increasing mitochondrial capacity and function.
   - *Lipid Metabolism*: mTORC1 influences lipid biosynthesis and storage, processes that are closely linked to mitochondrial function and energy metabolism.

5. Reactive Oxygen Species (ROS)

Mitochondria are a major source of ROS, which can act as signaling molecules:

- *ROS and mTORC1 Activation*: Moderate levels of ROS can activate mTORC1, promoting cell growth and proliferation. However, excessive ROS can lead to oxidative stress and inhibit mTORC1 activity, triggering protective cellular responses such as autophagy.

6. Cell Survival and Apoptosis
   Mitochondria and mTOR signaling coordinate cell survival and apoptosis:
   - *Survival Pathways*: mTORC1 promotes cell survival by enhancing mitochondrial function and ATP production, supporting the energy demands of growing cells.
   - *Apoptosis Regulation*: Dysfunctional mitochondria can release pro-apoptotic factors such as cytochrome c, triggering cell death pathways. mTOR signaling can modulate the balance between cell survival and apoptosis by regulating mitochondrial integrity and function.

Role of Lysosomes

Lysosomes play a critical role in regulating mTOR (mechanistic target of rapamycin) function, particularly mTORC1, a key protein complex that controls cell growth and metabolism in response to nutrient availability. Lysosomes are integral to mTORC1 function, serving as platforms for nutrient sensing and signaling integration. They regulate mTORC1 activity based on nutrient availability, control autophagy, influence lysosomal biogenesis, and participate in lipid and energy metabolism. This dynamic interplay ensures cellular growth and metabolic homeostasis in response to changing environmental conditions [24].

Here's an elaboration on the role of lysosomes in mTORC1 function:

1. *Nutrient Sensing and mTORC1 Activation:* Lysosomes are central hubs for nutrient sensing and mTORC1 activation. mTORC1 is recruited to the lysosomal surface, where it becomes activated in response to sufficient levels of amino acids, glucose, and other nutrients.

   - Amino Acids*:* Amino acids, particularly leucine and arginine, are sensed by the Rag GTPases on the lysosomal membrane. When amino acids are abundant, Rag GTPases become active and recruit mTORC1 to the lysosomal surface, where it interacts with Rheb (Ras homolog enriched in brain), a small GTPase that directly activates mTORC1.
   - Glucose*:* Lysosomes also play a role in glucose sensing, indirectly affecting mTORC1 activity through pathways that monitor cellular energy status.

2. Regulation of Autophagy: *Lysosomes are involved in autophagy, a cellular degradation process that* recycles damaged organelles and macromolecules. mTORC1 negatively regulates autophagy:

   - Autophagy Suppression*:* When nutrients are abundant, mTORC1 is active and suppresses autophagy by phosphorylating and inhibiting the ULK1 complex, a key initiator of autophagy.
   - Autophagy Activation*:* Under nutrient deprivation, mTORC1 activity decreases, leading to the activation of autophagy. This helps cells adapt to stress by degrading and recycling cellular components to maintain energy balance.

3. Lysosomal Biogenesis and Function: mTORC1 also regulates lysosomal biogenesis and function by controlling the transcription factor TFEB (Transcription Factor EB):

   - TFEB Activation*:* Under nutrient-rich conditions, mTORC1 phosphorylates TFEB, retaining it in the cytoplasm. Under nutrient starvation, dephosphorylated TFEB translocates to the nucleus, promoting the expression of genes involved in lysosomal biogenesis and autophagy.

4. Lipid and Energy Metabolism: *Lysosomes* and mTORC1 are involved in lipid metabolism and energy homeostasis:

   - Lipid Metabolism*:* mTORC1 activation influences lipid biosynthesis by regulating enzymes involved in lipid production. Lysosomes contribute to lipid catabolism through lipophagy, where lipid droplets are delivered to lysosomes for degradation.
   - Energy Homeostasis: Lysosomes help sense cellular energy status via AMPK (AMP-activated protein kinase) signaling. AMPK, activated under low energy conditions, inhibits mTORC1 to conserve energy.

Lysosomal Membrane Localization

mTOR and lysosomes [16, 18, 59, 61]: The relationship between the lysosome and mTORC1 is characterized by a bidirectional regulatory mechanism: The recruitment and activation of mTORC1 on the lysosomal surface are tightly regulated processes that act as an AND gate, integrating nutrient and growth factor signals. This mechanism ensures that mTORC1-mediated anabolic processes are only initiated under conditions that are favorable for cell growth and proliferation. By requiring both nutrient and growth factor signals, cells efficiently coordinate their metabolic activities with their external environment, optimizing resource utilization and maintaining cellular homeostasis.

In the context of cellular signaling and lysosomal function, an AND gate refers to a molecular mechanism where multiple conditions or inputs must be met simultaneously to trigger a specific downstream event, similar to the logical AND gate in computing. This concept is particularly relevant in the regulation of the mechanistic target of rapamycin complex 1 (mTORC1) at the lysosome.

- mTORC1 as an AND Gate in Lysosomal Function:

  Exercise influences mTOR (mechanistic target of rapamycin) activity depending on the type and intensity of the exercise. Endurance exercise typically inhibits mTORC1, promoting autophagy and cellular repair processes, while resistance training activates mTORC1, leading to increased protein synthesis and muscle growth. The balance between these responses helps regulate muscle adaptation, recovery, and overall metabolic health [80].

The activation of mTORC1 at the lysosomal membrane is a well-established example of an AND gate mechanism. mTORC1 integrates multiple inputs, such as:

1. Amino acid availability: Amino acids are sensed by the Rag GTPases, which bring mTORC1 to the lysosome.
2. Growth factor signals: Insulin or growth factors activate upstream pathways (such as the PI3K-AKT pathway), which also promote mTORC1 activation.
3. Energy status: The energy sensor AMP-activated protein kinase (AMPK) inhibits mTORC1 under low-energy conditions, so sufficient energy is required for mTORC1 activation.
4. Oxygen levels: mTORC1 can also respond to cellular oxygen levels, adding another layer of regulation.

All of these signals must be positive (active) for mTORC1 to become fully activated at the lysosome, thereby promoting processes such as protein synthesis, cell growth, and inhibition of autophagy.

AND Gate in Action:

- If any of these signals are missing (e.g., lack of amino acids, low energy, or absence of growth factors), mTORC1 remains inactive, and cellular growth processes are paused.
- When all conditions are met, mTORC1 is activated at the lysosomal surface, initiating downstream signaling.

This AND gate model ensures that mTORC1 only promotes growth when the cell has sufficient resources, preventing unnecessary energy expenditure under unfavorable conditions. Thus, lysosomes serve as central hubs where multiple metabolic signals converge, acting as the control point for this critical regulatory AND gate.

The mTOR pathway's ability to sense and respond to nutrient levels is critical for regulating cell growth and metabolic control. Specific recognition of nutrient inputs, such as amino acids, growth factors, and other nutrients, correlates to outputs of regulated cell growth and metabolic control. This regulation functions as a binary decision-making process, where the presence or absence of specific nutrients triggers distinct signaling cascades of mTOR.

- *Regulation by Nutrients*: mTORC1 is primarily regulated by nutrients, particularly amino acids. Amino acid availability leads to the recruitment of mTORC1 to the lysosomal surface.
- *Key Adapter Proteins*: The Regulator complex and the Rag GTPases are crucial adapter proteins that mediate the localization of mTORC1 to the lysosomal membrane. When amino acids are abundant, Rag GTPases become active and bind to the Regulator complex, which anchors them to the lysosomal surface. This positioning allows mTORC1 to interact with and be activated by the small GTPase Rheb, which is also located on the lysosome and is responsible for directly activating mTORC1.
- *Function*: Once activated at the lysosomal membrane, mTORC1 promotes anabolic processes, including protein synthesis, lipid synthesis, and nucleotide synthesis, while inhibiting catabolic processes like autophagy.
- *Lysosome Regulates mTORC1*:
  - *Nutrient Sensing*: Lysosomes sense nutrient levels, particularly amino acids, which activate mTORC1 through Rag GTPases.
  - *Signal Integration*: The lysosomal membrane acts as a platform where mTORC1 integrates signals related to growth factors, energy status, and stress.
- *mTORC1 Regulates Lysosome*:
  - *Autophagy Inhibition*: When active, mTORC1 inhibits autophagy by phosphorylating key autophagy-related proteins, preventing the lysosome from degrading cellular components.
  - *Catabolic Control*: In response to nutrient abundance, mTORC1 activity ensures that the lysosome's catabolic processes are downregulated.

This bidirectional control ensures cellular homeostasis, impacting processes such as growth, metabolism, and autophagy. The activation of mTORC1 on the lysosome is a highly regulated process that occurs under nutrient-replete conditions, ensuring that cells only engage in growth and anabolic processes when sufficient resources are available. This process involves the Rag–Regulator complex and the Rheb GTPase, acting as a coincidence detector or AND gate, requiring both nutrient and growth factor signals for full activation.

Mechanism of mTORC1 Activation on the Lysosome

Recruitment to the Lysosomal Surface

- *Rag GTPases*: Under nutrient-rich conditions, Rag GTPases (RagA/RagB and RagC/RagD) become active. RagA/RagB bind GTP, while RagC/RagD bind GDP.

- *Ragulator Complex*: The Rag GTPases interact with the Ragulator complex, a multi-protein complex that anchors them to the lysosomal membrane. This interaction is critical for recruiting mTORC1 to the lysosomal surface.

Proximity to Rheb GTPase

- *Rheb Localization*: Rheb (Ras homolog enriched in brain) is a small GTPase localized on the lysosomal membrane. Rheb is active when bound to GTP and inactive when bound to GDP.
- *Growth Factor Signaling*: Growth factors activate the PI3K/Akt pathway, leading to the inhibition of the TSC1/TSC2 complex, which is a GTPase-activating protein (GAP) for Rheb. Inhibition of TSC1/TSC2 allows Rheb to remain in its GTP-bound active state.

Activation as an AND Gate

- *Nutrient Signal*: The active Rag GTPases, through the Ragulator complex, recruit mTORC1 to the lysosomal surface in response to nutrient availability, particularly amino acids.
- *Growth Factor Signal*: Simultaneously, growth factor signaling activates Rheb by inhibiting its GAP, the TSC1/TSC2 complex, allowing Rheb to remain GTP-bound and active.
- *Coincidence Detection*: mTORC1 activation requires both signals. The recruitment of mTORC1 to the lysosome positions it near Rheb, but full activation of mTORC1 occurs only when Rheb is in its GTP-bound active state, responding to growth factor signals. This dual requirement ensures that mTORC1 is only active when both nutrients and growth factors are present, preventing unnecessary anabolic processes under suboptimal conditions.

Functional Outcomes

- *Protein Synthesis*: Once activated, mTORC1 phosphorylates substrates such as S6 kinase (S6K1) and 4E-BP1, leading to increased protein synthesis.
- *Lipid Biosynthesis*: mTORC1 activation promotes lipid biosynthesis, supporting membrane formation and energy storage.
- *Inhibition of Autophagy*: Active mTORC1 inhibits autophagy by phosphorylating and inactivating ULK1, a key initiator of the autophagy process.

Recruitment and Activation of mTORC1 on the Lysosome

Nutrient-Driven Recruitment

In the presence of nutrients, particularly amino acids, mTORC1 is recruited to the lysosomal surface through interactions with Rag GTPases (RagA, RagB, RagC, RagD). These Rag GTPases are anchored to the lysosomal membrane by the Ragulator complex, composed of five subunits (LAMTOR1–5). The precise mechanism by which nutrient availability drives the anchoring of Rag GTPases to the Ragulator and the concurrent recruitment of mTORC1 is not fully understood, but several key processes are involved:

1. *Amino Acid Sensing*:
   - Amino acids, such as leucine and arginine, activate the Rag GTPases by promoting the exchange of GDP for GTP on RagA or RagB and GDP binding on RagC or RagD. This nucleotide state (RagA/B•GTP–RagC/D•GDP) is essential for the active configuration of the Rag heterodimer.
2. *Ragulator Complex*:
   - The Ragulator complex acts as a scaffold, anchoring the active Rag GTPases to the lysosomal membrane. The interaction between the Rag GTPases and the Ragulator is crucial for the spatial regulation of mTORC1 recruitment.
3. *mTORC1 Recruitment*:
   - The active Rag GTPases (RagA/B•GTP–RagC/D•GDP) interact with the Raptor subunit of mTORC1, facilitating the translocation of mTORC1 to the lysosomal surface.

Cryo-EM Structure and Activation Mechanism

Translocation and Orientation on the Lysosome

- *Critical Role of Translocation*: Translocation of mTORC1 to the lysosomal surface is essential for its activation. This positioning allows mTORC1 to interact with the Rheb GTPase, which is anchored to the lysosomal membrane via a C-terminal farnesyl group.
- *Rheb GTPase*: Rheb is a small GTPase that activates mTORC1. It is membrane associated due to its C-terminal farnesyl group, which anchors it to the lysosomal surface.

Structural Insights from Cryo-EM (PDB ID 6BCU)

- *Structure of mTORC1 Bound to Rheb*: The cryo-EM structure (PDB ID 6BCU) provides a detailed view of mTORC1 in complex with Rheb [82]. This structure offers insights into how mTORC1 is oriented toward the lysosomal membrane when bound to Rheb.
- *Orientation and Interaction*: The structure indicates that mTORC1, when bound to Rheb, adopts an orientation that positions it optimally for activation by Rheb's GTPase activity.

Superimposition of Structural Models

- *Raptor Involvement*: Both the Rheb-bound mTORC1 structure and the Raptor-Rag-Ragulator complex contain the Raptor subunit. By superimposing these structures, researchers can generate a comprehensive model of mTORC1 activation.
- *Structural Model of Rheb-Activated mTORC1*: By superimposing the Rheb-bound mTORC1 structure onto the Raptor-Rag-Ragulator structure, a detailed model of the Rheb-activated mTORC1 dimer tethered to the lysosome is generated. This model shows how mTORC1 interacts with both the Rag GTPases and Rheb, positioning it for optimal activation.

Functional Implications

Activation of mTORC1

- *Dual Interaction*: The model highlights the importance of the dual interaction between mTORC1 and both the Rag GTPases and Rheb. This interaction ensures that mTORC1 is activated only when both nutrient and growth factor signals are present.
- *Kinase Activation*: The proximity of mTORC1 to Rheb on the lysosomal membrane allows Rheb to exert its kinase-activating effect on mTORC1, facilitating downstream signaling and promoting cell growth and metabolism.

The cryo-EM structure of mTORC1 bound to Rheb, combined with the Raptor-Rag-Ragulator complex, provides a comprehensive view of mTORC1 activation on the lysosomal surface. By superimposing these structures, a detailed model emerges that shows how mTORC1 is tethered to the lysosome and activated by Rheb. This structural model underscores the importance of the lysosomal localization of mTORC1 for its activation and highlights the intricate regulatory mechanisms that control cell growth and metabolism in response to nutrient and growth factor signals.

Sensing Intracellular Nutrients

- Fatty acids are metabolized in mitochondria through β-oxidation, producing energy in the form of ATP. AMPK (AMP-activated protein kinase) senses cellular energy levels and activates pathways to increase ATP production, including fatty acid oxidation. mTOR (mechanistic target of rapamycin) regulates cell growth and metabolism, promoting anabolic processes when energy is abundant. AMPK inhibits mTOR signaling under low energy conditions, thereby balancing energy production and consumption. This interplay ensures cellular energy homeostasis.
- Glucose and ATP are central to cellular energy metabolism and directly influence the mTOR (mechanistic target of rapamycin) pathway:

  1. *Glucose*: Glucose is metabolized via glycolysis and the TCA cycle, leading to the production of ATP. High glucose levels indicate abundant energy, activating mTORC1 through the PI3K-AKT pathway, promoting cell growth and proliferation.
  2. *ATP*: ATP serves as an energy currency. High ATP levels signal sufficient energy availability, supporting mTORC1 activation. Conversely, low ATP levels activate AMPK (AMP-activated protein kinase), which inhibits mTORC1 by activating the TSC1/2 complex, conserving energy by reducing anabolic processes.

Overall, glucose metabolism and ATP levels provide critical feedback to mTORC1, balancing energy production and consumption with cellular growth needs.

- Amino acids regulate mTOR signaling through the following pathway:

  1. *Amino Acid Sensing*: Cells sense amino acid availability through the Rag GTPases and the GATOR complexes.
  2. *Rag GTPases Activation*: When amino acids are abundant, Rag GTPases are activated.
  3. *mTORC1 Localization*: Activated Rag GTPases recruit mTORC1 to the lysosomal surface, where it interacts with Rheb, another small GTPase.
  4. *mTORC1 Activation*: This interaction leads to the activation of mTORC1, promoting protein synthesis, cell growth, and proliferation.

- In low amino acid conditions, Rag GTPases remain inactive, preventing mTORC1 activation and conserving cellular resources.

Cytosolic Nutrient Sensing

Amino Acid Sensing

- *Sestrin2 as a Leucine Sensor*:

  - *Function*: Sestrin2 acts as a cytosolic sensor for the amino acid leucine.
  - *Mechanism*: In the absence of leucine, Sestrin2 binds to and inhibits GATOR2 (GAP activity toward Rags 2), a component of the pathway that regulates the activity of the Rag GTPases.
  - *Activation*: When leucine levels increase, leucine binds to Sestrin2, causing a conformational change that releases GATOR2 from inhibition. This allows GATOR2 to activate the Rag GTPases, facilitating mTORC1 recruitment to the lysosomal membrane.

- *CASTOR1 as an Arginine Sensor*:

  - *Function*: CASTOR1 is a cytosolic sensor for the amino acid arginine.
  - *Mechanism*: In the absence of arginine, CASTOR1 binds to and inhibits GATOR2.
  - *Activation*: When arginine levels rise, arginine binds to CASTOR1, leading to the release of GATOR2 from inhibition. This enables GATOR2 to activate the Rag GTPases, promoting mTORC1 activation.

Integrated Nutrient and Growth Factor Sensing

- *Binary Decision and Signaling Cascades*:

  - *Nutrient Signals*: The presence of specific amino acids (e.g., leucine and arginine) triggers the release of GATOR2 from its inhibitors (Sestrin2 and CASTOR1), allowing the activation of Rag GTPases. Active Rag GTPases recruit mTORC1 to the lysosomal membrane.

Growth Factor Signals Growth factors activate the PI3K/Akt pathway, leading to the inhibition of the TSC1/TSC2 complex. This inhibition allows Rheb to remain GTP-bound and active, which is necessary for mTORC1 activation.

mTORC1 and Autophagy: The Key Points

Role of mTORC1 in Autophagy

Autophagy is a vital cellular process for degrading and recycling cellular components, ensuring cellular homeostasis and preventing diseases. This process, conserved from yeast to humans, relies on a set of autophagy-related (ATG) proteins.

Autophagy allows cells to break down and recycle damaged organelles and proteins through the autophagy-lysosome pathway, supporting survival under adverse conditions. Thus, mTORC1 acts as a critical switch between promoting anabolic processes and enabling catabolic processes like autophagy, maintaining cellular homeostasis [33].

There are many processes involving autophagy and mTORC1 in cellular biology. mTOR, through mTORC1, regulates autophagy, and the specific molecular interactions of GABARAPs in both autophagic and non-autophagic processes broaden the scope for potential therapeutic interventions [42]

- Elucidating the precise roles of GABARAPs in selective autophagy across various organelles.
- Investigating GABARAP-mediated receptor trafficking in disease contexts.
- Developing inhibitors or modulators targeting GABARAPs to influence disease outcomes, particularly in cancers and neurodegenerative diseases.

1. *GABARAPs in Selective Autophagy Processes*

   GABARAPs are critical mediators in selective autophagy, which targets specific organelles or protein aggregates for degradation. Below are the major selective autophagy processes where GABARAPs play an integral role:

   - *Mitophagy (Mitochondrial Autophagy)*: GABARAPs interact with mitophagy receptors like BNIP3 and NIX, which are responsible for tagging damaged mitochondria for degradation. GABARAPs recruit these receptors to nascent autophagosomes, facilitating mitochondrial turnover. Dysfunctional mitophagy is linked to diseases like *Parkinson's disease*, where the failure to clear damaged mitochondria leads to neuronal death.
   - *Reticulophagy (Endoplasmic Reticulum Autophagy)*: The ER is subject to autophagic degradation under stress conditions, such as in the unfolded protein response (UPR). GABARAPs assist in this process by binding to ER-localized autophagy receptors like FAM134B, which is essential for ER clearance. Impairment in this pathway is associated with neurodegenerative diseases and cancers, where ER stress plays a crucial role.
   - *Golgi Autophagy (Golgiphagy)*: GABARAPs also mediate the selective degradation of Golgi apparatus components, a process less understood but important for maintaining cellular organelle homeostasis. GABARAP interaction with Golgi-resident proteins during stress or damage could have implications for diseases such as *cancers* where protein trafficking is often dysregulated.
   - *Dorphagy (Degeneration of the Nuclear Envelope)*: The selective degradation of the nuclear envelope involves GABARAPs, especially during processes like nuclear envelope breakdown during cell division or damage. This form of autophagy is still under investigation but could provide insights into *cancer biology* and *aging-related disorders*.

2. *GABARAPs and Autophagy-Lysosome Fusion*

   The role of GABARAPs in autophagy-lysosome fusion is pivotal in maintaining autophagic flux, the continuous process from autophagosome formation to cargo degradation. GABARAP proteins, particularly through interaction with SNARE complexes, mediate the final steps where autophagosomes fuse with lysosomes. Without this function, autophagic degradation stalls, leading to the accumulation of undegraded materials. This is a hallmark of *neurodegenerative diseases* like *Alzheimer's disease*, where protein aggregates accumulate due to defective autophagy-lysosome fusion.

3. *GABARAPs in Non-autophagic Roles*

   In addition to autophagy, GABARAPs are involved in the trafficking of cell surface receptors, including:

   - *γ-GABAA Receptor*: GABARAPs are responsible for the intracellular trafficking of the γ-GABAA receptor, which is critical for inhibitory neurotransmission in the central nervous system. Dysfunction in this transport pathway can contribute to *neuropsychiatric disorders* like *schizophrenia* or *epilepsy*.
   - *Angiotensin II AT1 Receptor (AT1R)*: GABARAPs are also involved in the endocytosis and intracellular trafficking of AT1R, a key player in the *renin-angiotensin system*. Disruption in this process could contribute to *cardiovascular diseases*, such as *hypertension* and *heart failure*, by affecting the responsiveness of cells to angiotensin II.

4. *GABARAPs in Cancer*

   GABARAPs have gained attention in cancer research due to their role in tumor growth, metastasis, and therapeutic resistance. Here are some insights into their function:

   - *Tumor Growth and Survival*: GABARAPs promote cell survival by regulating autophagy, especially under nutrient-deprived or stressed conditions typical of tumor microenvironments. They can help cancer cells survive chemotherapy by maintaining autophagic flux, preventing apoptosis, and promoting cellular homeostasis.
   - *Metastasis*: GABARAP proteins are involved in the regulation of cellular motility through their interaction with cytoskeletal components. In *metastatic cancers*, GABARAP-mediated autophagy aids in the migration and invasion of cancer cells by remodeling the cytoskeleton and degrading cellular components that suppress movement.
   - *Clinical Implications and Biomarkers*: Elevated serum levels of GABARAP and GABARAPL1 in cancer patients suggest their potential as *biomarkers* for prognosis and therapeutic response. Targeting GABARAPs might improve treatment outcomes by inhibiting their support of autophagy-dependent survival mechanisms in cancer cells.

During macroautophagy, double-membrane vesicles called autophagosomes form around components to be degraded. Autophagosomes then fuse with lysosomes, where the enclosed components are degraded and recycled through various mechanisms. The dysregulation of mTOR signaling is a common feature in many cancers, making it a critical target for cancer research and treatment. The mechanistic target of rapamycin (mTOR) plays a significant role in cancer, influencing tumor growth, progression, and therapy resistance.

Autophagy is a critical quality control process essential for cellular homeostasis and the prevention of diseases. It is tightly regulated by various mechanisms, with mTORC1 serving as a primary regulator that balances anabolic and catabolic processes. Understanding how mTORC1 controls autophagy under different cellular conditions provides insights into its role in health and disease and may offer therapeutic targets for conditions associated with its dysregulation.

1. *Formation of Autophagosomes*: Autophagosomes encapsulate damaged organelles, misfolded proteins, and other cellular debris. This process is mediated by ATG proteins, which coordinate the formation and expansion of the autophagosome membrane.
2. *Fusion with Lysosomes*: Once formed, autophagosomes fuse with lysosomes, leading to the degradation of their contents by lysosomal enzymes. The resulting macromolecules are then recycled back into the cytoplasm for reuse.

Regulation of Autophagy

Autophagy occurs constitutively at basal levels but is upregulated in response to cellular stress, such as infection, nutrient starvation, or other adverse conditions. Due to its crucial role in maintaining cellular homeostasis, autophagy is tightly regulated, as both insufficient and excessive autophagy can have serious consequences.

mTORC1: A Key Regulator of Autophagy

The mechanistic target of rapamycin complex 1 (mTORC1) is a central regulator of cell growth that balances anabolic and catabolic metabolism. mTORC1 plays an essential role in controlling autophagy under various cellular conditions:

1. *Inhibition of Autophagy Initiation*: Under nutrient-rich conditions, mTORC1 is active and inhibits the initiation of autophagy. This is achieved by phosphorylating and inhibiting the ULK1 complex (comprising ULK1, ATG13, and FIP200), which is essential for the early stages of autophagosome formation.
2. *Regulation of Autophagy Maturation and Lysosomal Biogenesis*: mTORC1 also influences later stages of autophagy, including the maturation of autophagosomes and the formation of lysosomes. By modulating lysosomal biogenesis, mTORC1 ensures that sufficient lysosomes are available for the degradation and recycling of autophagic cargo.

Regulation of mTORC1 Activity

mTORC1 is a central regulator of cell growth and metabolism, integrating signals from growth factors and nutrients through a sophisticated coincidence detection system. Its regulation on the lysosomal surface ensures precise control of anabolic and catabolic processes, maintaining cellular homeostasis and preventing diseases associated with its dysregulation. Understanding the intricate mechanisms of mTORC1 activation and regulation provides valuable insights into therapeutic strategies for various conditions linked to its activity.

mTORC1 activity is tightly regulated by a network of signaling nodes located on the lysosomal surface. This regulation ensures that mTORC1 is activated only when both growth factors and nutrients are present, creating a coincidence detection system.

Growth Factors and Nutrients

- *Growth Factors*: Activation of mTORC1 by growth factors involves the PI3K/Akt pathway. Akt phosphorylates and inhibits the TSC1/TSC2 complex, which normally acts as a GAP (GTPase-activating protein) for Rheb, a small GTPase. Inhibition of TSC1/TSC2 allows Rheb to remain GTP-bound and active, thereby activating mTORC1.
- *Nutrients*: Nutrients, particularly amino acids, regulate mTORC1 through the Rag GTPases. These GTPases form heterodimers (RagA or RagB bound to RagC or RagD) that interact with the Ragulator complex on the lysosomal surface. Active Rag heterodimers recruit mTORC1 to the lysosome, where it can be activated by Rheb.

The activation of mTORC1 requires the simultaneous presence of both nutrients and growth factors, making it a sophisticated coincidence detection system:

- *Nutrient Signal*: When amino acids are abundant, the Rag GTPases become active and recruit mTORC1 to the lysosomal membrane.
- *Environment signals*:
  - Inflammation via interleukin signaling activates mTOR (mechanistic target of rapamycin) through a cascade involving the PI3K/AKT pathway. Interleukins bind to their receptors, activating PI3K (phosphoinositide 3-kinase), which then activates AKT (protein kinase B). AKT phosphorylates and inhibits the TSC1/2 (tuberous sclerosis complex), leading to the activation of mTOR. This pathway promotes cell growth, proliferation, and survival in response to immune signals [4].
  - *H*ypoxia, HIF-1 (hypoxia-inducible factor 1), is stabilized and activates the expression of genes including REDD1 (regulated in development and DNA damage responses 1). REDD1 inhibits the TSC1/2 complex (tuberous sclerosis complex 1/2), which in turn inhibits mTOR (mechanistic target of rapamycin) signaling. This pathway reduces cellular growth and metabolism in low oxygen conditions, conserving energy and promoting cell survival.
- *Growth Factor Signal*: Growth factors activate the PI3K/Akt pathway, leading to the activation of Rheb GTPase. Active Rheb then interacts with and activates mTORC1.

This dual requirement ensures that mTORC1 is only active under favorable conditions, preventing unnecessary anabolic activity and promoting cellular homeostasis.

Functional Outcomes of mTORC1 Activation

1. *Protein Synthesis*: mTORC1 promotes protein synthesis by phosphorylating S6 kinase (S6K1) and 4E-BP1, which enhances mRNA translation.
2. *Lipid Synthesis*: Activation of mTORC1 stimulates lipid biosynthesis, supporting membrane formation and energy storage.
3. *Inhibition of Autophagy*: mTORC1 inhibits autophagy by phosphorylating and inactivating ULK1, a key initiator of the autophagy process.
4. *Cell Growth and Proliferation*: By regulating anabolic processes, mTORC1 supports cell growth and proliferation.

Dysregulation of mTORC1 and its Implications

Interaction with the Rag GTPase-Ragulator Complex:

- *Rag GTPases*: These GTPases are essential for amino acid sensing and mTORC1 recruitment to the lysosome.
  - *Heterodimer Formation*: Rag GTPases form obligate heterodimers through their C-terminal roadblock domains (CRDs). The heterodimers consist of either RagA or RagB bound to RagC or RagD. This heterodimeric nature allows cross-talk between their GTPase domains, which is crucial for mTORC1 signaling to adapt quickly to changes in nutrient levels.
  - *GTP/GDP Binding*: In nutrient-rich conditions, RagA or RagB binds GTP, while RagC or RagD binds GDP, forming the active state that recruits mTORC1.
- *Ragulator Complex*: A five-subunit complex that is necessary for targeting the Rag GTPases to the lysosomal surface. It serves as a scaffold that anchors the Rag GTPases to the lysosome and facilitates their interaction with mTORC1.
  - *Components*: The five subunits of Ragulator include LAMTOR1, LAMTOR2, LAMTOR3, LAMTOR4, and LAMTOR5.

Docking and Activation

- *Raptor Interaction*: The Raptor subunit of mTORC1 directly interacts with the lysosome-associated Rag GTPase-Ragulator complex. This docking positions mTORC1 on the lysosomal surface, making it accessible to Rheb.

- *Rheb GTPase*: Rheb is a small GTPase localized on the lysosomal membrane. It is active when bound to GTP and inactive when bound to GDP. The presence of growth factors activates the PI3K/Akt pathway, which inhibits the TSC1/TSC2 complex (a GAP for Rheb), allowing Rheb to remain GTP-bound and active.

Nucleotide Configurations

The Rag heterodimer can exist in four different nucleotide configurations, but only one configuration, RagA/B•GTP–RagC/D•GDP, signals nutrient sufficiency and interacts with mTORC1. This specific configuration allows mTORC1 to dock on the lysosome and become activated by Rheb GTPase.

Structural Insights from Cryo-EM

- *Cryo-EM Structure*: Using cryo-electron microscopy (cryo-EM), researchers have determined the structure of the Raptor subunit of mTORC1 bound to the Rag-Ragulator complex. This structural information is critical for understanding how mTORC1 discriminates between different nucleotide states of the Rag GTPases.
- *Conformational Changes*: The cryo-EM structure reveals the conformational changes in the Rag GTPases that occur in response to nutrient levels. These changes are essential for the proper positioning of mTORC1 on the lysosome.

Structural Model of mTORC1 Docked on the Lysosome

The structural model of mTORC1 docked on the lysosome, informed by cryo-EM data, provides detailed insights into the molecular interactions and conformational dynamics that underlie nutrient sensing by mTORC1. This model highlights several key points:

- *Interaction Sites*: Specific interaction sites between the Raptor subunit of mTORC1 and the Rag-Ragulator complex are identified, explaining how mTORC1 is recruited to the lysosome.
- *Nucleotide State Discrimination*: The structure elucidates how mTORC1 discriminates between different nucleotide states of the Rag GTPases, ensuring activation only under nutrient-sufficient conditions.
- *Regulatory Mechanisms*: Understanding these structural details allows for a comprehensive view of the regulatory mechanisms controlling mTORC1 activity in response to nutrient availability.

The regulation of mTORC1 by Rag GTPases is a sophisticated process involving conformational changes regulated by nutrient-sensing GAPs and GEFs. The cryo-EM structure of the Raptor subunit of mTORC1 bound to the Rag-Ragulator complex provides crucial insights into how mTORC1 distinguishes between different nucleotide states of the Rag GTPases. This structural information enhances our understanding of the molecular basis for nutrient sensing and mTORC1 activation, enabling the development of detailed models of mTORC1 function and regulation.

The activation of mTORC1 is a highly regulated process that depends on its translocation to the lysosomal surface, where it interacts with its kinase activator, the Rheb GTPase. Recent structural insights from cryo-EM have provided a detailed view of this interaction and its orientation relative to the lysosomal membrane.

Functional Outcomes of mTORC1 Activation

Once activated, mTORC1 regulates cell growth and metabolism through several key mechanisms:

1. *Promotion of Protein Synthesis*:
   - *S6K1 Phosphorylation*: mTORC1 phosphorylates ribosomal S6 kinase 1 (S6K1), which enhances the translation of mRNA into proteins by phosphorylating the ribosomal protein S6.
   - *4E-BP1 Phosphorylation*: mTORC1 phosphorylates eukaryotic translation initiation factor 4E-binding protein 1 (4E-BP1), releasing it from eIF4E. This release allows eIF4E to initiate cap-dependent translation, further promoting protein synthesis.
2. *Inhibition of Autophagy*:
   - *Phosphorylation of ATG Proteins*: mTORC1 phosphorylates several autophagy-related (ATG) proteins involved in the initiation and maturation of autophagosomes. By inhibiting these proteins, mTORC1 prevents the initiation of autophagy under nutrient-rich conditions.
   - *Regulation of Lysosomal Biogenesis*: mTORC1 also influences the biogenesis of lysosomes, ensuring that lysosomal activity is coordinated with nutrient availability and cellular growth needs.

1. *mTORC1 as an Inhibitor of Autophagy:*
   - *Direct Inhibition:* mTORC1 (mTOR complex 1) is a master regulator that directly inhibits autophagy under nutrient-rich conditions. When nutrients are abundant, mTORC1 is active and phosphorylates several key proteins involved in the initiation of autophagy, such as ULK1 (Unc-51 like autophagy activating kinase 1). Phosphorylation of ULK1 by mTORC1 inhibits its activity, thereby preventing the initiation of the autophagic process.

- *Indirect Inhibition:* mTORC1 also regulates autophagy indirectly through its effects on other signaling pathways and metabolic processes. For example, mTORC1 promotes protein synthesis and inhibits catabolic processes, which are essential for autophagy induction.

2. *Nutrient Sensing and mTORC1 Regulation:*

   - *Amino Acids:* Amino acids, particularly leucine, activate mTORC1. In the presence of sufficient amino acids, mTORC1 remains active, inhibiting autophagy. Conversely, amino acid deprivation leads to mTORC1 inhibition, which promotes autophagy to provide the cell with necessary nutrients.
   - *Growth Factors and Energy Status:* Growth factors (e.g., insulin) and cellular energy levels (reflected by AMP/ATP ratio) also regulate mTORC1 activity. Low energy status and the absence of growth factors inhibit mTORC1, leading to the activation of autophagy.

Autophagy Regulation Mechanism

mTOR, particularly mTORC1, is a critical regulator of autophagy, acting as an inhibitor under nutrient-rich conditions. The balance between mTOR activity and autophagy is essential for cellular homeostasis, and dysregulation of this balance is implicated in various diseases, including cancer, neurodegeneration, metabolic disorders, and aging. Understanding the intricate relationship between mTOR and autophagy can lead to new therapeutic strategies for these conditions .

1. *Initiation:*

   - Under nutrient-rich conditions, active mTORC1 phosphorylates and inhibits ULK1, preventing the initiation of autophagy. When nutrients are scarce, mTORC1 is inhibited, leading to dephosphorylation and activation of ULK1, which then initiates the formation of the autophagosome. The interplay between mTORC1, AMPK, and ULK1 ensures a balanced regulation of autophagy according to the cell's nutritional and energy status:
   - *Under energy-stress Conditions,* AMPK is activated, which phosphorylates and activates ULK1, thereby promoting autophagy to generate energy and maintain cellular homeostasis.

   This regulatory network allows cells to adapt to varying environmental conditions by precisely controlling the autophagic process, ensuring survival and proper cellular function.

2. *Autophagosome Formation:*

   - The initiation complex, including ULK1, activates downstream proteins like Beclin-1 and the class III PI3K complex, which are essential for the nucleation of the autophagosome.

3. *Autophagosome Maturation and Degradation:*
   - The autophagosome matures by expanding and sealing to form a double-membrane structure. It then fuses with lysosomes to form the autolysosome, where the contents are degraded and recycled.

Implications for Health and Disease

1. *Cancer:*
   - Dysregulation of mTOR signaling and autophagy is common in cancer. Many cancer cells exhibit high mTORC1 activity, which suppresses autophagy and supports rapid cell growth. In some contexts, inducing autophagy through mTORC1 inhibition can reduce tumor growth, while in others, excessive autophagy can lead to cancer cell survival and resistance to therapy.
2. *Neurodegenerative Diseases:*
   - Proper autophagy is essential for neuronal health. mTOR inhibitors can potentially enhance autophagy and clear aggregated proteins associated with neurodegenerative diseases like Alzheimer's and Parkinson's.
3. *Metabolic Disorders:*
   - mTOR and autophagy are involved in the regulation of metabolic processes. Dysregulation can lead to conditions such as obesity, diabetes, and cardiovascular diseases. Enhancing autophagy through mTOR inhibition can improve metabolic health and reduce the risk of these disorders.
4. *Aging:*
   - mTOR inhibition has been associated with lifespan extension in various model organisms, possibly through enhanced autophagy. By promoting the removal of damaged cellular components, mTOR inhibitors may improve cellular function and longevity.

Amino acids play a crucial role in promoting the translocation of mTORC1 to the lysosomal surface, enabling its activation by the Rheb GTPase. This process involves several key components and interactions:

mTORC1 Composition and Activation

Components of mTORC1:

- *mTOR*: The central kinase
- *Raptor (Regulatory-associated protein of mTOR)*: Facilitates substrate binding and docking of mTORC1 on the lysosome
- *mLST8 (GβL)*: Stabilizes the mTOR complex

Functional Outcomes

Rapid Response to Nutrient Levels

- The obligate heterodimeric nature of the Rag GTPases ensures that mTORC1 can quickly respond to changes in amino acid levels. When amino acid levels are high, the active Rag GTPases recruit mTORC1 to the lysosome, where it can be activated by Rheb.

Regulation of Cell Growth and Metabolism

- *Protein Synthesis*: Activated mTORC1 phosphorylates substrates like S6K1 and 4E-BP1, leading to enhanced protein synthesis.
- *Lipid Biosynthesis*: mTORC1 promotes lipid biosynthesis, supporting membrane formation and energy storage.
- *Inhibition of Autophagy*: By phosphorylating and inhibiting ULK1, mTORC1 prevents autophagy, directing resources toward growth and proliferation.

Amino acids promote the translocation of mTORC1 to the lysosomal surface through the interaction of Raptor with the Rag GTPase-Regulator complex. The obligate heterodimeric nature of the Rag GTPases, along with the essential role of the Regulator complex, ensures that mTORC1 can respond quickly and efficiently to changes in nutrient levels. This precise regulation is crucial for maintaining cellular growth and metabolic homeostasis, allowing cells to adapt to their nutritional environment and optimize their anabolic processes.

The recruitment and activation of mTORC1 on the lysosomal surface are critical for regulating cell growth, protein synthesis, and autophagy. Nutrient availability and growth factor signaling converge on mTORC1 to ensure that it is activated only under favorable conditions, promoting anabolic processes while inhibiting catabolic autophagy. Understanding the detailed mechanisms of mTORC1 regulation, including the role of basal autophagy, remains an important area of research with implications for various diseases and cellular processes.

The regulation of mTORC1 by the Rag GTPases is a complex process involving several structural and functional elements. The Rag GTPases operate similarly to other GTPases, with their GTPase domains consisting of a network of secondary structural elements known as switches. These switches undergo conformational changes upon the exchange or hydrolysis of GDP or GTP, respectively. This process is tightly regulated by nutrient-regulated GTPase-activating proteins (GAPs) and guanine nucleotide exchange factors (GEFs).

Structural and Functional Insights into Rag GTPases and mTORC1 Activation

Rag GTPase Mechanism

- *Switch Mechanism*: The GTPase domains of the Rag GTPases undergo conformational changes in their switches upon binding to GDP or GTP. These changes are crucial for their function and interaction with mTORC1.
- *Regulation by GAPs and GEFs*: The activity of the Rag GTPases is controlled by various nutrient-regulated proteins, including:
  - *GATOR1*: Acts as a GAP, promoting the hydrolysis of GTP to GDP on RagA/B
  - *FLCN-FNIP*: Another GAP complex that regulates Rag GTPases
  - *SLC38A9*: Functions as a GEF, facilitating the exchange of GDP for GTP on RagA/B

Activation of mTORC1 by Growth Factors

Growth factors activate the Rheb GTPase on the lysosomal surface. Rheb, in its GTP-bound state, interacts directly with mTORC1, activating its kinase activity. This process involves the following steps:

1. *PI3K/Akt Pathway Activation*: Growth factors activate the PI3K/Akt signaling pathway, leading to the phosphorylation and inhibition of the TSC1/TSC2 complex. This inhibition allows Rheb to remain in its active GTP-bound state.
2. *Interaction with mTORC1*: When mTORC1 is recruited to the lysosome by Rag GTPases, it encounters active Rheb, which activates mTORC1's kinase activity.

Functional Outcomes of mTORC1 Activation

Once activated, mTORC1 regulates cell growth and metabolism by promoting protein synthesis and inhibiting autophagy:

1. *Promotion of Protein Synthesis*:
   - *Phosphorylation of S6K1*: Activated mTORC1 phosphorylates ribosomal S6 kinase 1 (S6K1), enhancing the translation of mRNA into proteins by phosphorylating the ribosomal protein S6.
   - *Phosphorylation of 4E-BP1*: mTORC1 phosphorylates eukaryotic translation initiation factor 4E-binding protein 1 (4E-BP1), releasing it from eIF4E. This release allows eIF4E to initiate cap-dependent translation, further promoting protein synthesis.

2. *Inhibition of Autophagy*:
   - *Phosphorylation of ATG Proteins*: mTORC1 phosphorylates several autophagy-related (ATG) proteins involved in the initiation and maturation of autophagosomes, thereby inhibiting autophagy under nutrient-rich conditions.
   - *Regulation of Lysosomal Biogenesis*: mTORC1 also influences lysosomal biogenesis, ensuring that lysosomal activity is coordinated with nutrient availability and cellular growth needs.

Regulation of Autophagy During Nutrient Scarcity

When nutrients are scarce, mTORC1 is inactivated, which allows autophagy to proceed. This process involves the following:

1. *Inactivation of mTORC1*: In the absence of nutrients, the Rag GTPases are in an inactive state, which prevents the recruitment of mTORC1 to the lysosome.
2. *Autophagy Initiation*: Inactivation of mTORC1 lifts its inhibitory effects on autophagy-related proteins, allowing the formation of autophagosomes and the degradation of cytoplasmic contents. This process helps replenish cellular nutrients and maintain homeostasis during periods of nutrient scarcity.

Insights from Studies on Nutrient Regulation of mTORC1 and Autophagy

Several studies have provided insights into how amino acids and other nutrients regulate mTORC1 and autophagy:

1. *Amino Acid Sensing*: Specific sensors, such as Sestrin2 for leucine and CASTOR1 for arginine, detect amino acid levels and regulate the activity of the Rag GTPases.
2. *Regulatory Mechanisms*: The precise mechanisms by which nutrients influence the anchoring of Rag GTPases to the Ragulator and the subsequent recruitment of mTORC1 remain areas of active research.

Role of MORG1 in mTORC1 Regulation and Autophagy

The WD-repeat protein mitogen-activated protein kinase organizer 1 (MORG1) has been identified as an important interactor of the selective autophagy receptor SQSTM1/p62. MORG1 plays a crucial role in regulating mTORC1 activity and enabling basal autophagy flux. Here, we delve into the mechanisms by which

MORG1 modulates mTORC1 activity and its interaction with other key components involved in nutrient sensing and autophagy.

MORG1 and Basal Autophagy

1. *Inhibition of mTORC1*:
   - MORG1 inhibits mTORC1 activity, which is essential for maintaining basal autophagy flux. By keeping mTORC1 activity in check, MORG1 ensures that autophagy continues to degrade and recycle cellular components under normal conditions.
2. *Interaction with Ragulator and Rag GTPases*:
   - MORG1 interacts directly with the Ragulator complex (LAMTOR1–5) and active Rag GTPases (RagA, RagB, RagC, RagD). This interaction is crucial for controlling the spatiotemporal localization of mTORC1 to the lysosomal surface.

Amino Acid Readdition and mTORC1 Activation

1. *Role of SQSTM1/p62*:
   - Upon readdition of amino acids following deprivation, SQSTM1/p62 interacts with MORG1 and Rag GTPases. This interaction counteracts MORG1-mediated inhibition of mTORC1, allowing mTORC1 to be recruited to the lysosomal surface and activated by Rheb GTPase.
2. *Nutrient Availability*:
   - MORG1 fine-tunes mTORC1 activity both during nutrient availability and scarcity. When amino acids are present, the interaction between SQSTM1/p62, MORG1, and Rag GTPases facilitates the activation of mTORC1, promoting anabolic processes such as protein synthesis and cell growth.

Mechanisms of mTORC1 Regulation by MORG1

MORG1 is a critical regulator of mTORC1 activity and autophagy. By inhibiting mTORC1 under basal conditions and facilitating its activation upon nutrient repletion, MORG1 ensures a balanced regulation of cellular metabolism and autophagy. The interaction of MORG1 with the Ragulator complex, Rag GTPases, and SQSTM1/p62 underscores its central role in the nutrient-sensing pathway, highlighting its importance in maintaining cellular homeostasis and responding to environmental changes. Understanding the precise mechanisms of MORG1's regulation of mTORC1 provides valuable insights into potential therapeutic targets for diseases associated with dysregulated mTORC1 activity and autophagy.

1. *Spatiotemporal Localization*:
   - MORG1 controls the localization of mTORC1 to the lysosomal surface by interacting with the Ragulator complex and Rag GTPases. This regulation ensures that mTORC1 is positioned correctly to be activated by Rheb when nutrients are available.
2. *Fine-Tuning mTORC1 Activity*:
   - By inhibiting mTORC1 under basal conditions and allowing its activation upon nutrient repletion, MORG1 ensures a balanced regulation of autophagy and anabolic processes. This fine-tuning is essential for cellular homeostasis and adaptation to changing environmental conditions.

Functional Implications

1. *Basal Autophagy*:
   - MORG1-mediated inhibition of mTORC1 under basal conditions enables continuous autophagy flux, which is vital for cellular maintenance and the turnover of damaged organelles and proteins.
2. *Nutrient-Responsive Activation*:
   - Upon nutrient repletion, the interaction between SQSTM1/p62, MORG1, and Rag GTPases allows the swift activation of mTORC1, facilitating a rapid response to changes in nutrient availability.
3. *Cell Growth and Metabolism*:
   - The dynamic regulation of mTORC1 by MORG1 affects various cellular processes, including protein synthesis, lipid biosynthesis, and autophagy, thereby influencing cell growth and metabolism.

mTOR plays a crucial role in the regulation of autophagy, a cellular process responsible for the degradation and recycling of damaged organelles, misfolded proteins, and other cellular components. Autophagy is essential for maintaining cellular homeostasis, especially under conditions of stress or nutrient deprivation. The relationship between mTOR and autophagy is complex and tightly regulated.

Role of mTOR in Cell Survival

mTOR (mechanistic target of rapamycin) plays a pivotal role in cell survival by integrating various signals from growth factors, nutrients, energy status, and stress conditions to coordinate cellular responses that promote survival and prevent apoptosis. Both mTOR complexes, mTORC1 and mTORC2, contribute to cell survival through distinct mechanisms.

mTORC1 and Cell Survival:

1. *Nutrient and Energy Sensing:*
   - mTORC1 is activated by sufficient levels of nutrients, particularly amino acids, and energy (high ATP levels). This activation ensures that cells have the necessary resources to sustain vital functions and growth.
2. *Protein Synthesis:*
   - mTORC1 promotes protein synthesis by activating S6K1 and inhibiting 4E-BP1, enhancing the translation of proteins involved in cell survival, growth, and repair.
3. *Lipid and Nucleotide Synthesis:*
   - By stimulating lipid and nucleotide biosynthesis, mTORC1 supports membrane production and DNA/RNA synthesis, which are crucial for cell survival and proliferation.
4. *Inhibition of Autophagy:*
   - Under nutrient-rich conditions, mTORC1 inhibits autophagy, preventing the degradation of cellular components. This inhibition is crucial for cells to focus on anabolic processes and growth.
5. *Regulation of Apoptosis:*
   - mTORC1 signaling can influence apoptosis by regulating the expression and activity of various pro-survival and anti-apoptotic factors. For instance, mTORC1 can increase the expression of anti-apoptotic proteins such as Bcl-2 and inhibit pro-apoptotic factors, thereby promoting cell survival.

mTORC2

mTOR Complex 2 (mTORC2)

Key Regulatory Components:

- *Rictor*: Essential for mTORC2's function, not sensitive to rapamycin
- *mSIN1*: Necessary for mTORC2 complex integrity and function
- *mLST8*: Also part of mTORC2, similar to its role in mTORC1
- *DEPTOR*: Similarly inhibits mTORC2 activity

Substrates and Outputs:

- *Akt/PKB*: Phosphorylation at Ser473 by mTORC2 activates Akt, promoting cell survival and growth by influencing various downstream targets like FoxO and GSK3.
- *SGK1*: Activation by mTORC2 leads to regulation of ion transport and cell survival.
- *PKCα*: Phosphorylation by mTORC2 affects the organization of the actin cytoskeleton, impacting cell shape and migration (Fig. 1.16).

mTORC2 and Cell Survival: mTOR plays a central role in cell survival by integrating various extracellular and intracellular signals to regulate anabolic and catabolic processes. Through its complexes, mTORC1 and mTORC2, it ensures that cells can survive under diverse conditions by promoting protein synthesis, lipid and nucleotide biosynthesis, and inhibiting apoptosis and autophagy as needed. Understanding the role of mTOR in cell survival provides insights into various physiological processes and diseases, offering potential avenues for therapeutic intervention [58].

1. *Activation of AKT (Protein Kinase B):*

   - mTORC2 phosphorylates and activates AKT, a key regulator of cell survival. Active AKT promotes survival by phosphorylating and inhibiting pro-apoptotic factors such as BAD (Bcl-2-associated death promoter) and procaspase-9, thereby preventing apoptosis.

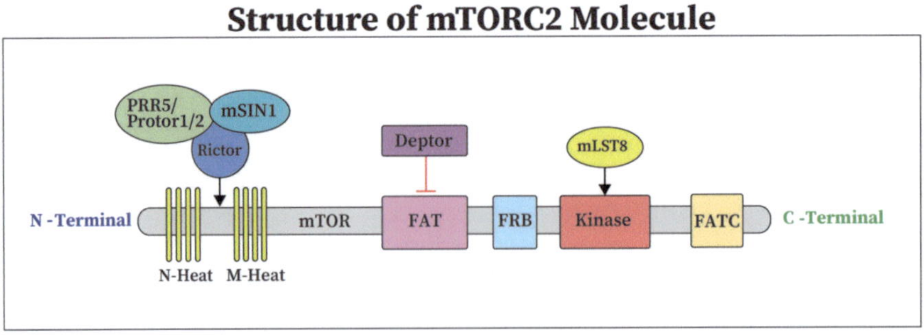

Fig. 1.16 The basic structure of mTORC2 with its components attached to specific sites of the mTOR molecule. Activators and inhibitors are represented by black arrows and a red t-bar

2. *Cytoskeleton Organization:*
   - mTORC2 regulates the actin cytoskeleton, which is important for cell shape, motility, and integrity. Proper cytoskeletal organization is essential for cell survival, particularly in dynamic environments.
3. *Regulation of Metabolism:*
   - mTORC2 influences cellular metabolism by regulating glucose uptake and glycolysis through AKT signaling. Enhanced glucose metabolism provides the energy necessary for cell survival, especially under stress conditions.

Integration of Survival Signals

1. *Growth Factors:*
   - Growth factors like insulin and IGF-1 activate the PI3K-AKT pathway, leading to mTORC1 and mTORC2 activation. This promotes cell survival by enhancing anabolic processes and inhibiting apoptosis.
2. *Nutrient Availability:*
   - Sufficient nutrients activate mTORC1, supporting biosynthetic processes necessary for cell survival. Nutrient sensing through the Rag GTPases and lysosomal localization of mTORC1 is crucial for this activation.
3. *Energy Status:*
   - High ATP levels inhibit AMPK (AMP-activated protein kinase), allowing mTORC1 to remain active. Conversely, low energy status activates AMPK, which inhibits mTORC1, reducing anabolic processes and promoting autophagy to maintain energy homeostasis.
4. *Stress Responses:*
   - Under stress conditions, such as hypoxia or DNA damage, mTOR signaling is modulated to enhance cell survival. For example, mTORC1 inhibition under hypoxia promotes autophagy, allowing cells to survive by degrading damaged components and recycling nutrients.

Clinical Implications:

1. *Cancer:*
   - mTOR signaling is often dysregulated in cancer, leading to enhanced cell survival, proliferation, and resistance to apoptosis. Targeting mTOR path-

ways with inhibitors like rapamycin and its analogs can reduce tumor growth and sensitize cancer cells to therapy.

2. *Neurodegenerative Diseases:*
   - mTOR signaling affects cell survival in neurons. Dysregulation can contribute to neurodegenerative diseases. Enhancing mTOR activity or modulating autophagy through mTOR pathways could offer therapeutic benefits in conditions like Alzheimer's and Parkinson's diseases.
3. *Metabolic Disorders:*
   - In metabolic diseases such as diabetes and obesity, mTOR signaling is crucial for maintaining cellular metabolism and survival. Modulating mTOR activity can improve insulin sensitivity and metabolic homeostasis, reducing the risk of metabolic complications.
4. *Aging:*
   - mTOR inhibition has been associated with lifespan extension and improved healthspan. By promoting autophagy and reducing age-related cellular damage, mTOR inhibitors may enhance cell survival and delay aging-related diseases.

Role of mTORc2 in Cancer

Summary of mEAK-7's Role in Normal Physiology and Cancer Development

Introduction:

- *mEAK-7 (mammalian EAK-7)*: A conserved lysosomal membrane protein
- *Expression*: Highly expressed in several cancer cells
- *Function*: Positive activator of mTOR signaling via an alternative mTOR complex

Key Roles of mEAK-7:

1. *mTOR Signaling Activation:*
   - mEAK-7 plays a crucial role in promoting cancer cell proliferation and migration.
   - Involved in the formation of an alternative mTOR complex.
   - Interaction with V-ATPase suggests a role in mTORC1 activation.
   - The C-terminal α-helix of mEAK-7 binds to the D and B subunits of V-ATPase, creating a pincer-like grip around the B subunit.
   - Binding is partially disrupted during ATP hydrolysis, potentially allowing mTOR to bind to mEAK-7.

2. *Chemoresistance and Radiation Resistance:*
   - mEAK-7 sustains DNA damage-mediated mTOR signaling through interactions with DNA-PKcs.
   - Promotes resistance to chemotherapy and radiation therapy.
3. *Potential as a Therapeutic Target:*
   - Given its role in cancer proliferation and therapy resistance, mEAK-7 is a promising target for cancer treatment.
   - Future research is needed to understand the precise molecular mechanisms and signal transduction pathways involving mEAK-7 (Fig. 1.17).

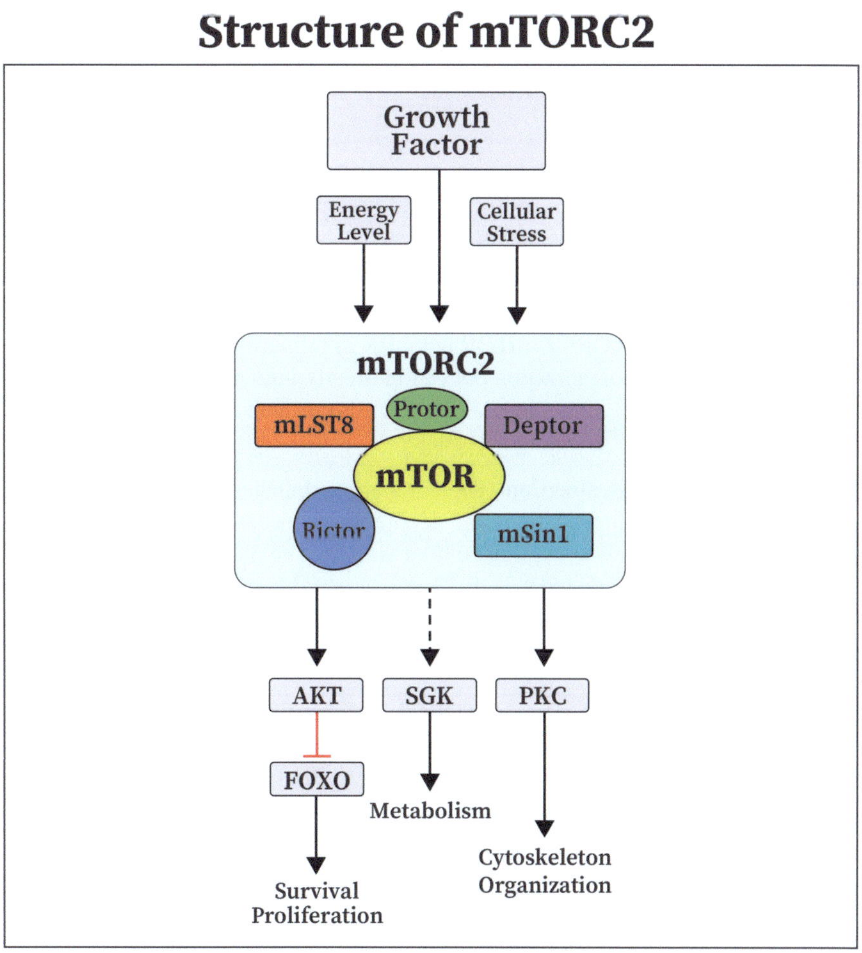

Fig. 1.17 The mTORC2 molecule's upstream pathways are shown above the image, while its downstream pathways are shown below

mTORC2 and Cellular Growth

1. *Actin Cytoskeleton Organization:*
   - mTORC2 regulates the organization of the actin cytoskeleton, which is critical for cell shape, motility, and division. This is achieved through the activation of Rho GTPases and the regulation of actin polymerization.
2. *Cell Survival and Proliferation:*
   - mTORC2 activates AKT (protein kinase B), a key player in promoting cell survival and proliferation. AKT activation by mTORC2 leads to the phosphorylation and inhibition of pro-apoptotic factors, thereby enhancing cell survival.
   - AKT also promotes cell growth by activating downstream effectors involved in protein synthesis and metabolism.
3. *Metabolism Regulation:*
   - mTORC2 influences cellular metabolism by regulating glucose uptake and glycolysis through AKT signaling. This ensures that cells have sufficient energy and metabolic intermediates to support growth and proliferation.
4. *mTORC2 and Autophagy:*
   - *Indirect Role:* mTORC2 (mTOR complex 2) primarily regulates cell survival and cytoskeletal organization but can indirectly influence autophagy through its effects on AKT signaling. AKT activation can lead to mTORC1 activation, thereby indirectly affecting autophagy.

Plasma Membrane Localization The compartmentalization of mTOR signaling via distinct membrane localizations and adapter proteins ensures precise regulation of its activity in response to varying cellular signals. The plasma membrane is crucial for growth factor-mediated mTORC2 activation. This spatial regulation enables mTOR to integrate multiple signals, coordinating cellular growth, metabolism, and survival effectively.

- *Regulation by Growth Factors*: mTORC2 is primarily regulated by growth factors, such as insulin and other growth signals.
- *Key Adapter Proteins*: mTORC2 is directed to the plasma membrane through interactions with various adapter proteins, including the mSIN1 subunit, which has a pleckstrin homology (PH) domain that binds to phosphatidylinositol (3,4,5)-trisphosphate (PIP3) at the plasma membrane. This localization is essential for mTORC2's activation in response to growth factor signaling.
- *Function*: Once activated at the plasma membrane, mTORC2 regulates cytoskeletal organization, cell survival, and metabolism. It phosphorylates and activates Akt, a critical kinase in the PI3K/Akt pathway, which promotes cell survival and growth.

Distinct Roles and Interactions

- *mTORC1 and mTORC2*: Although both complexes share the catalytic subunit mTOR, they have distinct regulatory proteins and functions. mTORC1 is primarily involved in promoting growth and inhibiting autophagy in response to nutrients, while mTORC2 is crucial for cell survival and metabolism in response to growth factors.
- *Cross-Talk and Feedback*: There is significant cross-talk and feedback between the two complexes. For example, mTORC1 activity can indirectly influence mTORC2 activity through regulatory pathways involving insulin signaling and feedback inhibition of IRS1.

mTORC2 Activators:

1. *Growth Factors*: Insulin, IGF-1 (insulin-like growth factor 1), EGF (epidermal growth factor)
2. *Hormones*: Insulin, estrogen
3. *PI3K (phosphoinositide 3-kinase)*: Activation via PIP3 production
4. *Ras GTPase*: Part of signaling cascade
5. *Nutrient Availability*: Amino acids, particularly leucine
6. *G-protein Coupled Receptors (GPCRs)*: Ligands like sphingosine-1-phosphate (S1P)
7. *Cell Adhesion*: Integrins
8. *Mechanical Stimuli*: Shear stress and mechanical stretch

mTORC2 Inhibitors:

1. *PI3K Inhibitors*: Wortmannin, LY294002
2. *TORC1 Feedback Loop*: S6K1 (a downstream target of mTORC1) can inhibit upstream PI3K/AKT signaling
3. *PP2A (Protein Phosphatase 2A)*: Dephosphorylates and inactivates AKT, indirectly affecting mTORC2
4. *Rictor-specific Inhibitors*: Compounds that target mTORC2-specific components
5. *Nutrient Deprivation*: Lack of amino acids, glucose, or lipids
6. *Pharmacological Inhibitors*: Torin1 (at higher concentrations affects both mTORC1 and mTORC2)
7. *Hypoxia*: Low oxygen levels can indirectly inhibit mTORC2
8. *Reactive Oxygen Species (ROS)*: Excessive levels can negatively impact mTORC2 signaling
9. *Stress Signals*: Cellular stress and DNA damage can downregulate mTORC2 activity through various mechanisms (Fig. 1.18)

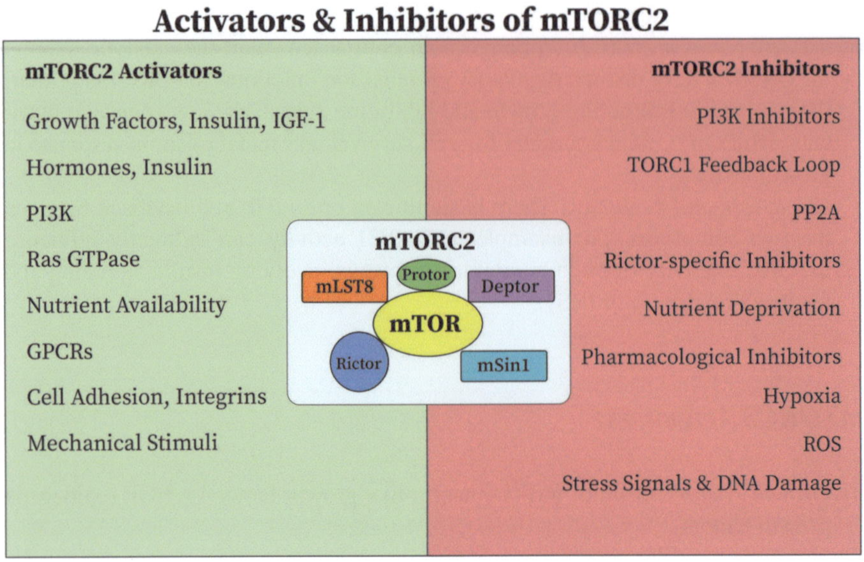

Fig. 1.18 The activators and inhibitors of mTORC2 molecule is categorized and presented in the table above

mTORC2: Key Functions and Impact on Cellular Signaling

mTORC2 (mechanistic target of rapamycin complex 2) plays a pivotal role in cellular signaling by phosphorylating and activating a subset of AGC family kinases, including AKT, PKC, and SGK1. These kinases have both shared and distinct substrates, which allows mTORC2 to regulate a variety of critical cellular processes:

1. *Macromolecule Biosynthesis*: mTORC2 influences the synthesis of proteins, lipids, and other macromolecules essential for cell structure and function.
2. *Angiogenesis*: It promotes the formation of new blood vessels, which is crucial for supplying nutrients and oxygen to growing tissues, especially in the context of tumor growth.
3. *Cell Survival*: By activating kinases like AKT, mTORC2 helps cells survive under stress conditions and resist apoptosis.
4. *Proliferation*: It stimulates cell division, contributing to tissue growth and repair.
5. *Mobility and Invasion*: mTORC2 enhances the motility and invasive capabilities of cells, which is particularly relevant in cancer metastasis.

Activation of AKT by mTORC2

The full activation of AKT, a key player in cell survival and growth, requires phosphorylation at two critical sites:

- *Ser308*: Phosphorylation by PDK1 (phosphoinositide-dependent kinase-1)
- *Thr473*: Phosphorylation by mTORC2

This dual phosphorylation is essential for AKT's maximal activity. When mTORC2 activity is increased, it accelerates the phosphorylation of AKT, thereby enhancing the PI3K-AKT-mTORC1 signaling pathway.

Positive Feedback Loop

The activation of AKT by mTORC2 creates a second positive feedback loop in the PI3K-AKT-mTOR signaling pathway. This feedback loop amplifies the signal, leading to sustained activation of downstream targets that promote cell growth, survival, and proliferation. Specifically:

- *PI3K Activation*: Initiates the signaling cascade by generating PIP3 (phosphatidylinositol-3,4,5-trisphosphate) at the cell membrane.
- *AKT Activation*: Full activation of AKT requires phosphorylation by both PDK1 and mTORC2.
- *mTORC1 Activation*: Activated AKT can then phosphorylate and inhibit TSC2 (tuberous sclerosis complex 2), leading to the activation of mTORC1.
- *mTORC1 Functions*: mTORC1 promotes protein synthesis and cell growth by phosphorylating key targets like S6K1 and 4E-BP1.

Implications for Cancer

The involvement of mTORC2 in activating AKT and forming a positive feedback loop with PI3K-AKT-mTORC1 signaling has significant implications for cancer. Increased mTORC2 activity can lead to hyperactivation of this pathway, driving tumor growth and survival. This makes mTORC2 a potential therapeutic target. Inhibiting mTORC2 could disrupt this feedback loop, reducing AKT activation and potentially suppressing tumor progression and resistance to therapies. Understanding the precise mechanisms and interactions within this signaling network is crucial for developing effective cancer treatments.

mTORC3

mTORC3 (Rapamycin-Insensitive mTOR Complex) [25]:
mTORC3 phosphorylates target proteins such as 4E-BP1, P70S6K, and AKT independent of Raptor or Rictor in the complex. The formation of mTORC3 is independent of ETV7's transcriptional activity, suggesting a non-canonical role for ETV7 in cellular signaling pathways (Fig. 1.19).

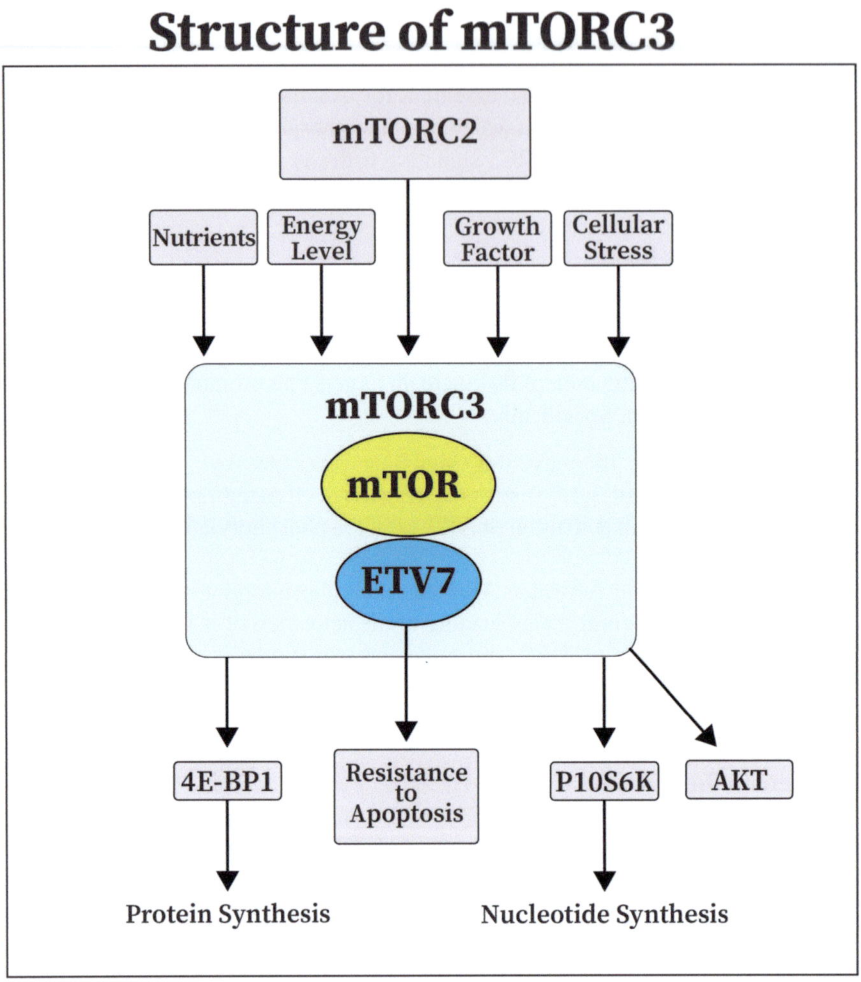

Fig. 1.19 The mTORC3 molecule's upstream pathways are shown above the image, while its downstream pathways are shown below

mTORC3 activation is influenced by a variety of factors related to nutrient availability, growth factors, energy status, stress responses, and key regulatory proteins such as mEAK-7 and V-ATPase. Understanding the precise mechanisms of mTORC3 activation and its role in cellular processes requires further investigation. Unraveling these details will provide insights into mTORC3's contribution to cell growth, proliferation, and its potential as a therapeutic target in cancer and other diseases.

The E26 transformation-specific (ETS) transcription factor ETV7 has been found to interact with the mechanistic target of rapamycin (mTOR) in the cytoplasm. This interaction leads to the assembly of a novel complex termed mTORC3. Notably, the formation of mTORC3 is independent of ETV7's transcriptional activity, suggesting a non-canonical role for ETV7 in cellular signaling pathways.

The interaction between ETV7 and mTOR represents an intriguing mechanism by which cellular processes such as growth, proliferation, and survival can be regulated. The discovery of mTORC3 adds another layer of complexity to our understanding of mTOR signaling, which traditionally involves mTORC1 and mTORC2 complexes.

While mTORC1 is primarily associated with the regulation of protein synthesis and cell growth in response to nutrient and energy status, and mTORC2 is involved in the regulation of the cytoskeleton and cell survival, the specific functions and regulatory mechanisms of mTORC3 remain to be fully elucidated. Further research into the role of ETV7 in mTORC3 assembly and its downstream effects could provide new insights into cellular homeostasis and potential therapeutic targets for diseases where mTOR signaling is dysregulated, such as cancer and metabolic disorders.

Activation and Influence of mTORC3

Overview of mTORC3

mTORC3 (mTOR Complex 3) is a proposed alternative complex in the mTOR signaling pathway, distinct from the well-characterized mTORC1 and mTORC2. The characterization of mTORC3 is still emerging, and its specific components and activation mechanisms are not yet fully understood. However, several potential activators and influencers have been suggested based on current research.

Potential Activators and Influencers of mTORC3:

1. *Nutrient Availability:*
    - *Amino Acids*: Like mTORC1, mTORC3 may be activated by the presence of amino acids, particularly leucine and arginine, which signal nutrient sufficiency.
    - *Glucose*: Adequate glucose levels can also contribute to mTORC3 activation by providing the necessary energy for cellular processes.
2. *Growth Factors and Hormones:*
    - *Insulin and IGF-1 (Insulin-Like Growth Factor 1)*: These growth factors activate upstream signaling pathways (e.g., PI3K-Akt) that can lead to mTORC3 activation.
    - *Other Cytokines*: Various cytokines and hormones that influence cell growth and metabolism may also impact mTORC3 activity.
3. *Energy Status:*
    - *ATP Levels*: High levels of cellular ATP can promote mTORC3 activation, signaling sufficient energy availability for anabolic processes.

- *AMPK (AMP-Activated Protein Kinase)*: When cellular energy is low, AMPK can inhibit mTORC complexes, potentially influencing mTORC3 activity indirectly by altering energy balance.

4. *Stress Responses:*
   - *Hypoxia*: Low oxygen levels can modulate mTORC signaling, with potential effects on mTORC3 activation and function.
   - *Oxidative Stress*: Reactive oxygen species (ROS) can influence signaling pathways upstream of mTOR, impacting mTORC3 activation.
5. *mEAK-7 (mammalian EAK-7):*
   - *Direct Activation*: mEAK-7 is proposed as a key component and activator of mTORC3, facilitating its formation and activation.
   - *Interaction with V-ATPase*: mEAK-7 interacts with V-ATPase, which regulates lysosomal function and pH homeostasis, potentially influencing mTORC3 activation.
6. *Lysosomal Function:*
   - *V-ATPase*: The interaction between mEAK-7 and V-ATPase suggests that lysosomal activity and pH regulation are critical for mTORC3 activation.
   - *Autophagy*: Autophagic processes can affect nutrient availability and lysosomal function, thereby influencing mTORC3 activity.
7. *Other Signaling Molecules:*
   - *Rag GTPases*: Similar to their role in mTORC1 activation, Rag GTPases may also contribute to amino acid sensing and to the activation of mTORC3 by Rapamycin.
   - *Rheb (Ras homolog enriched in brain)*: A small GTPase that directly activates mTORC1, Rheb may also influence mTORC3 activation under certain conditions.

mTORC4

mTORC4 mTORC4 is emerging as a critical player in tumorigenesis and the development of anticancer drug resistance. This complex exerts its influence through the regulation of the DNA damage response (DDR) and the physiology of cancer stem cells (CSCs). mTORC4 represents an emerging pathway in mTOR signaling with significant implications for cancer biology. Understanding its components, activation mechanisms, and functional roles will be crucial for developing novel therapeutic strategies targeting this pathway. Further research is essential to elucidate the precise molecular details of mTORC4 signaling and its potential as a therapeutic target [26] (Fig. 1.20)

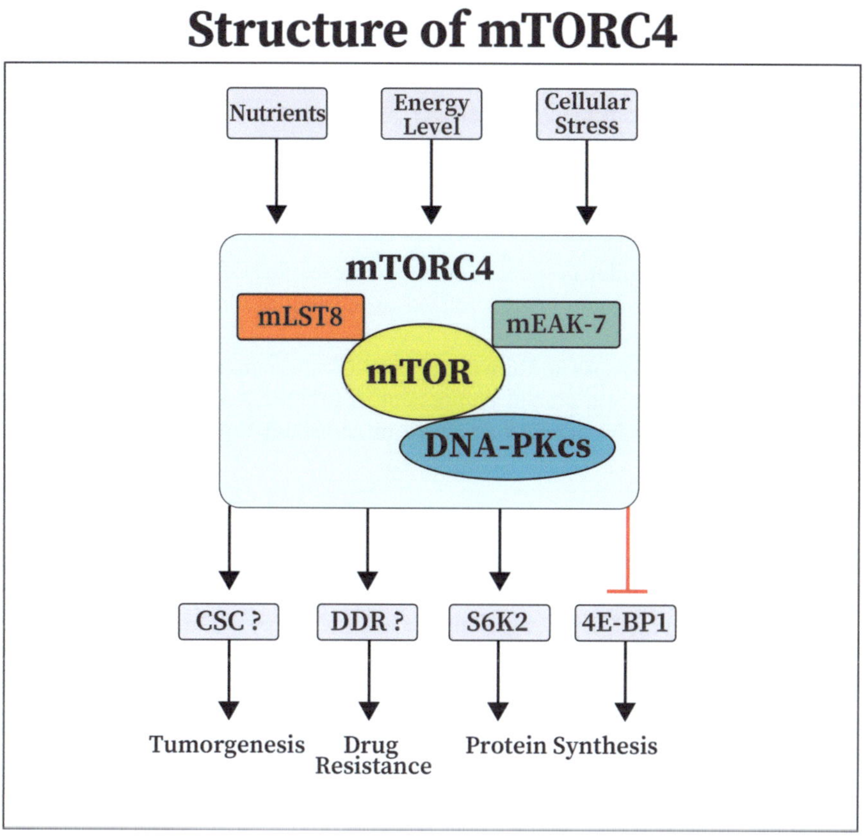

Fig. 1.20 The mTORC4 molecule's upstream pathways are shown above the image, while its downstream pathways are shown below

The emergence of mTORC4, potentially involved in cell proliferation and migration, presents another paradigm shift in the mTOR signaling landscape, particularly when linked to cancer biology. Through mEAK-7 and possibly other undiscovered pathways, mTORC4 might regulate downstream targets such as S6K2 and 4E-BP1, key effectors in protein synthesis and cell cycle control.

Given the essential role of DNA-PKcs (DNA-dependent protein kinase catalytic subunit) in DNA damage repair and cancer stem cell (CSC) maintenance, it is plausible that mTORC4 is integrated into this regulatory network. DNA-PKcs is essential for the repair of double-strand DNA breaks and the survival of CSCs, which are often resistant to conventional therapies. By controlling the DNA damage response and CSC physiology, mTORC4 could contribute to tumor progression and confer resistance to anticancer treatments.

This hypothesis positions mTORC4 as a critical player in tumorigenesis and drug resistance, particularly through its influence on CSCs, which are thought to drive recurrence and metastasis. Targeting mTORC4 may thus represent a novel therapeutic strategy, especially in cancers with high CSC populations or those exhibiting resistance due to faulty DNA repair mechanisms.

Signaling Pathways and Functions:

1. *mTORC4 Activation*:
   - *Mechanism*: Similar to other mTOR complexes, mTORC4 is believed to be activated by upstream signals related to nutrient availability, energy status, and cellular stress.
   - *Role of mEAK-7*: As a known activator of alternative mTOR complexes, mEAK-7 is likely a crucial component in mTORC4 activation, potentially interacting with lysosomal membrane proteins and V-ATPase to regulate its activity.
2. *Functional Roles*:
   - *Cell Proliferation and Growth*: mTORC4 is hypothesized to play roles in promoting cell proliferation and growth, particularly under conditions where mTORC1 and mTORC2 signaling are insufficient or inhibited.
   - *Cancer Progression*: Given the involvement of mEAK-7 in cancer, mTORC4 may contribute to tumorigenesis and metastasis through unique signaling pathways that promote cell survival and proliferation.
   - *Stress Response*: mTORC4 may also be involved in cellular stress responses, including DNA damage repair and resistance to chemotherapy and radiation, similar to mEAK-7's known functions.

Interactions with Other Signaling Molecules

1. *V-ATPase Interaction*:
   - mTORC4's interaction with V-ATPase suggests a role in pH homeostasis and lysosomal function, critical for cellular metabolism and nutrient sensing.
   - The binding dynamics of mEAK-7 with V-ATPase during ATP hydrolysis may facilitate mTORC4 activation and its downstream signaling effects.
2. *DNA-PKcs (DNA-Dependent Protein Kinase Catalytic Subunit)*:
   - mTORC4 may interact with DNA-PKcs to maintain DNA damage response and repair mechanisms, contributing to cellular survival under genotoxic stress (Fig. 1.21).

DNA Damage Response (DDR) mTORC4's involvement in the DDR is particularly significant as it helps maintain genomic stability by orchestrating the repair processes that follow DNA damage. By controlling key proteins and signaling pathways associated with DDR, mTORC4 ensures the proper repair of damaged DNA, thus preventing mutations that could lead to cancer progression. Dysregulation of mTORC4 in this context could lead to enhanced survival of can-

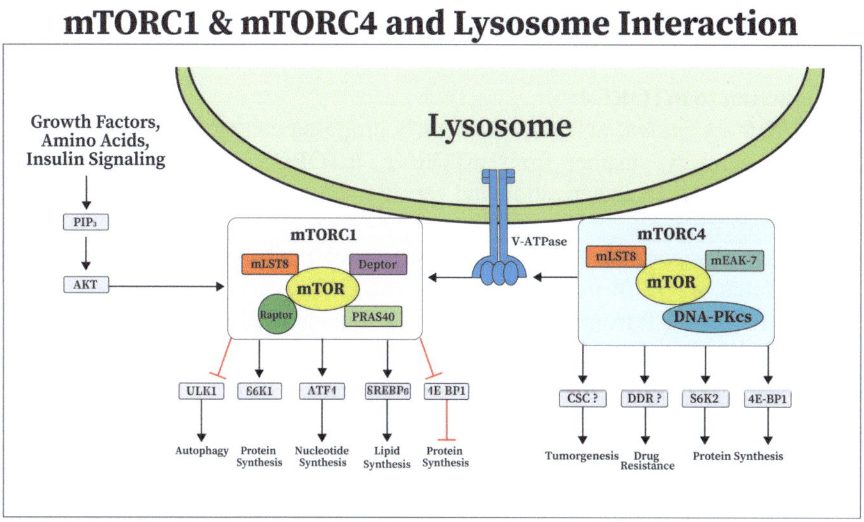

Fig. 1.21 There is a bidirectional regulatory mechanism between lysosome and mTORC1. In addition, mTORC4 activates V-ATPase which also activates mTORC1 and contols the pH of lysosome. Any function of mTORC1 is based on its attachment to the lysosome. Together this complex interaction between these molecules is essential for their various functions

cer cells despite the presence of DNA-damaging agents, contributing to resistance against therapies designed to induce DNA damage, such as certain chemotherapies and radiation.

Cancer Stem Cells (CSCs) CSCs are a subpopulation of cancer cells characterized by their ability to self-renew and differentiate into various cell types found in tumors. These cells are often resistant to conventional therapies, contributing to tumor recurrence and metastasis. mTORC4 influences the physiology of CSCs, potentially affecting their survival, proliferation, and differentiation. By modulating pathways critical to CSC maintenance and function, mTORC4 can impact tumorigenesis and therapeutic resistance.

Therapeutic Implications The role of mTORC4 in DDR and CSC physiology makes it a promising target for novel anticancer therapies. Inhibiting mTORC4 could sensitize cancer cells to DNA-damaging treatments and reduce the resilience of CSCs, thereby improving the efficacy of existing therapies and reducing the likelihood of relapse.

Understanding the precise mechanisms by which mTORC4 regulates these processes is crucial for developing targeted interventions that could disrupt its function in cancer cells while minimizing effects on normal cells. This dual role of mTORC4 underscores its potential as a pivotal target in the ongoing battle against cancer and drug resistance.

mTORC4 Signaling: An Emerging Pathway

Introduction to mTORC4:

- *mTORC4 Definition*: mTORC4 is a newly proposed complex in the mTOR signaling pathway, distinct from mTORC1, mTORC2, and the hypothesized mTORC3. The characterization and specific components of mTORC4 are still under investigation.
- *Potential Components*: While the exact makeup is not fully established, it is suggested that mTORC4 may include mTOR, mEAK-7, and other unique proteins that differentiate it from mTORC1, mTORC2, and mTORC3.

Signaling Pathways and Functions:

1. *mTORC4 Activation*:
    - *Mechanism*: Similar to other mTOR complexes, mTORC4 is believed to be activated by upstream signals related to nutrient availability, energy status, and cellular stress.
    - *Role of mEAK-7*: As a known activator of alternative mTOR complexes, mEAK-7 is likely a crucial component in mTORC4 activation, potentially interacting with lysosomal membrane proteins and V-ATPase to regulate its activity.
2. *Functional Roles*:
    - *Cell Proliferation and Growth*: mTORC4 is hypothesized to play roles in promoting cell proliferation and growth, particularly under conditions where mTORC1 and mTORC2 signaling are insufficient or inhibited.
    - *Cancer Progression*: Given the involvement of mEAK-7 in cancer, mTORC4 may contribute to tumorigenesis and metastasis through unique signaling pathways that promote cell survival and proliferation.
    - *Stress Response*: mTORC4 may also be involved in cellular stress responses, including DNA damage repair and resistance to chemotherapy and radiation, similar to mEAK-7's known functions.

Interactions with Other Signaling Molecules

1. *V-ATPase Interaction*:
    - mTORC4's interaction with V-ATPase suggests a role in pH homeostasis and lysosomal function, critical for cellular metabolism and nutrient sensing.
    - The binding dynamics of mEAK-7 with V-ATPase during ATP hydrolysis may facilitate mTORC4 activation and its downstream signaling effects.
2. *DNA-PKcs (DNA-Dependent Protein Kinase Catalytic Subunit)*:
    - mTORC4 may interact with DNA-PKcs to maintain DNA damage response and repair mechanisms, contributing to cellular survival under genotoxic stress.

Implications for Cancer Therapy:

- *Targeting mTORC4*: Inhibitors or modulators of mTORC4 components, including mEAK-7, could be developed to disrupt cancer cell growth and survival pathways.
- *Resistance Mechanisms*: Understanding mTORC4's role in chemoresistance and radiation resistance can lead to the development of combination therapies to overcome these barriers in cancer treatment.

Future Research Directions

- *Characterization of mTORC4 Components*: Identifying the specific proteins involved in mTORC4 and understanding their interactions will provide insights into its unique signaling mechanisms.
- *Mechanistic Studies*: Detailed investigation into how mTORC4 is activated and regulated, particularly by mEAK-7 and V-ATPase.
- *Functional Analysis in Cancer*: Studying the role of mTORC4 in different cancer types and stages to identify potential therapeutic targets.
- *Therapeutic Development*: Designing drugs that specifically target mTORC4 components or its regulatory mechanisms to inhibit cancer progression and overcome therapy resistance.

Bibliography

1. Abudu. MORG1 limits mTORC1 signaling by inhibiting Rag GTPases. Affiliations Notes. 2024; https://doi.org/10.1016/j.molcel.2023.11.023.
2. Akbay. Modulation of mTORC1 signaling pathway by HIV-1. Cells. 2020; https://doi.org/10.3390/cells9051090.
3. Akbay. Double-edge effects of leucine on cancer cells. Life Sci. 2024; https://doi.org/10.20944/preprints202409.0126.v1.
4. Ali. Upstream signalling of mTORC1 and its hyperactivation in type 2 diabetes (T2D). BMB Rep. 2017; https://doi.org/10.5483/BMBRep.2017.50.12.206.
5. Allard. mTORC1 in energy expenditure: consequences for obesity. Nat Rev Endocrinol. 2024; https://doi.org/10.1038/s41574-023-00934-0.
6. Amin. The journey of metformin from glycaemic control to mTOR inhibition and the suppression of tumour growth. Br J Clin Pharmacol. 2018; https://doi.org/10.1111/bcp.13780.
7. Amin. The Janus face of HIF-1α in ischemic stroke and the possible associated pathways. Neurochem Int. 2024; https://doi.org/10.1016/j.neuint.2024.105747.
8. An. PI3K/AKT signaling pathway associates with pyroptosis and inflammation in patients with endometriosis. J Reprod Immunol. 2024; https://doi.org/10.1016/j.jri.2024.104213.
9. Avital-Cohen. Resveratrol induces myotube development by altering circadian metabolism via the SIRT1-AMPK-PP2A axis. Cells. 2024; https://doi.org/10.3390/cells13121069.
10. Babiec. Inhibition of purinergic P2 receptors prevents synaptic and behavioral alterations in a rodent model of autism spectrum disorders. Res Autism Spectr Disord. 2024; https://doi.org/10.1016/j.rasd.2024.102353.

11. Bai. Epigenetic regulation of autophagy in neuroinflammation and synaptic plasticity. Front Immunol. 2024; https://doi.org/10.3389/fimmu.2024.1322842.
12. Ballesteros-Álvarez. mTORC2: The other mTOR in autophagy regulation. Aging Cell. 2021; https://doi.org/10.1111/acel.13431.
13. Barzegar A. The obesity-autophagy-cancer axis: Mechanistic insights and therapeutic perspectives. Sem Cancer Biol. 2024; https://doi.org/10.1016/j.semcancer.2024.01.003.
14. Begagic. Understanding the significance of Hypoxia-Inducible Factors (HIFs) in glioblastoma: a systematic review. Cancers. 2024; https://doi.org/10.3390/cancers16112089.
15. Burke. Skeletal muscle hypertrophy: cell growth is cell growth. Am J Physiol. 2024; https://doi.org/10.1152/ajpcell.00418.2024.
16. Carosi. The mTOR–lysosome axis at the centre of ageing. FEBS Open Bio. 2022; https://doi.org/10.1002/2211-5463.13347.
17. Casciano. The role of the mTOR pathway in diabetic retinopathy. Front Med. 2022; https://doi.org/10.3389/fmed.2022.973856.
18. Chang. Targeting of lysosomal-bound protein mEAK-7 for cancer therapy. Front Oncol. 2024; https://doi.org/10.3389/fonc.2024.1375498.
19. Choudhury. Polyploidy and mTOR signaling: a possible molecular link. Cell Commun Signal. 2024; https://doi.org/10.1186/s12964-024-01526-9.
20. Condon. Nutrient regulation of mTORC1 at a glance. J Cell Sci. 2019; https://doi.org/10.1242/jcs.222570.
21. Davoody. mTOR signaling and Alzheimer's disease: What we know and where we are? CNS Neurosci Ther. 2023; https://doi.org/10.1111/cns.14463.
22. De-Leon-Covarrubias. Unlocking the potential: caloric restriction, caloric restriction mimetics, and their impact on cancer prevention and treatment. Metabolites. 2024; https://doi.org/10.3390/metabo14080418.
23. Deleyto-Seldas N, Efeyan A. The mTOR–autophagy axis and the control of metabolism. Front Cell Dev Biol. 2021; https://doi.org/10.3389/fcell.2021.655731.
24. Gargalionis. mTOR signaling: recent progress. Int J Mol Sci. 2024; https://doi.org/10.3390/ijms25052587.
25. Harwood. ETV7 is an essential component of a rapamycin-insensitive mTOR complex in cancer. Sci Adv. 2018; https://doi.org/10.1126/sciadv.aar3938.
26. He. Regulation of DNA duplication by the mTOR signaling pathway. Cell Cycle. 2021; https://doi.org/10.1080/15384101.2021.1897271.
27. He C. Notch signaling regulates Th17 cells differentiation through PI3K/AKT/mTORC1 pathway and involves in the thyroid injury of autoimmune thyroiditis. J Endocrinol Investig. 2024; https://doi.org/10.1007/s40618-023-02293-z.
28. Hobby. A treasure from a barren island: the discovery of rapamycin. Natl Library Med. 2022; https://doi.org/10.1093/ckj/sfac116.
29. Iranpanah. Exploiting new strategies in combating head and neck carcinoma: a comprehensive review on phytochemical approaches passing through PI3K/Akt/mTOR signaling pathway. Phytother Res. 2024; https://doi.org/10.1002/ptr.8228.
30. Islam. Endothelial cell-specific reduction in mTOR ameliorates age-related arterial and metabolic dysfunction. Cancer Aging. 2023; https://doi.org/10.1111/acel.14040.
31. Jin. TSC1 and DEPDC5 regulate HIV-1 latency through the mTOR signaling pathway. Emerg Microb Infect. 2018; https://doi.org/10.1038/s41426-018-0139-5.
32. Kasowanjete. A review of photobiomodulation on PI3K/AKT/mTOR in wound healing. J Photochem Photobiol. 2024; https://doi.org/10.1016/j.jpap.2023.100215.
33. Kim. mTOR: a pharmacologic target for autophagy regulation. J Clin Invest. 2015; https://doi.org/10.1172/JCI73939.
34. Klute. Friends and foes: the ambivalent role of autophagy in HIV-1 infection. Viruses. 2024; https://doi.org/10.3390/v16040500.
35. Kseniia. mTOR pathway occupies a central role in the emergence of latent cancer cells. Cell Death Dis. 2024; https://doi.org/10.1038/s41419-024-06547-3.

36. Lee JW. Targeting ageing with rapamycin and its derivatives in humans: a systematic review. The Lancet. February. www.thelancet.com/healthy-longevity Vol. 2024;(5 February 2024)
37. Legon. Dissecting mTOR-dependent gene and protein networks in normal and neurodegenerative states. University od East London, PHD Thesis. 2024, July 02. https://doi.org/10.15123/uel.8xy8w.
38. Leiphrakpam. PI3K/Akt/mTOR signaling pathway as a target for colorectal cancer treatment. Int J Mol Sci. 2024; https://doi.org/10.3390/ijms25063178.
39. Li. The mechanistic effects of acupuncture in rodent neurodegenerative disease models: a literature review. Front Neurosci. 2024; https://doi.org/10.3389/fnins.2024.1323555.
40. Liang. Echinacoside regulates PI3K/AKT/HIF-1α/VEGF cross signaling axis in proliferation and apoptosis of breast cancer. Anal Biochem. 2024; https://doi.org/10.1016/j.ab.2023.115360.
41. Lim S. Molecular mechanisms of autophagy decline during aging. Cells. 2024; https://doi.org/10.3390/cells13161364.
42. Liu J. Selective autophagy in cancer: mechanisms, therapeutic implications, and future perspectives. Mol Cancer. 2024; https://doi.org/10.1186/s12943-024-01934-y.
43. Lu L. Postmenopausal osteoporosis coexisting with sarcopenia: the role and mechanisms of estrogen. J Endocrinol. 2023; https://doi.org/10.1530/JOE-23-0116.
44. Maiese. The mechanistic target of Rapamycin (mTOR): novel considerations as an antiviral treatment. Curr Neurovasc Res. 2020; https://doi.org/10.2174/1567202617666200425205122.
45. Mao. Overview of research into mTOR inhibitors. Molecules. 2022; https://doi.org/10.3390/molecules27165295.
46. Martin-Bocanegra. Involvement of mTOR signaling in physiopathology and its potential therapeutic interventions. Redox Exper Med. 2024; https://doi.org/10.1530/REM-23-0024.
47. Matsuda. HIV reservoirs and treatment strategies toward curing HIV infection. Int J Mol Sci. 2024; https://doi.org/10.3390/ijms25052621.
48. Mo. HIF-1α affects sperm autophagy and motility. Andrologia. 2024; https://doi.org/10.1155/2024/4575305.
49. Moghbeli. PI3K/AKT pathway as a pivotal regulator of epithelial-mesenchymal transition in lung tumor cells. Cancer Cell Int. 2024; https://doi.org/10.1186/s12935-024-03357-7.
50. Morgos. Targeting PI3K/AKT/mTOR and MAPK signaling pathways in gastric cancer. Int J Mol Sci. 2024; https://doi.org/10.3390/ijms25031848.
51. Mu. Examining chronic inflammation, immune metabolism, and T cell dysfunction in HIV infection. Viruses. 2024; https://doi.org/10.3390/v16020219.
52. Neto. Unveiling the molecular landscape of cognitive aging: insights from polygenic risk scores, DNA methylation, and gene expression. Hum Genom. 2024; https://doi.org/10.1186/s40246-024-00640-6.
53. Nixon. Mechanisms of autophagy–lysosome dysfunction in neurodegenerative diseases. Nat Rev Mol Cell Biol. 2024;(August 06) https://doi.org/10.1038/s41580-024-00757-5.
54. Nouwen. Pathogens MenTORing macrophages and dendritic cells: manipulation of mTOR and cellular metabolism to promote immune escape. Cells. 2020; https://doi.org/10.3390/cells9010161.
55. Onaka. Exercise, mTOR activation, and potential impacts on the liver in rodents. Biology. 2024; https://doi.org/10.3390/biology13060362.
56. Panwar. Multifaceted role of mTOR (mammalian target of rapamycin) signaling pathway in human health and disease. Nature. 2023; https://doi.org/10.1038/s41392-023-01608-z.
57. Papadopoli. mTOR as a central regulator of lifespan and aging. F1000Res. 2019; https://doi.org/10.12688/f1000research.17196.1.
58. Ragupathi. The mTORC2 signaling network: targets and cross-talks. Biochem J. 2024; https://doi.org/10.1042/BCJ20220325.
59. Ratto. Direct control of lysosomal catabolic activity by mTORC1 through regulation of V-ATPase assembly. Nature. 2022; https://doi.org/10.1038/s41467-022-32515-6.
60. Ravizza. mTOR and neuroinflammation in epilepsy: implications for disease progression and treatment. Nat Rev Neurosci. 2024; https://doi.org/10.1038/s41583-024-00805-1.

61. Rogala. Structural basis for the docking of mTORC1 on the lysosomal surface. Science. 2019; https://doi.org/10.1126/science.aay0166.
62. Sharma. Targeting crosstalk of signaling pathways among muscles-bone-adipose tissue: a promising therapeutic approach for sarcopenia. Aging Dis. 2024; https://doi.org/10.14336/AD.2023.00903.
63. Si-Chen. DEPDC1 as a metabolic target regulates glycolysis in renal cell carcinoma through AKT/mTOR/HIF1α pathway. Cell Death Dis. 2024; https://doi.org/10.1038/s41419-024-06913-1.
64. Smiles. New developments in AMPK and mTORC1 cross-talk. Essays Biochem. 2024; https://doi.org/10.1042/EBC20240007.
65. Song C. Bioenergetic dysfunction in the pathogenesis of intervertebral disc degeneration. Pharmacol Res. 2024; https://doi.org/10.1016/j.phrs.2024.107119.
66. Stephens C. The host cytoskeleton: a key regulator of early HIV-1 infection. Cancer Metabol. 2022; https://doi.org/10.1111/febs.16706.
67. Sun. mTORC2: a multifaceted regulator of autophagy. Cell Commun Signal. 2021; https://doi.org/10.1186/s12964-022-00859-7.
68. Sun X-G. Aerobic glycolysis induced by mTOR/HIF-1α promotes early brain injury after subarachnoid hemorrhage via activating M1 microglia. Transit Stroke Res. 2022; https://doi.org/10.1007/s12975-022-01105-5.
69. Surviladze. Cellular entry of human papillomavirus type 16 involves activation of the phosphatidylinositol 3-kinase/Akt/mTOR pathway and inhibition of autophagy. Am Soc Microbiol. 2013; https://doi.org/10.1128/jvi.02319-12.
70. Thomas. Exercise-specific adaptations in human skeletal muscle: molecular mechanisms of making muscles fit and mighty. Free Rad Biol Med. 2024; https://doi.org/10.1016/j.freeradbiomed.2024.08.010.
71. Tovilovic. mTOR-independent autophagy counteracts apoptosis in herpes simplex virus type 1-infected U251 glioma cells. Microb Infect. 2017; https://doi.org/10.1016/j.micinf.2013.04.012.
72. Wang B. OCRL regulates lysosome positioning and mTORC1 activity through SSX2IP-mediated microtubule anchoring. EMBO Rep. 2021; https://doi.org/10.15252/embr.202052173.
73. Wang T. KIRREL promotes the proliferation of gastric cancer cells and angiogenesis through the PI3K/AKT/mTOR pathway. 2023; https://doi.org/10.1111/jcmm.18020.
74. Wang H. Autophagy in disease onset and progression. Aging Dis. 2024a; https://doi.org/10.14336/AD.2023.0815.
75. Wang N. Autophagy: Playing an important role in diabetes and its complications. Med Drug Discov. 2024b; https://doi.org/10.1016/j.medidd.2024.100188.
76. Wang Y. Targeting mTOR signaling pathways in multiple myeloma: biology and implication for therapy. Cell Commun Signal. 2024c; https://doi.org/10.1186/s12964-024-01699-3.
77. Winden. Abnormal mTOR Activation in Autism. Ann Rev Neurosci. 2018; https://doi.org/10.1146/annurev-neuro-080317-061747.
78. Wu N. Autophagy in aging-related diseases and cancer: Principles, regulatory mechanisms and therapeutic potential. Ageing Res Rev. 2024; https://doi.org/10.1016/j.arr.2024.102428.
79. Xie X. Mammalian AKT, the emerging roles on mitochondrial function in diseases. Aging Dis. 2022; https://doi.org/10.14336/AD.2021.0729.
80. Zeng Z. Exercise-induced autophagy suppresses sarcopenia through Akt/mTOR and Akt/FoxO3a signal pathways and AMPK-mediated mitochondrial quality control. Front Physiol. 2020; https://doi.org/10.3389/fphys.2020.583478.
81. Zhan. Assembly of mTORC3 involves binding of ETV7 to two separate sequences in the mTOR kinase domain. BioRxiv. 2024; https://doi.org/10.1101/2024.03.19.583970.
82. Zhang S. Cryo-EM structures of the mammalian endo-lysosomal TRPML1 channel elucidate the combined regulation mechanism. Protein Cell. 2017; https://doi.org/10.1007/s13238-017-0476-5.

83. Zhang X. Baicalein induces apoptosis of rheumatoid arthritis synovial fibroblasts through inactivation of the PI3K/Akt/mTOR pathway. Evidence-Based Complement Alternat Med. 2022; https://doi.org/10.1155/2022/3643265.
84. Zhao. Thymoquinone affects hypoxia-inducible factor-1α expression in pancreatic cancer cells via HSP90 and PI3K/AKT/mTOR pathways. World J Gastroenterol. 2024a; https://doi.org/10.3748/wjg.v30.i21.2793.
85. Zhao P. Celastrol inhibits mouse B16-F10 melanoma cell survival by regulating the PI3K/AKT/mTOR signaling pathway and repressing HIF-1α expression. Discov Oncol. 2024b; https://doi.org/10.1007/s12672-024-01045-6.
86. Zhilin. mTOR signaling pathway and mTOR inhibitors in cancer: progress and challenges. Cell Biosci. 2020; https://doi.org/10.1186/s13578-020-00396-1.
87. Zhu Y. Recent progresses in the late stages of autophagy. Cell Insight. 2024; https://doi.org/10.1016/j.cellin.2024.100152.

Chapter 2
mTOR Signaling Pathways

Contents

Abstract As discussed in the previous chapter, the mechanistic target of rapamycin (mTOR) is a central regulator of cellular growth, metabolism, and survival. mTOR integrates signals from a variety of upstream pathways and is organized into distinct complexes: mTORC1, mTORC2, mTORC3, and mTORC4, with mTORC1 and mTORC2 being the most extensively studied in relation to growth factor signaling. In this chapter, we will explore the critical signaling pathways associated with the mTOR complexes, their specific signal transductions, and the resulting cellular outcomes. This analysis will provide a comprehensive understanding of how mTOR regulates key cellular processes through its diverse and complex signaling network.

K. T. Moazed, *mTOR Signaling in Ophthalmology*,
https://doi.org/10.1007/978-3-032-05044-1_2

Discussions

Understanding the Foundations of mTOR Signaling

At the heart of cellular regulation, particularly in processes like autophagy, growth, and survival, lies mTOR. This protein is a linchpin in signaling pathways that dictate the fate of cells, influencing everything from nutrient uptake to the response to stress and damage. The terms in molecular biology encompass various components and mechanisms involved in cellular signaling pathways.

To understand how mTOR affects the eye, it's crucial to grasp some general key concepts and components involved in its signaling pathways.

mTOR integrates a wide array of signals from growth factors, energy levels, and environmental stress to control cellular processes like growth, proliferation, metabolism, and survival. mTORC1 is primarily regulated by growth factor signals (via Akt and ERK), nutrient levels, and energy status, while mTORC2 is primarily linked to growth factor signaling and cytoskeletal regulation. mTORC 3 and 4 are involved in proliferation and survival and a critical player in tumor genesis. Together, these pathways ensure that mTOR activity is finely tuned to the cell's internal and external conditions.

We begin with an overview of the mTOR transcription process, followed by a brief introduction to the key pathways associated with each of its complexes. Last, we delve into each pathway in detail.

There is *upstream signaling,* which refers to external stimulus to the cell including hormones, nutrients, hypoxia, energy level, and stress signals. Then there is the process of *signal transduction* inside the cell, which is the activation of the receptors by the upstream signals and the domino effect of enzymes phosphorylation of the protein messengers to activate or suppress the mTOR molecule. Next is the *downstream signaling,* which refers to the outcome of the previous steps such as autophagy, protein and lipid synthesis, and ribosome biogenesis.

Overview of mTOR Signaling Pathway [7]

1. *Upstream Signaling*

   This stage involves *external stimuli* that influence the cell's internal processes. These signals include:

   - *Stress signals* (such as oxidative stress or DNA damage)
   - *Hypoxia* (low-oxygen conditions)
   - *Nutrients* (such as amino acids, glucose, and lipids)
   - *Hormones* (like insulin or growth factors)
   - *Energy levels* (often sensed via ATP/AMP ratios)
   - *Oncogenesis factors*

These signals are detected by cell surface receptors or intracellular sensors, initiating the transmission of information into the cell.

2. *Signal Tranduction*

   This process involves the activation of *receptors* by the upstream signals, triggering a cascade of intracellular reactions. A key mechanism is phosphorylation, where enzymes (like kinases) add phosphate groups to proteins, modulating their activity. This creates a domino effect, where the activation or suppression of one protein leads to the regulation of downstream proteins.

   mTOR is a central player, receiving and integrating signals from multiple pathways. Depending on the type and strength of the input, mTOR either activates or inhibits further processes; few examples are:

   - *AMPK* pathway inhibits energy-consuming pathways (e.g., mTOR) and stimulates energy-producing pathways like fatty acid oxidation and glucose uptake.
   - *JAK/STAT3* pathway promotes survival and immune evasion.
   - *MAPK/ERK* pathway.
   - *P53* pathway induces cell cycle arrest, DNA repair, or apoptosis.
   - *PI3K/AKT* pathway converts PIP2 to PIP3; activating AKT promotes cell survival, proliferation, and metabolism by phosphorylating downstream targets like mTOR.
   - *Wnt* pathway controls cell fate, proliferation, differentiation, and calcium signaling.

3. *Downstream Signaling*

   The activation or suppression of *mTOR* affects several critical cellular functions:

   - *Autophagy regulation*: mTOR suppresses autophagy under nutrient-rich conditions and allows it during starvation or stress.
   - *Protein and lipid synthesis*: mTOR promotes biosynthesis, which supports cell growth and proliferation.
   - *Ribosome biogenesis*: The production of ribosomes is enhanced, boosting the cell's protein-making capacity.

Together, these outcomes determine whether the cell grows, divides, or conserves resources through processes like autophagy.

mTOR Location in the Cell

The diverse subcellular localization of mTOR reflects its multifaceted roles in cellular processes. The dual presence of mTOR in the cytoplasm and nucleus indeed broadens the scope for understanding its functional dynamics in both physiological and pathological states [14].

Here are some key aspects and emerging perspectives related to mTOR's localization that might further refine this discussion:

Cytoplasmic and Membrane-Associated Roles

- *Lysosomal Localization*: mTORC1 is primarily activated at the lysosomal surface, where it integrates nutrient availability signals via interactions with the Rag GTPases and the Ragulator complex [60].
- *ER and Golgi*: mTOR's presence at the ER and Golgi apparatus links it to processes such as protein synthesis, folding, and trafficking. This is particularly important in maintaining cellular homeostasis under stress conditions.
- *Mitochondria*: Localization to mitochondria implicates mTOR in regulating energy metabolism, mitochondrial dynamics, and apoptosis.

Nuclear Localization of mTOR [59]

- *Mechanisms of Nuclear Import*: Nuclear import of mTOR may be mediated through its interaction with nuclear transport proteins, although the specifics of these pathways remain an active area of investigation.
- *Regulation of Gene Expression*: Nuclear mTOR is implicated in the transcriptional regulation of ribosomal RNA (rRNA) synthesis, thereby linking it directly to the control of cellular biosynthesis.
- *DNA Damage Response*: mTOR in the nucleus may also participate in DNA damage repair mechanisms, particularly in response to genotoxic stress.

mTOR Gene Transcription

The transcription of mTOR is a tightly regulated process influenced by multiple transcription factors, signaling pathways, and environmental cues. It begins with transcription factor binding to the mTOR promoter, followed by RNA polymerase II-mediated transcription, RNA processing, and eventual regulation by microRNAs. This dynamic control ensures that mTOR expression and activity align with cellular needs, such as growth, nutrient availability, and stress response. The following is a detailed overview of this process [53]:

1. *Gene Structure and Regulation*
    - The *mTOR gene* (MTOR in humans) is located on chromosome 1 and contains multiple exons and introns, with its expression being tightly regulated at both transcriptional and post-transcriptional levels.
    - The *promoter region* of the mTOR gene contains binding sites for various transcription factors that are sensitive to external signals like nutrients, growth factors, stress, and energy availability.
2. *Transcription Initiation*
    - *Transcription factors* involved in mTOR regulator bind to the promoter region of the MTOR gene and initiate the transcription process. Some key transcription factors that regulate mTOR transcription include:
        - *c-Myc*: A well-known transcription factor that enhances mTOR expression by binding to its promoter in response to growth signals.

- *HIF-1α* (Hypoxia-inducible factor-1α): Under low-oxygen conditions, HIF-1α can increase mTOR transcription, linking mTOR activity to hypoxic responses.
- *NF-κB* (Nuclear factor-kappa B): Activated during stress or inflammation, NF-κB can promote mTOR transcription, integrating mTOR signaling with immune responses.
- *STAT3* (Signal transducer and activator of transcription 3): Often activated by cytokines and growth factors, STAT3 can also increase mTOR expression, particularly in cancer and inflammation contexts.

• *RNA Polymerase II*, the enzyme responsible for transcribing protein-coding genes, is recruited to the promoter region and begins synthesizing a complementary RNA strand using the DNA template of the MTOR gene.

3. *Transcription Elongation*

• Once RNA polymerase II is properly recruited, it begins the elongation phase, moving along the DNA template strand and synthesizing the primary mTOR mRNA transcript (pre-mRNA) in a 5′ to 3′ direction.
• *Histone modifications* and other chromatin remodeling factors help loosen the chromatin structure around the mTOR gene, facilitating smooth transcription. Acetylation and methylation of histones can positively or negatively influence mTOR transcription depending on cellular context and external signals.

4. *Transcription Termination*

• As the RNA polymerase II reaches the termination sequence at the end of the mTOR gene, it stops synthesizing RNA, and the nascent pre-mRNA is released from the DNA template.
• After transcription, the pre-mRNA undergoes several processing steps, including 5′ capping, 3′ polyadenylation, and splicing to remove introns and produce a mature mTOR mRNA transcript.

5. *Post-transcriptional Regulation*

• The mature mTOR mRNA is exported from the nucleus to the cytoplasm, where it can be translated into the mTOR protein.
• However, the expression of mTOR can be further regulated by microRNAs (miRNAs), which can bind to the 3′ untranslated region (3′ UTR) of mTOR mRNA, inhibiting its translation or leading to its degradation. For example, miR-99a and miR-199a are known to target mTOR mRNA for downregulation.

6. *Regulation by Signaling Pathways*

• The transcription of mTOR is also influenced by major signaling pathways, particularly:

  - *PI3K/AKT Pathway*: Growth factors such as insulin or IGF-1 activate the PI3K/AKT pathway, which promotes mTOR transcription and activation.

AKT can activate transcription factors like c-Myc, increasing mTOR transcription.
  - *AMPK Pathway*: When energy levels are low, AMPK (AMP-activated protein kinase) inhibits mTOR signaling by downregulating mTOR transcription and activity, conserving energy resources [1].
  - *p53 Pathway*: Under conditions of DNA damage or cellular stress, p53 can negatively regulate mTOR transcription to limit cell growth and allow for DNA repair or apoptosis.

7. Environmental and Metabolic Regulation

   - mTOR transcription is sensitive to external conditions like nutrient availability (especially amino acids), oxygen levels, and energy status. For instance:

     - *Amino Acids*: Amino acids, particularly leucine, are critical in mTOR activation. When nutrients are plentiful, mTORC1 is activated, promoting anabolic processes like protein and lipid synthesis, necessary for cell growth and proliferation. Low nutrient levels inhibit mTOR activity, leading cells to adopt catabolic states such as autophagy, conserving resources under nutrient scarcity.
     - *Energy Status*: mTOR senses cellular energy through the AMP-activated protein kinase (AMPK). Low ATP levels activate AMPK, which in turn inhibits mTOR activity, signaling the cell to shift away from energy-intensive processes. High energy levels favor mTOR activation, supporting biosynthetic pathways.
     - *Oxygen Level*: Hypoxia or low-oxygen levels can increase mTOR transcription via HIF-1α, coupling oxygen sensing to mTOR-driven processes like angiogenesis and metabolism. mTOR is responsive to oxygen availability. Hypoxia (low oxygen) suppresses mTOR activity via hypoxia-inducible factor (HIF)-dependent pathways, which adapt cellular processes to limited oxygen, reducing energy consumption and promoting survival under stress.

MicroRNA and mTOR

There is a significant relationship between mTOR signaling and microRNAs (miRNAs). mTOR, a key regulator of cellular growth, proliferation, metabolism, and survival, can influence miRNA expression and function, while miRNAs can in turn modulate mTOR signaling pathways. This bidirectional regulation plays a crucial role in various physiological and pathological processes.

MicroRNAs (miRNAs) are small, non-coding RNA molecules typically about 20–24 nucleotides long, which play a critical role in regulating gene expression. They function by binding to complementary sequences of messenger RNA (mRNA) transcripts, primarily leading to mRNA degradation or inhibition of translation. This regulatory process is crucial for controlling a wide range of cellular activities, including development, differentiation, proliferation, and apoptosis.

The biogenesis of miRNAs involves several steps.

First, they are transcribed by RNA polymerase II or III as primary miRNAs (pri-miRNAs), which are then processed into precursor miRNAs (pre-miRNAs) by the Drosha-DGCR8 complex in the nucleus. The pre-miRNAs are exported to the cytoplasm, where they are further processed by Dicer, another RNase, into mature miRNAs. These mature miRNAs are incorporated into the RNA-induced silencing complex (RISC), guiding the complex to target mRNAs [4].

1. *mTOR Regulation of miRNAs*

   mTOR controls several cellular processes that affect miRNA biogenesis and function. For instance:

   - *Transcriptional Regulation*: mTOR can influence the expression of transcription factors such as Myc or HIF-1α, which are involved in the transcription of miRNA genes. Under certain conditions, mTOR activation or inhibition can modulate the levels of specific miRNAs.
   - *Regulation of Biogenesis*: mTORC1 (mTOR Complex 1) signaling may influence the miRNA biogenesis machinery, particularly through its effect on RNA-binding proteins or enzymes like Drosha and Dicer, which are responsible for processing pri-miRNAs into mature miRNAs.
   - *Nutrient Availability*: As a sensor of nutrient status, mTORC1 regulates gene expression in response to energy levels, amino acids, and growth factors, which can alter the expression profiles of specific miRNAs in various tissues.

2. *miRNAs Regulating mTOR Signaling*

   Several miRNAs have been identified as direct regulators of mTOR signaling. These miRNAs either target mTOR itself or components of its upstream regulators and downstream effectors:

   - *miRNAs Targeting mTOR mRNA*: Some miRNAs, such as miR-99a, miR-100, and miR-199a, can bind to the 3′ untranslated region (UTR) of mTOR mRNA, suppressing its translation and thereby downregulating mTOR signaling.
   - *Upstream Regulators of mTOR*: Certain miRNAs can regulate upstream components of the mTOR pathway, such as TSC1/TSC2 (tuberous sclerosis complex), PTEN (phosphatase and tensin homolog), or Akt, thus modulating the overall mTOR pathway activity. For example, miR-21 has been shown to target PTEN, a negative regulator of the PI3K/Akt/mTOR pathway, leading to enhanced mTOR signaling.
   - *Downstream Targets of mTOR*: miRNAs can also affect downstream effectors of mTOR, including the regulation of proteins involved in autophagy, protein synthesis, and cell metabolism.

3. *Pathophysiological Implications*

   The interplay between mTOR and miRNAs has been observed in various diseases:

   - *Cancer*: In many cancers, dysregulation of mTOR signaling and miRNA expression is common. For example, overexpression of miR-21, which inhibits PTEN, can lead to hyperactivation of the mTOR pathway, promoting tumor growth.

- *Metabolic Disorders*: miRNAs can modulate mTOR signaling in insulin resistance and diabetes, where the balance between miRNAs and mTOR activity affects glucose homeostasis and lipid metabolism.
- *Neurodegenerative Diseases*: In conditions like Alzheimer's disease, miRNAs and mTOR signaling are involved in regulating autophagy, a key process for clearing protein aggregates.

Key mTOR Signaling Pathways

The *mTOR (mechanistic Target of Rapamycin)* signaling network consists of two key complexes, *mTORC1* and *mTORC2*, which regulate cellular growth, metabolism, and survival in response to nutrients, energy, and growth signals, and recently suggested two other complexes, *mTORC3* and *mTORC4* (Fig. 2.1).

The mTOR signaling process initiates with activation of the assigned receptors by their specific ligands such as hormones.

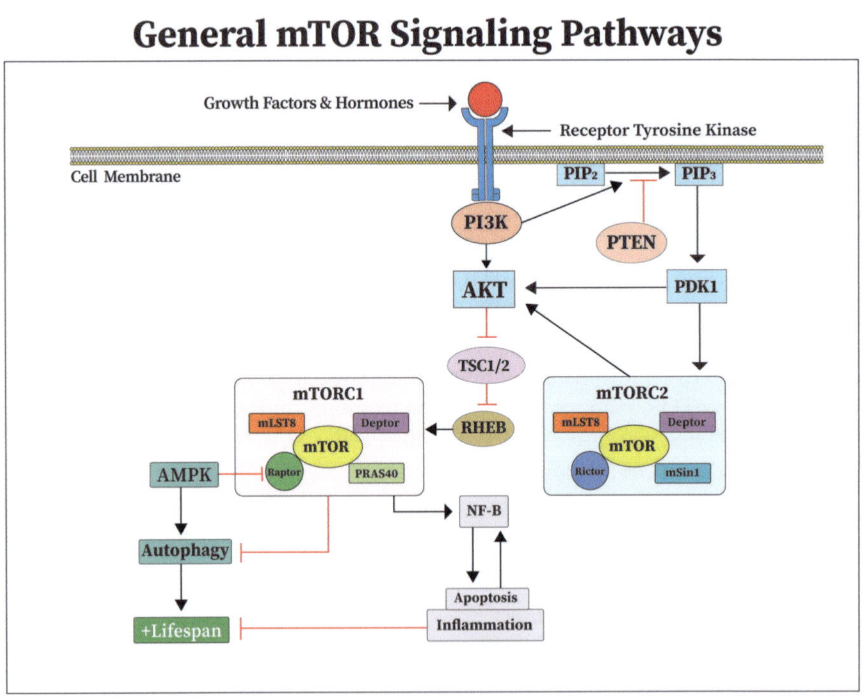

Fig. 2.1 General and simplified overview of mTOR pathways, highlighting the activation of mTOR complexes 1 and 2 and their resulting biological effects

mTOR Receptors

There are multiple receptors on the cell surface that attach to the specific ligand such as growth factors. These receptors act upstream of mTOR, integrating signals related to growth, metabolism, nutrient availability, immune responses, energy status, and environmental stresses. Their activation and cross-talk ensure that the mTOR signaling pathway adjusts cellular processes to maintain homeostasis and respond appropriately to environmental changes [52].

Here, we discuss the most influential receptors involved in mTOR function:

Amino Acid Sensors and Nutrient Receptors [30]

These receptors monitor nutrient availability and modulate mTORC1 activity.

- SLC38A9 (amino acid transporter) acts as an arginine sensor on the lysosome, activating mTORC1 during amino acid abundance.
- CASTOR proteins are arginine sensors that suppress mTORC1 under nutrient-poor conditions.
- Sestrins act as leucine sensors that regulate mTORC1 activity at the lysosome.
- G-protein-coupled receptors (GPCRs) respond to extracellular signals like nutrients and hormones, influencing mTOR indirectly through second messengers.

Cytokine Receptors [32]

Receptor Tyrosine Kinases (RTKs)

- Extracellular Ligand-Binding Domain: This domain is located outside the cell and has high affinity for specific ligands such as growth factors, cytokines, and hormones. Upon ligand binding, this domain undergoes a conformational change.
- Transmembrane Domain: This is a hydrophobic segment that anchors the receptor in the cell membrane, facilitating the transmission of signals from the extracellular environment to the cell's interior.
- Intracellular Tyrosine Kinase Domain: This domain has enzymatic activity that catalyzes the transfer of a phosphate group from ATP to tyrosine residues on target proteins, including the RTK itself (autophosphorylation) and other downstream signaling molecules.

Growth Factor and Hormone Receptors [3]

These receptors trigger mTOR activation through the PI3K-Akt pathway (Fig. 2.2).

1. Insulin Receptor (IR)
    - Activated by insulin, promoting glucose uptake and mTORC1 activation.
    - Involves the PI3K-Akt pathway to enhance anabolic processes.

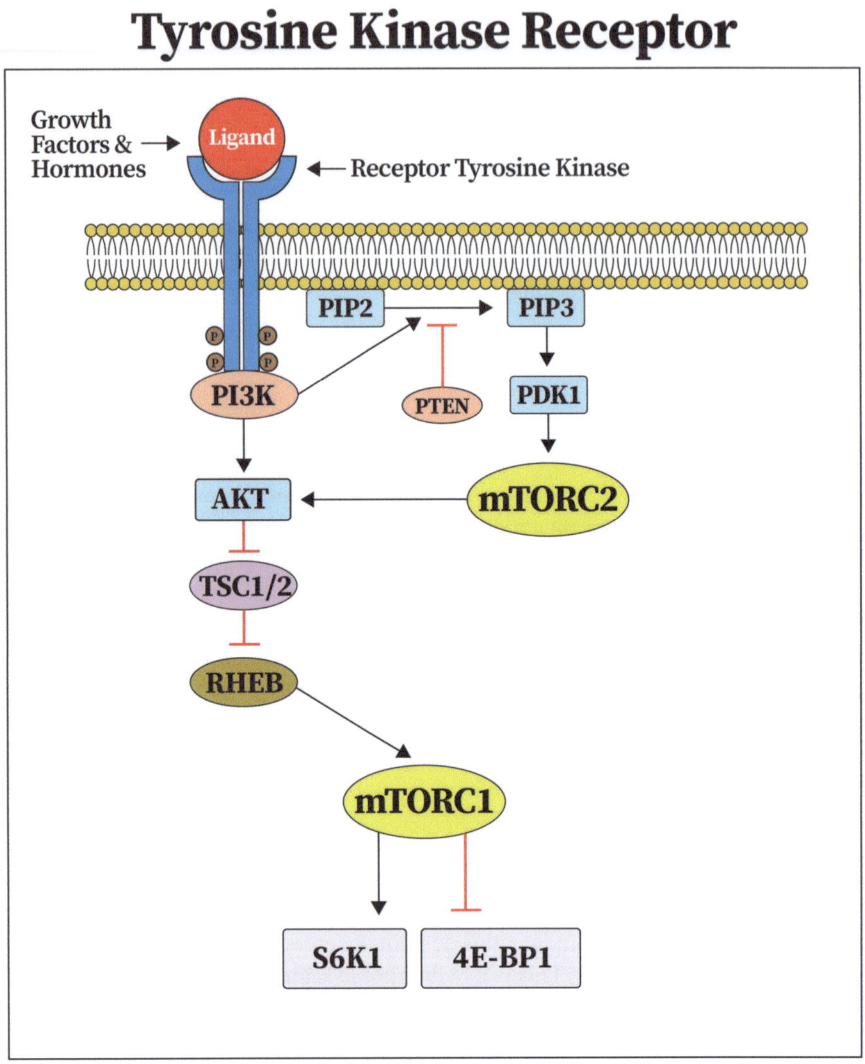

Fig. 2.2 Simplified overview of tyrosine kinase receptor with their effect on mTOR complexes 1 and 2

2. Insulin-like Growth Factor Receptor (IGF-1R)
   - Binds to IGF-1 and activates mTORC1 to promote growth and protein synthesis.
   - Stimulates the PI3K-Akt-mTOR axis.
3. Epidermal Growth Factor Receptor (EGFR)
   - Responds to EGF, enhancing cell proliferation through mTOR activation.
   - Stimulates both mTORC1 and mTORC2 via Ras-PI3K pathways (Fig. 2.3).

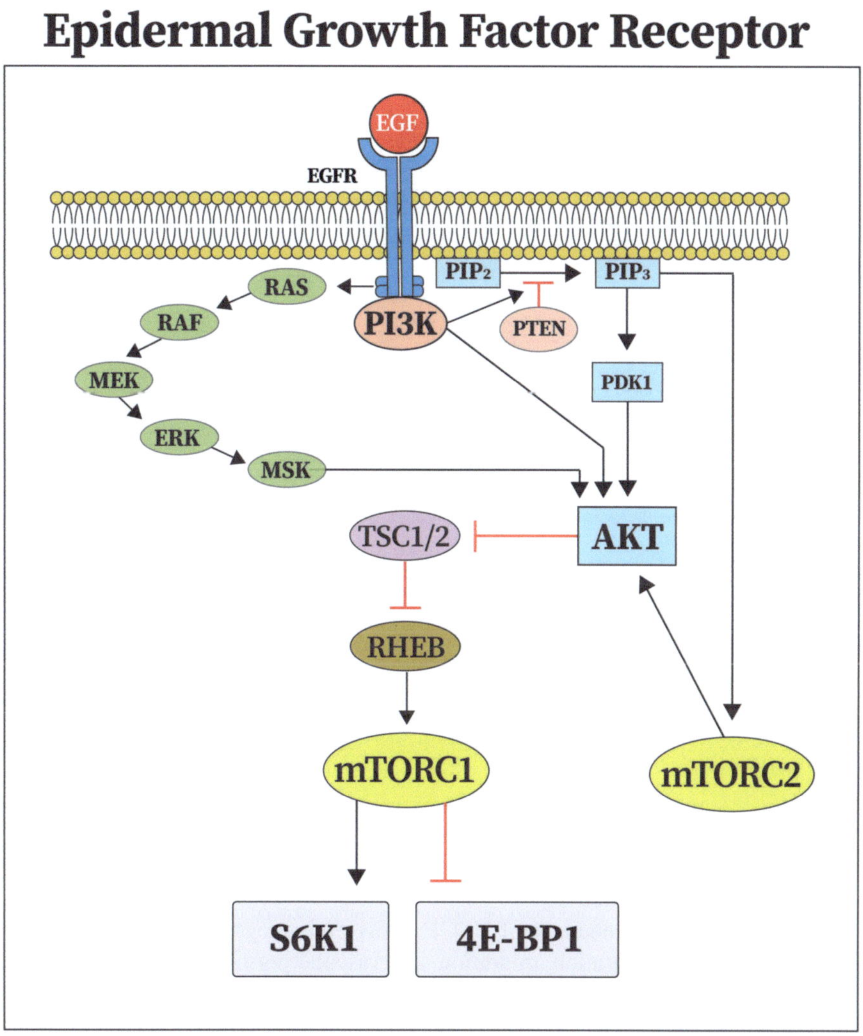

Fig. 2.3 The EGF pathway functions through the RAS-PI3K signaling pathways to modulate cellular growth and proliferation, affecting both mTORC1 and mTORC2

4. Platelet-Derived Growth Factor Receptor (PDGFR)
   - Activates mTOR via PI3K/Akt to stimulate cellular proliferation, migration, and angiogenesis.
5. Vascular Endothelial Growth Factor Receptor (VEGFR)
   Responds to VEGF, promoting angiogenesis through activation of the mTOR pathway. VEGF Receptors are a family of tyrosine kinase receptors critical for vascular and lymphatic development, as well as pathological processes like cancer and inflammation.

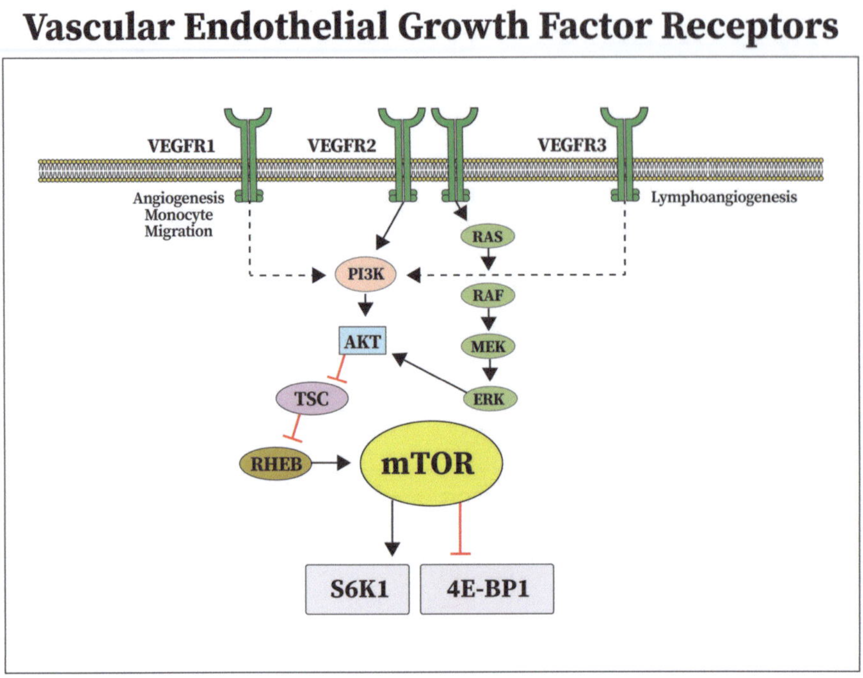

Fig. 2.4 VEGF receptors promote angiogenesis and lymphangiogenesis by activation of mTOR signaling pathway, which regulates cell growth and the formation of new blood and lymphatic vessels

- *VEGFR1*: High-affinity receptor for VEGF-A, VEGF-B, and PlGF; regulates angiogenesis and inflammation. Acts as a signaling receptor or a decoy, modulating VEGFR2 activity.
- *VEGFR2*: Main mediator of VEGF-A-driven angiogenesis; promotes endothelial cell proliferation, migration, and vascular permeability through strong tyrosine kinase activity.
- *VEGFR3*: Primary receptor for VEGF-C and VEGF-D; regulates lymphangiogenesis and lymphatic vessel maintenance, critical for fluid balance and immune trafficking (Fig. 2.4).

Immune Responses and Metabolic Pathway Receptors [48]

1. Interleukin Receptors (e.g., IL-6R, IL-2R)
   - Activate mTORC1 via JAK-STAT and PI3K pathways, regulating immune cell proliferation and metabolism.
2. Tumor Necrosis Factor Receptor (TNFR)
   - Involved in stress response and immune regulation, indirectly influencing mTOR through the NF-κB and PI3K pathways.

Energy and Stress Receptors and Sensors [57]

1. AMP-Activated Protein Kinase (AMPK)
   - Although not a classical receptor, AMPK senses energy depletion and inhibits mTORC1 to conserve energy.
2. Hypoxia-Inducible Factor (HIF) Receptors and Sensors
   - Activated by low-oxygen levels, they inhibit mTORC1 to reduce metabolic demand under hypoxia.

Frizzled Receptors [8]

Frizzled receptors are part of the Wnt signaling pathway, crucial for developmental processes, tissue homeostasis, and stem cell maintenance.

- Wnt signaling, mediated by Frizzled receptors, can crosstalk with the PI3K/Akt pathway, a key upstream regulator of mTOR.
- Activation of Wnt/β-catenin may influence mTORC1 activity indirectly through Akt phosphorylation.

In certain ocular diseases, Wnt signaling and mTOR pathways might converge on processes like retinal cell survival or angiogenesis.

IRS Receptors [46]

Insulin receptor substrates (IRS) are key adaptor proteins in insulin and IGF-1 signaling. Upon activation by receptor tyrosine kinases, IRS proteins facilitate downstream signaling cascades, including the PI3K-AKT-mTOR pathway. This pathway regulates cell growth, metabolism, and survival. Dysregulation of IRS or mTOR signaling is implicated in conditions like insulin resistance, cancer, and metabolic disorders.

TGF-β Receptors [49, 56]

Transforming growth factor-beta (TGF-β) receptors are key components of the TGF-β signaling pathway, mediating its effects on cell growth, differentiation, apoptosis, and extracellular matrix production. These receptors belong to the serine/threonine kinase receptor family and function as heteromeric complexes.

There are three main types of TGF-β receptors:

1. TGF-β Type I Receptor (TGF-βRI)
   - A transmembrane serine/threonine kinase receptor.
   - Approximately 55 kDa in size.

- Contains an extracellular ligand-binding domain, a transmembrane region, and an intracellular kinase domain.
- Phosphorylated and activated by TGF-βRII upon ligand binding.
- Directly phosphorylates receptor-regulated SMADs (R-SMADs: SMAD2 and SMAD3).
- Essential for initiating canonical (SMAD-dependent) TGF-β signaling.

2. TGF-β Type II Receptor (TGF-βRII)

- A transmembrane serine/threonine kinase receptor.
- Approximately 75 kDa in size.
- Similar structural organization to TGF-βRI.
- Constitutively active kinase that binds TGF-β ligands with high affinity.
- Recruits and phosphorylates TGF-βRI upon ligand binding.
- Required for both canonical and non-canonical (e.g., MAPK, PI3K/AKT) TGF-β signaling.

3. TGF-β Type III Receptor (TGF-βRIII or Betaglycan)

- A large proteoglycan receptor.
- Lacks intrinsic kinase activity but modulates ligand binding.
- Acts as a co-receptor, enhancing the binding of TGF-β ligands to TGF-βRII.
- Important for efficient signal transduction, especially in tissues with low TGF-β levels (Fig. 2.5).

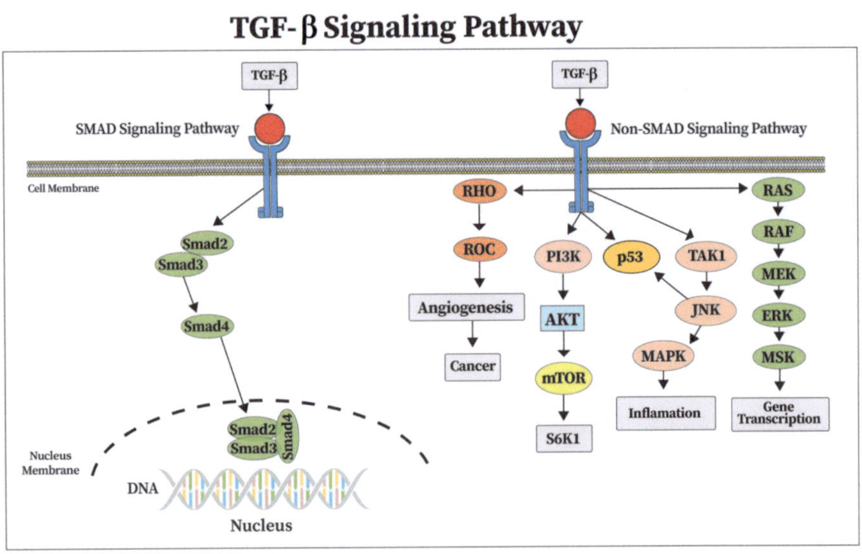

Fig. 2.5 Illustration of transforming growth factor beta (TGF-B) receptors, which are essential components of TGF-ß signaling pathways. These pathways include SMAD signaling and non-SMAD signaling, each leading to different gene transcription outcomes. The receptors regulate key cellular processes such as growth, differentiation, apoptosis, and extracellular matrix production

TNF Family Receptors [13]

Tumor necrosis factor (TNF) family receptors are critical components of cellular signaling networks that influence a wide array of cellular processes, including immune responses, apoptosis, proliferation, and inflammation. These receptors also have intricate crosstalk with the mechanistic target of rapamycin (mTOR) pathway, which plays a central role in regulating cell growth, metabolism, autophagy, and survival.

Tumor necrosis factor-alpha (TNF-α), either in its soluble or membrane-bound form, activates two distinct receptors: TNFR1 and TNFR2. Upon TNF-α binding, TNFR1 recruits adaptor molecules such as TRAF2 and TRADD to its intracellular death domain, initiating three key signaling pathways: NF-κB signaling, MAPK/C-Jun signaling, and caspase-mediated apoptotic signaling. In contrast, TNFR2, activated by membrane-bound TNF-α, triggers the PI3K/Akt pathway and promotes proangiogenic signaling, such as VEGF/VEGFR2 activation, while also modulating NF-κB signaling.

- TNF receptors, such as TNFR1 and TNFR2, are activated by TNF ligands and initiate downstream signaling cascades.
- TNFR signaling can influence mTOR activity through the activation of intermediates like NF-κB, PI3K/Akt, and MAPKs.
- Akt phosphorylates and inhibits TSC2 (tuberous sclerosis complex 2), leading to mTORC1 activation and subsequent promotion of protein synthesis, cell growth, and inhibition of autophagy.
- TNF-induced NF-κB signaling influences mTOR activity indirectly by modulating inflammatory and metabolic gene expression.
- NF-κB can regulate autophagy, a process heavily controlled by mTOR signaling, creating a dynamic interplay between inflammation and cellular homeostasis.

mTOR Signal Transduction and Crucial Signaling Pathways

Akt (Ak Strain transforming or Protein Kinase B (PKB)) Pathway

The *AKT pathway* is a key signaling pathway regulating cell growth, survival, metabolism, and proliferation. Activated by PI3K and mTORC2, AKT phosphorylates downstream targets like mTORC1 and GSK3 to promote cellular functions and inhibit apoptosis.

AKT Activators

1. *Growth Factors*: EGF (epidermal growth factor), IGF-1 (insulin-like growth factor 1), PDGF (platelet-derived growth factor)
2. *Insulin*: Activates the PI3K-AKT pathway

3. *Cytokines*: IL-2, IL-4
4. *G-protein Coupled Receptors (GPCRs) Ligands*: Sphingosine-1-phosphate (S1P)
5. *Cell Adhesion Molecules*: Integrins
6. *Hormones*: Estrogen
7. *Nutrients*: Amino acids

AKT Inhibitors

1. *PTEN (Phosphatase and Tensin Homolog)*: Dephosphorylates PIP3, counteracting PI3K activity
2. *PP2A (Protein Phosphatase 2A)*: Dephosphorylates AKT directly
3. *SHIP (SH2-containing Inositol Phosphatase)*: Hydrolyzes PIP3 to PIP2
4. *TRB3 (Tribbles Pseudokinase 3)*: Binds to and inhibits AKT activation
5. *AMPK*: Inhibits mTORC1 and indirectly affects AKT signaling
6. *mTORC1*: Negative feedback loop inhibits AKT
7. *IKK (IκB Kinase)*: Inhibits AKT through various downstream effectors
8. *Pharmacological Inhibitors*: Wortmannin, LY294002 (PI3K inhibitors), MK-2206 (AKT inhibitor) (Fig. 2.6)

Akt and Cell Apoptosis and Survival

Akt significantly enhances cell survival by modulating several proapoptotic proteins and signaling processes:

Inhibition of Bcl-2 Family Members

- Bax and Bim Proteins: These are proapoptotic members of the Bcl-2 family. Akt can phosphorylate these proteins, leading to their inactivation or degradation, which prevents them from promoting apoptosis
- By inhibiting these proteins, Akt helps to maintain the integrity of the mitochondrial outer membrane, thereby preventing the release of cytochrome c and other proapoptotic factors that lead to cell death.

Suppression of BH3-Only Proteins

- Akt can inhibit the expression of BH3-only proteins, which are another category of proapoptotic molecules. It does this primarily by modulating the activity of transcription factors that control the expression of these proteins.
- FOXO Transcription Factors: Akt phosphorylates FOXO family members, leading to their exclusion from the nucleus. This prevents them from transcribing genes that promote apoptosis, including those encoding BH3-only proteins.
- p53 Tumor Suppressor: p53 is a critical regulator of the cell response to DNA damage and stress, often inducing apoptosis if the cell is severely damaged. Akt can promote the phosphorylation and activation of MDM2, an E3 ubiquitin ligase that tags p53 for proteasomal degradation, thereby inhibiting p53-mediated apoptotic pathways.

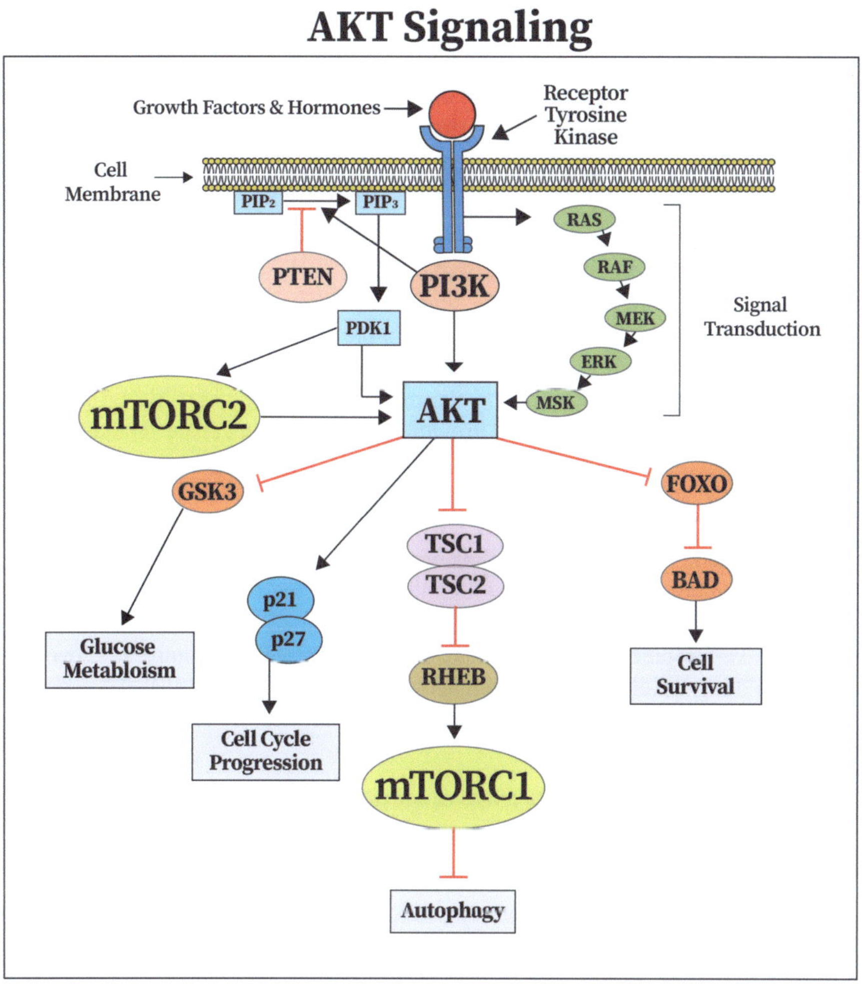

Fig. 2.6 A simplified overview of the AKT pathway, highlighting its complexity, interactions with upstream regulators, signal transduction mechanisms, and resulting biological outcomes

Regulation of GSK3

- GSK3 Isoforms: Akt phosphorylates and inactivates Glycogen Synthase Kinase 3 (GSK3) isoforms at a conserved N-terminal regulatory site. This inactivation plays a role in preventing apoptosis and also affects glucose metabolism.
- By inhibiting GSK3, Akt contributes to the stabilization and activation of various proteins and transcription factors involved in cell survival and metabolic processes.

Akt and TSC1 and TSC2 (Tuberous Sclerosis Complex 1 & 2)

These are tumor suppressor proteins that form a functional complex to regulate cell growth and proliferation by inhibiting the mechanistic target of rapamycin complex 1 (mTORC1).

Their primary functions are:

- Inhibition of mTORC1: TSC1 and TSC2 form a complex that acts as a GTPase-activating protein (GAP) for the small GTPase Rheb. The TSC1/TSC2 complex converts Rheb from its active GTP-bound state to its inactive GDP-bound state, thereby inhibiting mTORC1 activity. This prevents mTORC1 from promoting protein synthesis, cell growth, and other anabolic processes.
- Regulation of Cell Growth and Proliferation: By inhibiting mTORC1, the TSC1/TSC2 complex helps control cell growth and proliferation, ensuring that cells do not grow uncontrollably. This function is crucial for maintaining normal cellular homeostasis and preventing tumor formation.
- Response to Cellular Stress: The TSC1/TSC2 complex is sensitive to various cellular stress signals, including low energy levels, hypoxia, and DNA damage. Under such conditions, the complex inhibits mTORC1 to conserve energy and resources, aiding in cell survival and repair.
- Role in Development and Differentiation: The TSC1/TSC2 complex is involved in regulating developmental processes and cell differentiation. It helps ensure that cells differentiate properly, and that tissue architecture is maintained during development.

Mutations in either TSC1 or TSC2 can lead to uncontrolled mTORC1 activity, resulting in the development of tuberous sclerosis complex (TSC), a genetic disorder characterized by the growth of benign tumors in various organs.

Akt and Protein Synthesis and Cell Growth

Akt promotes protein synthesis and cell growth, largely by interacting with the mTOR pathway by activation of S6K and 4E-BP1.

- S6 Kinase (S6K): Once activated by mTORC1, S6K phosphorylates the ribosomal protein S6, enhancing the translation of mRNAs that encode components of the protein synthesis apparatus.
- 4E-BP1: mTORC1 also phosphorylates and inactivates the eukaryotic initiation factor 4E-binding protein 1 (4E-BP1), which normally binds and inhibits eIF4E. Phosphorylation of 4E-BP1 releases eIF4E, allowing it to initiate the cap-dependent translation of mRNA into protein.

Akt Role on Cell Proliferation and Cell Cycle Regulation

Akt influences cell proliferation and the cell cycle by phosphorylating key cyclin-dependent kinase inhibitors such as phosphorylation of P21 and P27:

- P21(Waf1/Cip1) and P27(Kip1): These proteins are cyclin-dependent kinase inhibitors that can arrest the cell cycle in the G1 phase. Akt phosphorylates P21 and P27, leading to their retention in the cytoplasm.
- This phosphorylation prevents P21 and P27 from inhibiting cyclin-dependent kinases in the nucleus, thereby promoting the progression of the cell cycle from G1 to S phase and facilitating cell proliferation.

Akt summary of its functions include:

1. *Cell Survival and Anti-apoptosis*: AKT promotes cell survival by inhibiting apoptotic processes. It phosphorylates and inactivates several pro-apoptotic proteins, including Bad and caspase-9.
2. *Cell Growth and Proliferation*: AKT stimulates cell growth and proliferation by activating mTORC1 through the inhibition of the TSC1/TSC2 complex. This promotes protein synthesis and cellular growth.
3. *Glucose Metabolism*: AKT enhances glucose uptake and metabolism by promoting the translocation of glucose transporter 4 (GLUT4) to the cell membrane and by phosphorylating key enzymes involved in glycolysis.
4. *Protein Synthesis*: AKT activates mTORC1, which then stimulates protein synthesis by phosphorylating downstream targets such as S6 kinase (S6K) and 4E-BP1.
5. *Cell Cycle Progression*: AKT facilitates cell cycle progression by phosphorylating and inhibiting cell cycle inhibitors, such as p21 and p27, and by promoting the degradation of p53, a tumor suppressor protein.
6. *Angiogenesis*: AKT promotes angiogenesis by enhancing the expression of vascular endothelial growth factor (VEGF) and other angiogenic factors.

AMPK Pathway

AMP-activated protein kinase (AMPK) is a sensor of cellular energy levels. When energy is low, AMPK phosphorylates and activates TSC2, inhibiting mTOR and reducing anabolic processes to conserve energy [25].

The AMPK pathway ensures that, during energy stress, the cell conserves energy by inhibiting mTORC1, thus halting growth and proliferation until energy levels are restored. AMP-activated protein kinase (AMPK) is a critical energy sensor in cells that help to maintain energy homeostasis. Its interaction with mTOR is a key regulatory mechanism, especially under conditions of low energy.

AMPK is activated in response to increases in the AMP/ATP ratio, which occurs when a cell's energy is depleted. This activation can be triggered by low glucose levels, hypoxia, and other metabolic stresses that deplete cellular ATP.

AMPK and REDD1 Under conditions of low energy or stress such as hypoxia, AMPK (activated by increases in AMP/ATP ratio) and REDD1 are activated. These proteins enhance the activity of the TSC complex, promoting the inhibition of mTORC1. Additionally, AMPK can directly inhibit mTORC1 by phosphorylating RAPTOR, a component of mTORC1.

Activated AMPK works to restore energy balance by switching off anabolic processes (which consume energy) and switching on catabolic processes (which produce energy). It phosphorylates and activates TSC2 and also directly phosphorylates Raptor, a component of mTORC1. By activating TSC2, AMPK enhances the inhibitory effect of the TSC complex on Rheb, thus turning off mTORC1 activity.

AMPK also directly phosphorylates Raptor, leading to the suppression of mTORC1.

This dual inhibition ensures that, when energy levels are low, mTOR is turned off, preventing energy-consuming processes like protein synthesis (Fig. 2.7).

AMPK Pathway

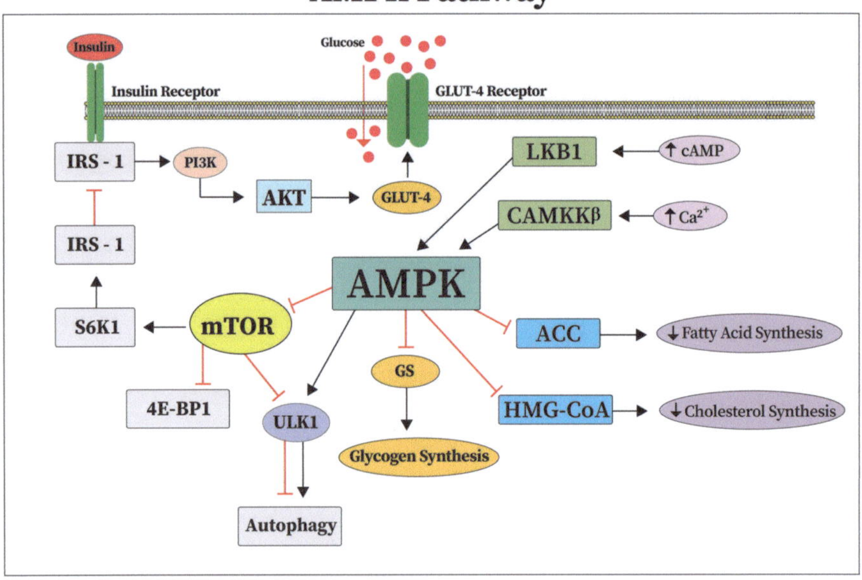

Fig. 2.7 A simplified representation of the AMPK pathway, showcasing its upstream receptors, regulatory influences, signal transduction mechanisms, and resulting biological outcomes

cAMP-Dependent Pathway

In humans, the cyclic AMP (cAMP)-dependent pathway is primarily mediated by the activation of Protein Kinase A (PKA). When signaling molecules (e.g., hormones) bind to G-protein-coupled receptors (GPCRs), an enzyme called adenylyl cyclase is activated, leading to the production of cAMP from ATP [26].

- cAMP binds to and activates PKA. Activated PKA then phosphorylates target proteins, leading to varied cellular responses, such as changes in metabolism, gene expression, or ion channel activity.
- The downstream effects of this pathway depend on the cell type and the proteins phosphorylated by PKA.
- This pathway is involved in processes such as glucose metabolism, heart rate regulation, and memory formation.

JAK-STAT Pathway (Janus Kinases- Signal Transducer and Activator of Transcription)

The JAK-STAT pathway is a key signaling cascade for cytokine and growth factor responses, indirectly linking to mTOR activation. Cytokines or growth factors bind to their receptors (e.g., IL-6 receptor). JAK phosphorylates the receptor, creating docking sites for STAT, which JAK-STAT signaling enhances expression of molecules like PI3K or IRS-1, which activate the PI3K-AKT-mTORpathway [42].

JNK/MAPK Pathway

The JNK/MAPK pathway interacts with mTOR signaling through crosstalk that regulates cell survival, growth, and stress responses. JNK activation can influence mTOR by modulating upstream regulators like TSC2 (tuberous sclerosis complex 2) and AMPK, often in response to stress. This interaction typically inhibits mTORC1 activity during cellular stress to conserve energy and promote autophagy, helping cells adapt to adverse conditions [23] (Fig. 2.8).

IP3/DAG Pathway

The Inositol Triphosphate (IP3)/Diacylglycerol (DAG) pathway is activated by Phospholipase C (PLC), which cleaves the membrane phospholipid phosphatidylinositol 4,5-bisphosphate (PIP2) into two signaling molecules [55]:

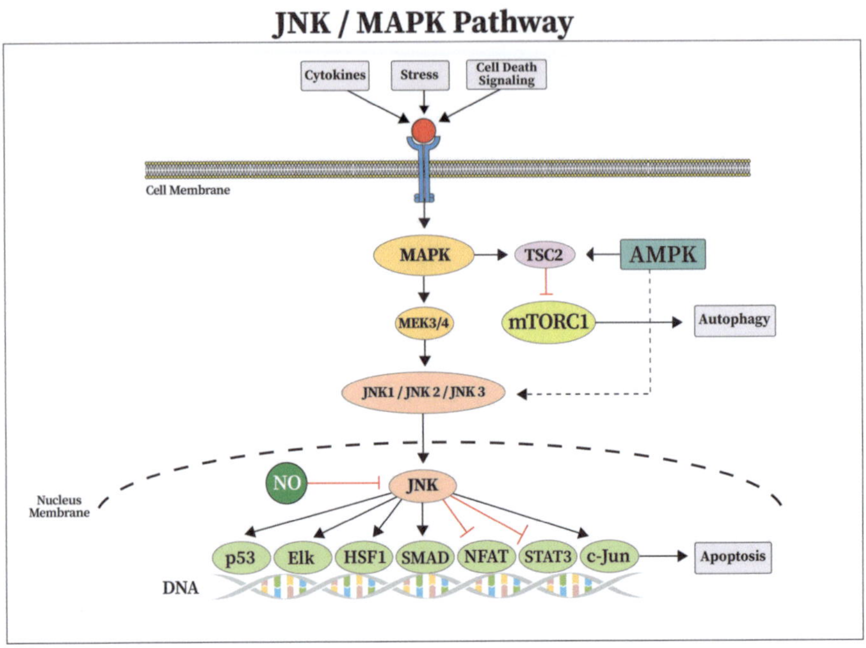

Fig. 2.8 The pathway shown above illustrates the final outcome of stress leading to cell apoptosis. The interaction of JNK and MAPK with mTORC1 plays a key role, as JNK activation can influence mTOR by modulating TSC2 and AMPK, often in response to stress. This interaction inhibits mTORC1 activity during cellular stress, helping to conserve energy and promote autophagy

1. Diacylglycerol (DAG)—remains in the membrane.
2. Inositol 1,4,5-trisphosphate (IP3)—Released into the cytosol.

   - IP3 binds to specific calcium channels on the endoplasmic reticulum (ER), causing the release of calcium ions into the cytosol. This surge in calcium concentration triggers various calcium-dependent processes.
   - DAG, along with calcium, activates Protein Kinase C (PKC), which phosphorylates target proteins to alter cellular functions.

This pathway regulates numerous processes, including taste perception, mood regulation (e.g., manic depression), and tumor promotion.

MAPK/ERK Pathway

Mitogen-activated protein kinase (MAPK) or extracellular signal-regulated kinase (ERK) pathway stimulates mTOR through the phosphorylation and inhibition of TSC2, promoting protein synthesis and cell proliferation [34].

MAPK/ERK pathway links extracellular signals, such as growth factors, to intracellular responses. When growth factors bind to cell surface receptors (e.g., receptor tyrosine kinases), a cascade of phosphorylation events is initiated. This cascade involves multiple key proteins, such as RAS, RAF, MEK, and ERK. Once activated, ERK translocates to the nucleus, where it can regulate gene expression and promote cell division.

In many cell types, activation of this pathway drives cell proliferation. Dysregulation or mutations in components of this pathway are implicated in numerous cancers due to uncontrolled cell growth.

P38/MAPK Pathway

p38 MAPK is typically activated by stress stimuli such as inflammation, oxidative stress, and DNA damage. p38 can suppress mTOR activity under stress by inhibiting upstream activators like TSC2 or by directly influencing mTOR complex components [9].

p53 Pathway

The p53 pathway and mTOR signaling are interconnected through several regulatory mechanisms that influence cell growth, metabolism, and survival. p53, a tumor suppressor, primarily acts to prevent tumor formation by promoting DNA repair, cell cycle arrest, or apoptosis under stress conditions. Its interaction with mTOR influences cellular responses to energy stress, nutrient availability, and growth stimuli [41].

Key Interactions Between p53 and mTOR

- Inhibition of mTOR by p53.
- p53 can indirectly suppress mTOR activity by activating the AMPK pathway. p53 induces the transcription of Sestrin1 and Sestrin2, which activate AMPK. Activated AMPK then inhibits mTOR by phosphorylating and activating TSC2 (tuberous sclerosis complex 2).
- Additionally, p53 can increase the expression of PTEN (phosphatase and tensin homolog), a negative regulator of the PI3K-Akt pathway. This reduces Akt activation, thus inhibiting mTOR activity.
- Nutrient stress and autophagy regulation.
- Under nutrient stress, p53 promotes autophagy by inhibiting mTOR. Autophagy is a catabolic process that degrades cellular components to maintain energy homeostasis. The inhibition of mTOR by p53 is essential in facilitating this process.
- Regulation of cell growth and metabolism.

- In normal conditions, mTOR promotes anabolic processes such as protein and lipid synthesis to support cell growth. However, under stress, p53-mediated inhibition of mTOR shifts the balance toward catabolic processes (like autophagy), thereby conserving energy and preventing uncontrolled growth.
- p53 mutations and mTOR activation.
- Loss or mutation of p53, which is common in various cancers, leads to unchecked mTOR activation. This contributes to increased cell growth and reduced apoptosis, promoting tumorigenesis (Fig. 2.9).

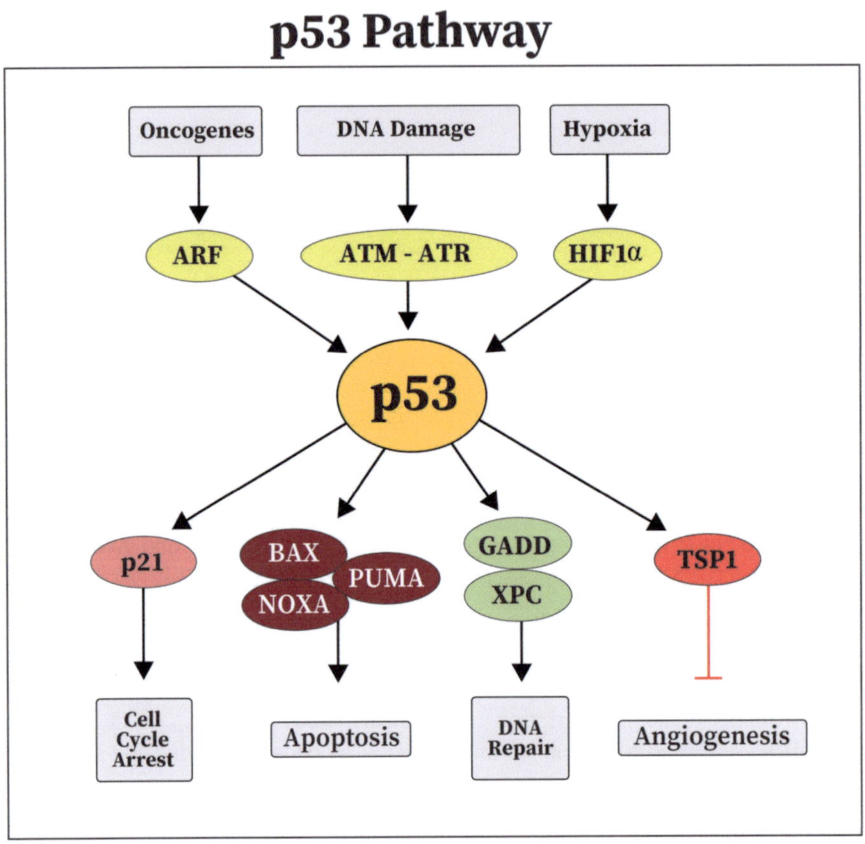

Fig. 2.9 The p53 pathway, as shown above, is interconnected through various regulatory mechanisms that influence cellular survival. The final outcomes of this pathway include cell cycle arrest, apoptosis, DNA repair, and tumor suppression, which also involves the regulation of angiogenesis

PI3K Pathway (Phosphatidylinositol 3-Kinase)

Regulation by the PI3K/Akt Pathway [15]

Phosphoinositide 3-kinase (PI3K) is a key enzyme involved in various cellular processes, primarily through its role in signal transduction pathways. PI3K is a critical enzyme that integrates extracellular signals to regulate multiple cellular functions, including growth, survival, metabolism, protein synthesis, motility, and immune responses. Dysregulation of PI3K signaling is associated with various diseases, including cancer, metabolic disorders, and immune deficiencies. Given its pivotal role in cellular signal transduction, we will explore it in greater detail.

PI3K is a heterodimer composed of two primary subunits:

1. *Catalytic subunit (p110)*: This subunit is responsible for the enzymatic activity of PI3K. It exists in several isoforms (e.g., p110α, p110β, and p110δ), each with distinct tissue distributions and functions.
2. *Regulatory subunit (p85)*: This subunit stabilizes and regulates the activity of p110. It contains SH2 domains that mediate interactions with phosphorylated tyrosine residues on activated receptors or adaptor proteins.

Activation Mechanisms

PI3K can be activated through multiple mechanisms:

1. *Receptor Interaction*:
   - Activation occurs directly when the regulatory subunit (p85) binds to phosphorylated tyrosine residues on activated receptor tyrosine kinases (RTKs) or cytokine receptors.
   - This binding positions the catalytic subunit (p110) near the membrane, where its substrate, phosphatidylinositol, is located.
2. *Adaptor Molecules*:
   - PI3K can also be activated indirectly via adaptor proteins like insulin receptor substrates (IRS). Upon phosphorylation by insulin receptors, IRS proteins recruit PI3K to the membrane.
3. *RAS Protein*:
   - Activation of PI3K can be facilitated by RAS, a small GTPase. Active, GTP-bound RAS interacts with the p110 catalytic subunit, enhancing its enzymatic activity. This provides a link between PI3K and other growth factor signaling pathways.

The primary functions and roles of PI3K in the cell follow.

1. Signal Transduction
   PI3K is activated by various extracellular signals such as growth factors, hormones, and cytokines. Upon activation, PI3K phosphorylates the 3′ hydroxyl group of the inositol ring of phosphoinositide, producing PIP3 (phosphatidylinositol-3,4,5-trisphosphate). PIP3 serves as a second messenger, recruiting and activating downstream signaling proteins that contain pleckstrin homology (PH) domains, such as AKT.
2. Cell Growth and Proliferation
   PI3K signaling is crucial for cell growth and proliferation. PIP3 activates AKT, which in turn phosphorylates and regulates various targets involved in cell cycle progression, survival, and metabolism. This pathway promotes the transcription of genes necessary for cell cycle progression and inhibits apoptotic pathways.
3. Cell Survival
   PI3K-AKT signaling promotes cell survival by inhibiting apoptotic pathways. AKT phosphorylates and inactivates several pro-apoptotic proteins, such as BAD and caspase-9, enhancing cell survival and resistance to stress.
4. Metabolism
   PI3K plays a significant role in regulating cellular metabolism. Through the activation of AKT, PI3K signaling enhances glucose uptake and glycolysis by promoting the translocation of glucose transporters (such as GLUT4) to the cell membrane. AKT also regulates glycogen synthesis by phosphorylating and inhibiting glycogen synthase kinase 3 (GSK-3).
5. Protein Synthesis
   PI3K-AKT signaling is involved in protein synthesis through the activation of the mTOR pathway. mTORC1 (mechanistic target of rapamycin complex 1) promotes protein synthesis and cell growth by phosphorylating downstream targets such as S6 kinase and 4E-BP1.
6. Cell Motility and Cytoskeleton Organization
   PI3K influences cell motility and cytoskeletal reorganization by regulating actin filament formation and cell adhesion molecules. This is crucial for processes like cell migration, invasion, and tissue remodeling [24].
7. Immune Response
   In immune cells, PI3K signaling is essential for various functions, including the activation and differentiation of T cells, B cells, and other immune cells. PI3K also regulates the production of cytokines and other immune mediators.
8. Angiogenesis
   PI3K signaling promotes angiogenesis, the formation of new blood vessels, by regulating the expression of vascular endothelial growth factor (VEGF) and other angiogenic factors. This is important for tissue growth and repair.

PI3K-AKT Signaling Pathway

In general, the function of PI3K-AKT signaling pathway is to stimulate cell to proliferation and growth and simultaneously inhibit cell apoptosis. Phosphoinositide 3-kinase (PI3K) activates Akt (protein kinase B) through phosphorylation [35].

The pathway typically starts with the activation of PI3K by growth factors, insulin, or other stimuli through receptor tyrosine kinases (RTKs) or G-protein-coupled receptors (GPCRs).

Activated PI3K phosphorylates PIP2 (phosphatidylinositol-4,5-bisphosphate) to produce PIP3 (phosphatidylinositol-3,4,5-trisphosphate), a lipid second messenger.

PIP3 recruits AKT (also known as protein kinase B) to the cell membrane, where it is phosphorylated and activated by PDK1 (phosphoinositide-dependent kinase-1) and mTOR complex 2 (mTORC2) [21].

Activated AKT phosphorylates and inhibits the TSC1/TSC2 (tuberous sclerosis complex) complex, a negative regulator of mTOR complex 1 (mTORC1). This inhibition allows Rheb (Ras homolog enriched in brain), a small GTPase, to activate mTORC1, once activated, promotes protein synthesis, lipid synthesis, and other anabolic processes by phosphorylating downstream targets such as S6K (ribosomal protein S6 kinase) and 4E-BP1 (eukaryotic translation initiation factor 4E-binding protein 1).

Feedback Mechanisms There are feedback loops within the PI3K/AKT/mTOR pathway. For example, S6K can negatively feedback to inhibit insulin receptor substrate (IRS) proteins, which can reduce PI3K signaling.

One of the critical targets of AKT is the TSC (Tuberous Sclerosis Complex), specifically TSC2.

AKT phosphorylates TSC2, leading to the inhibition of the TSC1/2 complex, a negative regulator of mTOR.

With TSC1/2 inhibited, the small GTPase Rheb becomes active. Rheb, in its GTP-bound form, directly activates mTORC1, leading to increased protein synthesis, cell growth, and proliferation.

Akt also phosphorylates PRAS40, which, when released from mTORC1, alleviates its inhibitory effect on the complex, further promoting mTORC1 activation (Fig. 2.10).

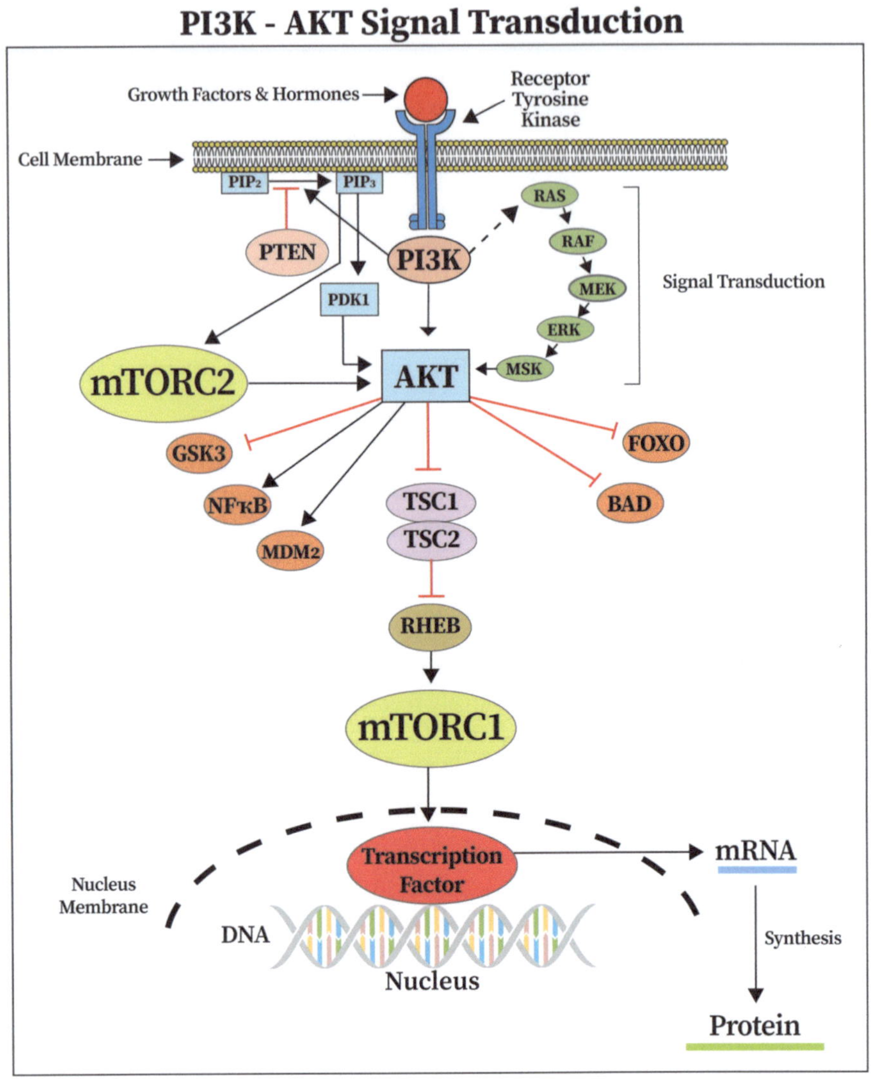

Fig. 2.10 This pathway begins with the activation of PI3K by growth factors, which leads to the phosphorylation of PIP2 to PIP3. PIP3 then activates AKT through PDK1. Additionally, PIP3 directly activates mTORC2, which further activates AKT. AKT, in turn, inhibits TSC1 and TSC2, which normally inhibit RHEB. This inhibition of TSC1/2 prevents RHEB from activating mTORC1

General Impact of the PI3K-AKT Signaling Pathway [38]

Overall, the PI3K-AKT signaling pathway plays a crucial role in stimulating cell proliferation and growth while simultaneously inhibiting cell apoptosis. This pathway ensures that cells can respond appropriately to growth signals by enhancing their survival, increasing protein synthesis, and facilitating progression through the cell cycle. Dysregulation of this pathway is often associated with various cancers and other diseases, making it a critical target for therapeutic intervention.

Once active, Akt could translocate from the plasma membrane to the cytoplasm and nucleus, where many of its substrates reside. Phosphorylation by Akt can be inhibitory or stimulatory, either suppressing or enhancing the activity of target proteins. Depending on the target protein, Akt can regulate different cell functions, here we discuss several main effects of PI3K-Akt pathway.

Other Feedback Mechanisms in PI3K-AKT Signaling

1. *Positive Feedback Loop*
   - *NF-κB and PPARβ/δ:*
     - *Transcription Factor NF-κB Activation*: AKT can activate the NF-κB pathway, which plays a role in cell survival and inflammatory responses. Once activated, NF-κB translocates to the nucleus and can induce the expression of many genes.
     - *Regulation of PPARβ/δ*: Among the genes activated by NF-κB are those encoding peroxisome proliferator-activated receptor delta (PPARβ/δ) agonists. These agonists can promote the expression of survival and metabolic genes.
     - *Downregulation of PTEN*: Both NF-κB and PPARβ/δ can lead to the transcriptional repression of PTEN, creating a positive feedback loop that enhances PI3K-AKT signaling by reducing the levels of PTEN and thus increasing PIP3 availability.
2. *Negative Feedback Loop*
   - *mTORC1-S6K1 Axis:*
     - *mTORC1 Activation*: The activation of AKT leads to the stimulation of mTORC1, a downstream effector that promotes protein synthesis and cell growth.
     - *S6K1 Activation*: One of the key targets of mTORC1 is S6 Kinase 1 (S6K1), which is involved in protein synthesis and also plays a role in feedback inhibition.
     - *Phosphorylation of IRS-1*: S6K1 phosphorylates Insulin Receptor Substrate 1 (IRS-1) on serine residues. This phosphorylation reduces the ability of IRS-1 to associate with and activate the insulin receptor and RTKs, leading to a decrease in PI3K activation.
     - *Suppression of PI3K Activity*: The result is a dampening of the PI3K-AKT signaling pathway, forming a negative feedback loop that prevents excessive activation.

Rag GTPase Pathway for Amino Acid Sensing

mTOR responds to amino acid availability through Rag GTPases, which recruit mTOR to lysosomes where it can be activated by Rheb, another small GTPase regulated by TSC2 [44].

Rheb and TSC Complex

The interaction between Rheb, a small GTPase, and the TSC complex is central to the direct regulation of mTOR activity [6].

TSC Complex
The TSC complex is composed of TSC1 (hamartin), TSC2 (tuberin), and TBC1D7. TSC2 has a GTPase-activating protein (GAP) domain that catalyzes the conversion of Rheb-GTP to Rheb-GDP. When TSC2 is active, it converts Rheb into its inactive GDP-bound state, thereby inhibiting mTORC1 activity.

Regulation by Signals
The TSC complex is regulated by multiple signals, including those from the PI3K/AKT pathway (via phosphorylation of TSC2 by AKT), AMPK (which activates TSC2), and growth factors.

When growth factors are abundant, and energy levels are high, TSC is inhibited, leading to the activation of Rheb.

Role of Rheb Rheb and the TSC complex form a critical regulatory node that directly modulates mTORC1 activity based on upstream signals, including nutrient availability, growth factors, and cellular energy status.

Rheb, When in Its GTP-Bound Form (Rheb-GTP), Directly Activates mTORC1
The exact mechanism by which Rheb activates mTORC1 is not fully understood but is believed to involve promoting the localization of mTORC1 to the lysosomal membrane where it becomes fully active.

TGF-β Pathway

The TGF-β signaling pathway regulates cell growth, differentiation, apoptosis, and extracellular matrix (ECM) production [16].

- Canonical Pathway: Signals through SMAD proteins
  TGF-β binds to its receptors (TGF-βRI and TGF-βRII), activating receptor-SMADs (R-SMADs: SMAD2/3), which form complexes with SMAD4 and translocate to the nucleus to regulate gene expression

- Non-canonical Pathway: Activates other pathways, such as PI3K/AKT/mTOR, Rho/ROCK, and MAPK, to regulate cytoskeletal dynamics, cell migration, and survival.

Interplay Between TGF-β and mTOR

The TGF-β pathway interacts with the mTOR signaling network at multiple levels, influencing diverse cellular outcomes

1. TGF-β Activation of PI3K/AKT/mTOR
   - Non-canonical TGF-β Signaling
     - TGF-β activates PI3K via TGF-β receptors or intermediates like Src
     - PI3K activation leads to phosphorylation of AKT, which directly activates mTORC1 by inhibiting TSC2, a negative regulator of mTOR
     - This results in increased protein synthesis, cell survival, and ECM production
2. SMAD-Dependent mTOR Regulation
   - SMAD and mTOR Transcriptional Control
     - SMAD proteins, activated by TGF-β, can regulate the transcription of genes encoding components of the mTOR pathway, such as RHEB (activates mTORC1) or autophagy-related genes
     - TGF-β can suppress or enhance mTORC1 activity depending on cellular context (e.g., during fibrosis versus in nutrient deprivation).
3. mTORC1 Feedback Inhibition
   - mTORC1 activity can suppress upstream signals (e.g., via negative feedback on IRS-1) that dampen TGF-β-induced PI3K/AKT activation, creating a complex regulatory loop (Fig. 2.5).

Wnt Pathway (Wingless/Integration1)

The Wnt pathway inhibits the GSK3β-TSC2 interaction, promoting mTOR activity. Wnt signaling thus regulates mTOR in processes such as stem cell proliferation and differentiation. It, mediated by Frizzled receptors, can crosstalk with the PI3K/Akt pathway. Wnt signaling can enhance cancer cell growth via mTOR activation, suggesting therapeutic targets in their intersection [47].

mTORC1 Signal Transduction Pathways

mTOR Complex 1 (mTORC1)

Role and Function [43]

- *Anabolic Processes*: mTORC1 is primarily responsible for promoting anabolic metabolism, including protein synthesis and lipid synthesis. These processes contribute to cell growth and proliferation by generating the necessary building blocks and energy.
- *Inhibition of Catabolic Pathways*: mTORC1 inhibits catabolic processes such as autophagy and lysosome biogenesis. Autophagy is a mechanism where the cell degrades and recycles its components, particularly under starvation or stress conditions. By inhibiting autophagy, mTORC1 ensures that cells do not consume essential components when nutrients are plentiful.
- *Nutrient and Growth Factor Signaling*: mTORC1 integrates signals from catabolic pathways like lysosome biogenesis and autophagy, crucial for balancing synthesis and degradation within the cell. Growth factors activate Receptor Tyrosine Kinases (RTKs), which initiate downstream signaling cascades such as PI3K/AKT and Ras/Erk. These pathways ultimately lead to the inhibition of the Tuberous Sclerosis Complex (TSC), a critical negative regulator of mTORC1.
- *Activation Mechanism*: Growth factors initiate receptor tyrosine kinases (RTKs), which activate the PI3K/AKT and Ras/Erk pathways. These pathways converge to inhibit the TSC complex, a GTPase-activating protein (GAP) for Rheb, which is an essential upstream effector of mTORC1. Inhibition of TSC leads to the activation of Rheb, which in turn activates mTORC1. The TSC complex functions as a GTPase-activating protein (GAP) for Rheb, a small GTPase that is an upstream effector of mTORC1. When TSC is inhibited, Rheb is active (GTP-bound), which directly activates mTORC1.

Regulation by Cellular Stress

- *Activation by AMPK and REDD1*: Cellular stressors such as low-energy levels and hypoxia can activate the TSC complex through AMP-activated protein kinase (AMPK) and REDD1 (regulated in development and DNA damage responses 1). This activation inhibits mTORC1, conserving energy and resources under stress conditions.
- *Direct Inhibition by AMPK*: Besides activating TSC, AMPK directly inhibits mTORC1 by phosphorylating RAPTOR, a component of mTORC1. This serves as a rapid response to low energy levels.

Amino Acids and mTORC1 Localization

- *Rag GTPases and Lysosomal Recruitment*: In the presence of amino acids, Rag GTPases facilitate the recruitment of mTORC1 to the lysosomal surface. This localization is essential for mTORC1 activation, as it allows Rheb to activate mTORC1 in this compartment.

Upstream mTORC1 Signaling Pathways

mTORC1(Mechanistic Target of Rapamycin Complex 1) Its role is essential in cellular stress response. This complex also plays a pivotal role in inhibiting mTOR Complex 2 (mTORC2)

The mTORC1 complex is one of the two main mTOR complexes, with Raptor (Regulatory-associated protein of mTOR) as a crucial component. This complex plays a central role in regulating cell growth and metabolism by integrating various environmental and intracellular signals [37] (Fig. 2.11).

Key Inputs That Regulate mTORC1 Activity

1. *Stress Signals; DNA Damage, Reactive Oxygen Species (ROS), and Hypoxia*

   - *DNA damage* triggers stress response pathways, often leading to the inhibition of mTORC1 to conserve energy for DNA repair.
   - *Reactive oxygen species (ROS)*, when elevated, indicate oxidative stress, prompting the cell to adjust metabolic processes, including the suppression of mTORC1 to promote autophagy and protect against further damage.

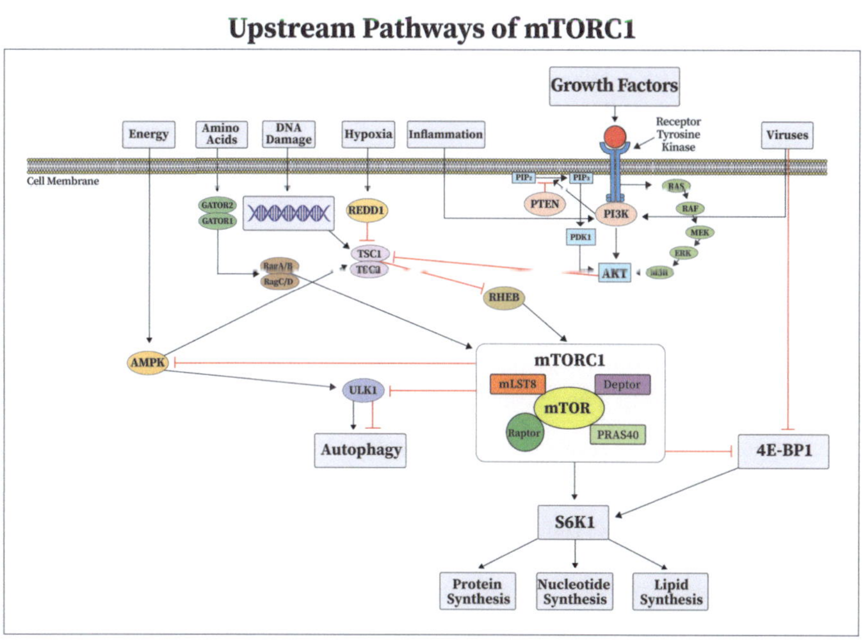

Fig. 2.11 The upstream signaling pathway of mTORC1 is primarily activated by growth factors, nutrients, and cellular stress signals. Key players include the PI3K/AKT pathway, which promotes mTORC1 activation through TSC1/2 inhibition, and the RAS/RAF/MEK pathway, which also influences mTORC1 activity. These signals converge to regulate cell growth, metabolism, and protein synthesis

- *Hypoxia* triggers a cellular stress response, primarily mediated by HIF-1α (Hypoxia-Inducible Factor 1-alpha), which helps cells adapt to low-oxygen levels by altering gene expression.

2. *Nutrient Signals: Amino Acid Abundance, Glucose, and Lipids*

- Amino acids (especially *leucine, arginine, and glutamine*) directly activate mTORC1 by interacting with lysosomal sensors (e.g., Sestrins, CASTOR, and the GATOR complex), signaling the availability of nutrients for protein synthesis and growth.
- Glucose fluctuation activates AMPK and affects glycolysis to influence mTORC1.
- Lipids: mTORC1 senses lipids via multiple mechanisms, which will be discussed later.

3. *Growth Factors*

- Insulin activates the PI3K-Akt pathway, which positively regulates mTORC1 activity, driving processes like protein and lipid synthesis to support cell proliferation.
- IGF-1

4. *Energy Levels from Glucose and Other Sources*

- mTORC1 also senses the cell's energy status via AMP-activated protein kinase (AMPK). When energy is low (e.g., during glucose deprivation), AMPK inhibits mTORC1 to conserve energy, shifting the cell into a catabolic state by promoting autophagy.

Downstream mTORC1 Signaling and Protein Synthesis

mTORC1 regulates protein synthesis through two key targets, which together these mechanisms allow mTORC1 to tightly regulate protein production, aligning cellular growth and metabolism with nutrient availability and energy status [11].

1. Eukaryotic initiation factor 4E-binding protein 1 (4E-BP1)
   Role of 4E-BP1 and Cap-Dependent Translation:

- mTORC1 phosphorylates 4E-BP1, causing it to dissociate from eIF-4E (eukaryotic initiation factor 4E).
- Once released, eIF-4E binds to eIF-4G, forming the eIF-4F complex.
- This complex promotes cap-dependent translation, a critical process for initiating the translation of many mRNAs.

2. p70 ribosomal S6 kinase 1 (S6K1)
   Role of S6K1 in Translation Initiation and Elongation:

- mTORC1 phosphorylates and activates S6K1, which in turn targets several substrates involved in translation.
- Activated S6K1:
  - Enhances mRNA translation initiation and elongation.
  - Promotes ribosome biogenesis, ensuring adequate ribosomal machinery for protein synthesis.

mTORC1 and Autophagy Suppression: The following breakdown is to clarify the molecular mechanisms and their implications for autophagic regulation:

- Inhibition of ULK1 and Atg13

  mTORC1 phosphorylates ULK1 (unc-51-like kinase 1) and Atg13 (autophagy-related protein 13), preventing the initiation of autophagy. These proteins are crucial components of the ULK1 complex, which is required for autophagosome formation.
- Inhibition of TFEB

  mTORC1 inhibits TFEB (Transcription Factor EB) and related family members (e.g., TFE3), which regulate the expression of lysosomal and autophagy-related genes. TFEB activity increases the cell's degradative capacity by enhancing lysosome biogenesis and autophagy.

- CLEAR Motifs and Gene Regulation:
  - Many autophagy and lysosome-related genes contain CLEAR (Coordinated Lysosomal Expression and Regulation) sequences in their promoters.
  - When TFEB is active (due to mTORC1 inhibition), it binds to CLEAR motifs, promoting the expression of autophagy and lysosomal genes, thereby enhancing cellular degradative capacity.
- Energy and Nutrient Regulation: mTORC1 suppression of anabolism (e.g., protein and lipid synthesis) reduces the demand for energy and nutrients, aligning with the catabolic processes driven by autophagy.
- Lysosome-derived nutrients (like leucine and arginine) can reactivate mTORC1 signaling via the Rag GTPase pathway, creating a feedback loop that modulates nutrient availability and mTORC1 activity.
- mTORC2 and Autophagy (distinct from mTORC1) and its downstream AGC kinases (e.g., Akt and SGK1) also limit autophagy:
  - Transcription-dependent: mTORC2 can influence transcription factors that regulate autophagy-related gene expression.
  - Transcription-independent: mTORC2 may also inhibit autophagy via phosphorylation of proteins involved directly in autophagic processes.
  - FoxO Transcription Factors: mTORC2 indirectly suppresses autophagy by maintaining FoxO transcription factors in the cytoplasm preventing their nuclear activity [54].

– FoxO targets include proteins essential for various steps of autophagy and lysosomal function. When FoxO activity is restricted, autophagic flux and catabolism are reduced.

Forkhead box O (FoxO) proteins represent a highly versatile family of transcription factors that orchestrate cellular responses to a wide range of stimuli, thereby playing crucial roles in maintaining cellular homeostasis and organismal longevity [45].

FOXO and p53 are critical transcription factors that cooperate in cellular stress responses, regulating apoptosis, senescence, and metabolism. They co-regulate genes like sestrins to activate AMPK and inhibit mTORC1 during stress. Both enhance pro-apoptotic pathways (e.g., PUMA, BIM) and contribute to senescence by inducing cell cycle inhibitors (p21 and p27). While FOXO primarily manages oxidative stress and metabolism, p53 focuses on DNA damage repair and tumor suppression. Their interplay balances cell survival and death, influencing cancer, aging, and metabolic diseases.

Structural and Functional Characteristics

- *Forkhead Domain*: The defining feature of FoxO proteins, the Forkhead domain, facilitates DNA binding to specific response elements, allowing these transcription factors to regulate a diverse set of target genes.
- *Post-Translational Modifications (PTMs)*: FoxO proteins are heavily regulated by PTMs, including phosphorylation, acetylation, and ubiquitination. These modifications influence their localization (nuclear or cytoplasmic), stability, and activity.

Cellular Processes Regulated by FoxO Proteins

FoxO proteins influence several critical pathways:

1. *Cell Proliferation and Cell Cycle*: By inducing cell cycle inhibitors like p27(Kip1) and p21(Cip1), FoxO proteins contribute to cell cycle arrest under stress conditions.
2. *Metabolism*: FoxO transcription factors regulate glucose and lipid metabolism, playing a significant role in energy homeostasis, particularly during fasting.
3. *Apoptosis*: FoxO proteins promote apoptosis through upregulation of pro-apoptotic genes such as BIM and FasL, in response to severe cellular stress.
4. *Autophagy*: They enhance autophagy by inducing expression of autophagy-related genes, particularly during nutrient deprivation.
5. *Oxidative Stress Resistance*: FoxO proteins, including FOXO3a, regulate genes like catalase and superoxide dismutase (SOD), enhancing cellular defenses against reactive oxygen species (ROS).
6. *Stem Cell Maintenance*: By mitigating oxidative damage, FoxO proteins preserve the quiescence and self-renewal capacity of stem cells, which is essential for tissue regeneration (Fig. 2.12).

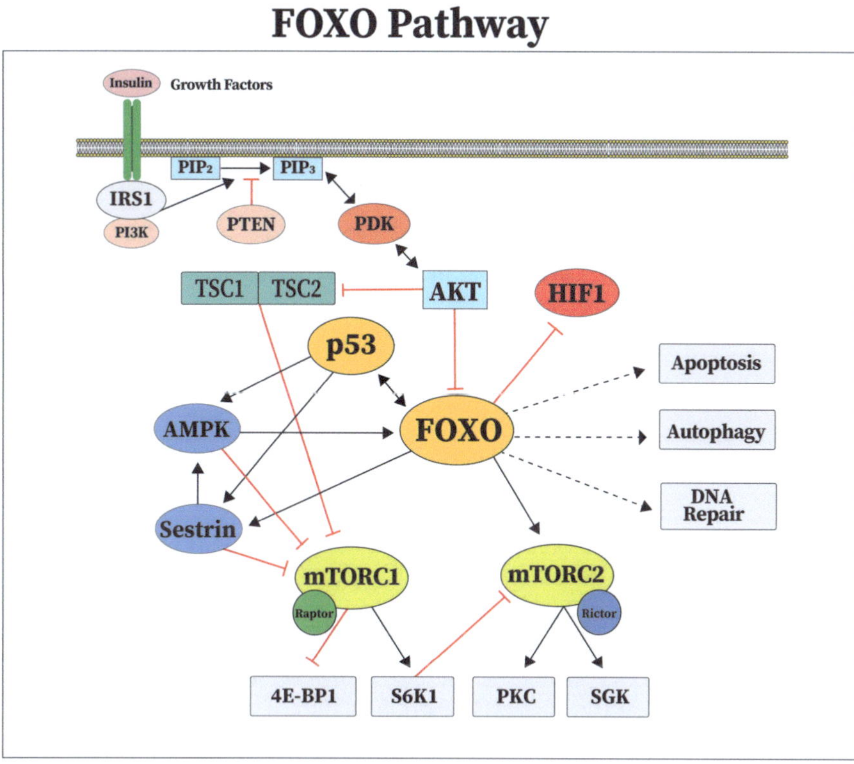

Fig. 2.12 The image represents a highly versatile family of transcription factors that orchestrate cellular responses to a wide range of stimuli. FOXO and p53 are critical transcription factors that work together to regulate key cellular processes, including apoptosis, autophagy, DNA repair, senescence, and metabolism

The FOXO (Forkhead box O) family consists of four members in humans:

1. FOXO1 (also known as FKHR)
2. FOXO3 (also known as FKHRL1)
3. FOXO4 (also known as AFX)
4. FOXO6

These transcription factors are characterized by a conserved Forkhead DNA-binding domain and play critical roles in various cellular processes, including metabolism, apoptosis, cell cycle regulation, and oxidative stress response.

FoxO transcription factors have been implicated in oncogenic processes through fusion events in various cancers. Specifically:

- FoxO1: Found in pediatric alveolar rhabdomyosarcomas as chimeric fusion proteins involving the DNA-binding domains of PAX3 or PAX7. These fusions disrupt normal transcriptional regulation, contributing to tumorigenesis.

- FoxO3 and FoxO4: Identified as fusion partners of the mixed-lineage leukemia (MLL) gene in acute myeloid leukemias (AML). These fusions likely alter the transcriptional activity of MLL, promoting leukemic transformation.

Interaction Between FOXO3a and mTOR

The interaction between FOXO3a and mTOR reflects a balance between growth/survival and stress resistance/autophagy.

FOXO3a Inhibition of mTORC1

mTOR, through *AKT phosphorylation*, inhibits FOXO3a by promoting its nuclear exclusion.

- *AKT-mediated phosphorylation* of FOXO3a (e.g., at Ser253) prevents its transcriptional activity by retaining it in the cytoplasm. This leads to a suppression of FOXO3a-mediated transcription of genes involved in autophagy and apoptosis.
- *REDD1* (Regulated in Development and DNA Damage Response 1) Negatively regulates mTORC1 by stabilizing the TSC1-TSC2 complex.
- *Sestrins*: Activate AMPK, Activated AMPK inhibits mTORC1 by phosphorylating TSC2 (tuberous sclerosis complex 2) or directly phosphorylating Raptor, a component of mTORC1. This reduces anabolic processes like protein and lipid synthesis, aligning with stress responses.

FOXO3a Activation of mTORC2

- FoxO can elevate Rictor, a defining component of mTORC2.
- Increased Rictor enhances the assembly and activity of mTORC2.
- mTORC2 then phosphorylates and activates AKT (at Ser473), a kinase involved in promoting cell survival, growth, and metabolism.

Summary Diagram of the Pathway

1. *Growth Signal* → PI3K → AKT → mTOR ↑, FOXO3a ↓ (Cytoplasmic)
2. *Stress Signal* → AMPK ↑, REDD1 ↑ → mTOR ↓, FOXO3a ↑ (Nuclear)

The position of *FOXO3* in cellular signaling processes depends on the specific pathway or context being considered. However, in general, FOXO3 functions primarily as a downstream effector in signaling cascades, particularly those related to stress responses, autophagy, apoptosis, and metabolism.

FOXO3 Pathway Overview [17]

1. *Upstream Signals*
   - FOXO3 activity is influenced by upstream regulators, primarily kinases like:
     - *AKT/PKB*: Phosphorylates FOXO3, causing its nuclear exclusion and inactivation.
     - *AMPK*: Activates FOXO3 by counteracting AKT and promoting nuclear localization under low energy/nutrient conditions.
     - *mTORC1/2*: Indirectly modulates FOXO3 via AKT and other intermediates.
     - *JNK*: Activates FOXO3 in response to oxidative stress by enhancing nuclear translocation.
2. *Signal Transduction*
   - FOXO3 acts as a transcription factor, meaning it lies downstream of transduction pathways but functions as a signal integrator to modulate gene expression. Its role is pivotal in converting upstream signals into specific cellular outcomes.
   - Example: Growth factors signal through the PI3K/AKT/mTOR pathway, which regulates FOXO3 phosphorylation, localization, and activity.
3. *Downstream Foxo3*
   - FOXO3 is downstream in signaling pathways, acting as a critical effector and regulator.
   - It serves as a transducer of upstream signals into gene expression changes, effectively bridging transduction and execution phases.
   - The relationship between FOXO3a (Forkhead box O3a) and mTOR is a crucial axis in regulating cellular processes such as metabolism, autophagy, stress resistance, and survival.

Downstream and Regulatory Impact of mTORC1

Once activated, mTORC1 promotes several anabolic processes and inhibits catabolic ones, including:

- *Inhibition of Autophagy*: mTORC1 blocks autophagy by phosphorylating components like ULK1, preventing the recycling of cellular components during times of nutrient abundance .
- *Protein and Lipid Synthesis*: It enhances biosynthetic processes to support cell growth and division.
- *Ribosome Biogenesis*: mTORC1 stimulates the production of ribosomes, increasing the cell's protein synthesis capacity.

***Hypoxia* (Low-Oxygen Levels) and Its Effect on mTORC1**

- Hypoxia triggers a cellular stress response, primarily mediated by HIF-1α (Hypoxia-Inducible Factor 1-alpha), which helps cells adapt to low-oxygen levels by altering gene expression.
- Inhibition of mTORC1 during hypoxia occurs to conserve energy and resources. The inhibition mainly involves:

    1. REDD1 (Regulated in Development and DNA Damage Response 1): A hypoxia-inducible protein that suppresses mTORC1 by activating TSC2 (Tuberous Sclerosis Complex 2), a negative regulator of mTORC1.
    2. AMPK Activation: Hypoxia can reduce ATP production, leading to the activation of AMPK, which further inhibits mTORC1 to prevent energy-consuming processes.

- Autophagy Induction: mTORC1 suppression under hypoxia promotes autophagy, helping cells recycle components to maintain survival.

The TSC Complex and Regulation of mTORC1

TSC complex functions as a metabolic gatekeeper for mTORC1, linking upstream signals to the control of cellular growth and metabolism. Disruptions in TSC function, such as in tuberous sclerosis complex disease, lead to uncontrolled mTORC1 activation, resulting in abnormal cell growth and proliferation [18].

- The TSC complex is a heterotrimeric complex consisting of:

    – TSC1 (Hamartin)
    – TSC2 (Tuberin)
    – TBC1D7

- TSC2 acts as a GTPase-activating protein (GAP), inhibiting Ras homolog enriched in brain (Rheb) by hydrolyzing its bound GTP.
- Rheb, a small GTPase, plays a key role by binding to mTORC1 on the lysosomal surface and activating it. Thus, TSC acts as a negative regulator of mTORC1 signaling by maintaining Rheb in its inactive GDP-bound form.
- Although TSC2 contains the functional GAP domain, TSC1 is required for its stabilization. The cooperation of both TSC1 and TSC2 is essential for the proper functioning of the complex (Fig. 2.13).

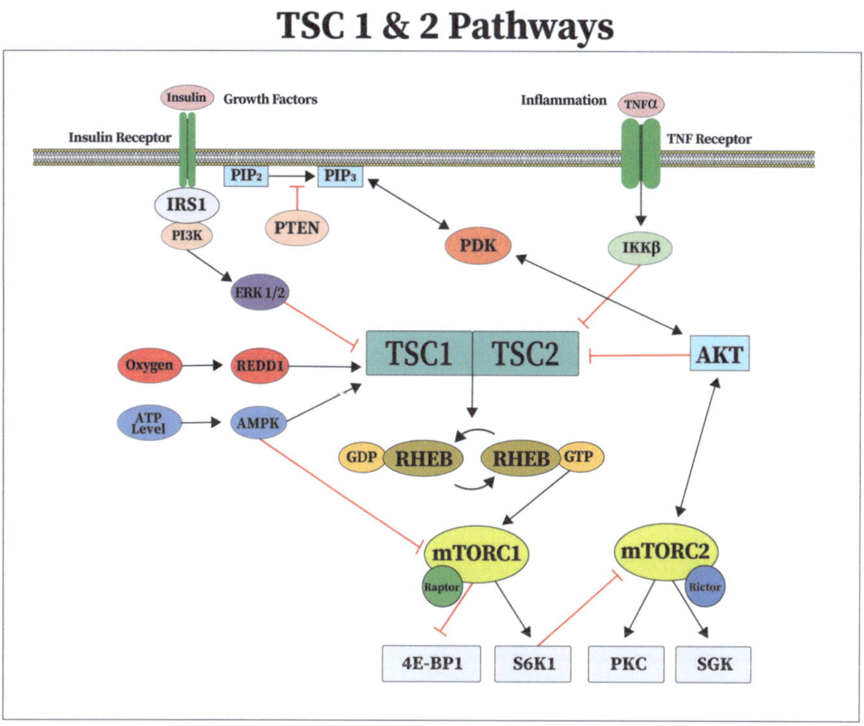

Fig. 2.13 This pathway involves multiple interactions with other signaling pathways and acts as a metabolic gatekeeper for mTORC1, linking upstream signals to regulate cell growth and metabolism. It functions as a GTPase-activating protein (GAP) and has a direct effect on RHEB. RHEB plays a key role in binding to mTORC1 on the lysosomal surface, facilitating its activation

mTORC1 and Autophagy Inhibition

Phosphorylation-Dependent Inhibition

- ULK1 and Atg13: mTORC1 directly inhibits the initiation of autophagy by phosphorylating Unc-51 Like Autophagy Activating Kinase 1 (ULK1) and autophagy-related 13 (Atg13). ULK1 is part of a protein complex including Atg13 that is essential for the nucleation of autophagosomes, the vesicles that engulf cellular components to be degraded.
  - When nutrients are plentiful, mTORC1 is active and phosphorylates ULK1 and Atg13, preventing their participation in autophagy initiation.
  - Under nutrient deprivation, mTORC1 activity decreases, leading to the dephosphorylation and activation of the ULK1-Atg13 complex, thereby promoting autophagy.

Inhibition of TFEB

- TFEB and Lysosomal Biogenesis: mTORC1 also inhibits the transcription factor EB (TFEB) and related family members, which are master regulators of lysosomal biogenesis and function.
  - TFEB controls the expression of a variety of genes involved in lysosome formation and function through the Coordinated Lysosomal Expression and Regulation (CLEAR) network. These genes contain a CLEAR motif in their promoters and are activated by TFEB to increase the cell's degradative capacity.
  - Active mTORC1 phosphorylates TFEB, leading to its cytoplasmic sequestration and inhibition. This reduces the expression of lysosomal and autophagy-related genes, diminishing the cell's capacity to degrade and recycle materials.

Autophagic Degradation and mTORC1 Reactivation

Nutrient Sensing and mTORC1 Activation

- Lysosome-Derived Nutrients: The degradation of cellular components via autophagy releases nutrients, such as amino acids (notably leucine and arginine), back into the cytosol. These nutrients can reactivate mTORC1, forming a regulatory feedback loop [31].
  - Amino acids and other metabolites like glucose-derived DHAP (dihydroxyacetone phosphate), cholesterol, and S-adenosylmethionine (SAM), can activate Rag GTPases.
  - Activated Rag GTPases then recruit mTORC1 to the lysosomal surface where it can be reactivated by Rheb, in the presence of amino acids, thus linking nutrient availability directly to mTORC1 activity.

mTORC1 and Lipid Signaling

mTORC1 plays a pivotal role in regulating *lipid metabolism* by promoting the synthesis and storage of lipids in response to nutrient availability and energy demands. This regulation ensures that cells have sufficient membrane components and energy reserves for growth and survival [39].

Key Roles of mTORC1 in Lipid Signaling

1. Lipogenesis (Lipid Synthesis):
   - mTORC1 activates sterol regulatory element-binding proteins (SREBPs), which are transcription factors that promote the expression of enzymes involved in:
     - Fatty acid synthesis (e.g., acetyl-CoA carboxylase, fatty acid synthase)
     - Cholesterol synthesis
   - This ensures an adequate supply of lipids for cell membranes and energy storage.

2. Adipogenesis (Fat Cell Formation):

    - mTORC1 promotes the differentiation of pre-adipocytes into mature adipocytes, facilitating fat storage in tissues.

3. Lipid Storage and Energy Balance:

    - mTORC1 regulates lipid droplet formation and lipid storage, which is crucial for maintaining energy balance during periods of nutrient fluctuation.

4. Regulation of Lipid Catabolism:

    - mTORC1 inhibits autophagy and lipid breakdown processes, such as lipophagy (the degradation of lipid droplets via autophagy), to prevent excessive lipid degradation during nutrient-rich conditions.

    Through these mechanisms, mTORC1 integrates nutrient sensing with lipid metabolism, ensuring cells efficiently manage lipid synthesis and storage to support growth and energy needs. Disruptions in mTORC1-mediated lipid signaling can contribute to metabolic disorders such as obesity, fatty liver disease, and diabetes.

    How mTOR Senses Lipids

mTORC1 directly integrates signals from cellular lipid levels to adjust metabolism, balancing lipid synthesis, storage, and degradation. Here's how mTORC1 senses lipids:

1. *Role of Lysosomal Positioning and Rheb Activation*

    - mTORC1 is localized on the lysosomal surface, where it interacts with Ras homolog enriched in brain (Rheb) for activation.
    - Lipids, such as cholesterol and phosphatidic acid (PA), influence the lysosomal membrane composition and mTORC1's activity.
    - Cholesterol accumulation on lysosomal membranes promotes mTORC1 activation by stabilizing the interaction between Rag GTPases and mTORC1.
    - Phosphatidic acid (PA), a lipid intermediate, also binds directly to mTOR, enhancing its kinase activity.

2. *SREBP Pathway and Lipid Availability*

    - mTORC1 regulates the sterol regulatory element-binding proteins (SREBPs), which control lipid synthesis. When intracellular cholesterol or fatty acid levels are low, mTORC1 fine-tunes lipid metabolism accordingly:
    - In response to lipid abundance, mTORC1 promotes SREBP activation, enhancing fatty acid, phospholipid, and cholesterol synthesis.

3. *Amino Acids and Lipid Sensors*

    - mTORC1 interacts with Rag GTPases and V-ATPase on lysosomes, which help sense amino acids, but some of these components are also modulated by lipid signals. For instance fatty acid metabolites influence the lysosomal machinery that activates mTORC1, bridging nutrient sensing with lipid metabolism.

4. *Lipid Metabolites Affecting mTORC1*

   - Ceramides (sphingolipid metabolites) and *fatty acids* have been shown to modulate mTORC1 either positively or negatively, depending on the context, such as nutrient stress or insulin signaling, for example, excess palmitate (a saturated fatty acid) can impair mTORC1 signaling, leading to insulin resistance, whereas unsaturated fatty acids may support mTORC1 activity.

Regulation by Oxygen Availability (Hypoxia) [22]

- *HIF-1 and REDD1*: Under hypoxic conditions, the transcription factor HIF-1 (hypoxia-inducible factor 1) upregulates REDD1 (regulated in development and DNA damage response 1).
- *REDD1 Activates TSC1/2*: REDD1 promotes the activation of the TSC1/2 complex, which in turn inhibits mTORC1.
- *Additional Inhibition via Akt and PP2A*: REDD1 can also bind to Akt and PP2A (protein phosphatase 2A), leading to the inhibition of Akt and consequently reducing mTORC1 activity.

Regulation by Energy Stress and AMPK

- *AMPK Activation*: Under conditions of energy stress, AMPK (AMP-activated protein kinase) is activated.
- *Phosphorylation of Raptor*: AMPK phosphorylates raptor (a component of mTORC1) on S792, which directly inhibits mTORC1 activity.
- *Phosphorylation of TSC2*: Additionally, AMPK phosphorylates TSC2, enhancing the inhibitory function of the TSC1/2 complex on Rheb, thereby suppressing mTORC1 activity.

Regulation by Bnip3

- *Bnip3 and HIF-1*: Bnip3 (BCl2/adenovirus E1B 19 kDa protein-interacting protein) can be regulated by HIF-1 and serves as another mechanism to inhibit mTORC1.
- *Direct inhibition of Rheb*: Bnip3 directly inhibits Rheb, providing yet another layer of control over mTORC1 activity.

These pathways and their interactions highlight the complexity and tight regulation of mTORC1, ensuring that its activity is appropriately modulated in response to various cellular conditions, including growth signals, oxygen availability, and energy status.

mTORC1 and HIPPO Signaling

Hippo signaling pathway is interconnected regulatory networks with mTORC1, which influence cellular growth, proliferation, metabolism, and survival. Their interplay is critical in maintaining tissue homeostasis and responding to environmental cues. The Hippo signaling pathway, a highly conserved regulatory network that controls organ size, tissue growth, postnatal organ development, and regeneration by regulating cell proliferation, apoptosis, and stem cell behavior. Although the pathway itself is named "Hippo," there isn't a single receptor explicitly called the "Hippo receptor." Instead, the pathway integrates signals from various receptors and cell-surface proteins [10].

The term *HIPPO* does not stand for an acronym in the context of the Hippo signaling pathway. Instead, it is derived from a gene initially identified in Drosophila melanogaster (fruit flies), where mutations in the *hippo* gene led to excessive tissue growth resembling the size of a hippopotamus. The pathway was named "Hippo" due to this characteristic phenotype.

Key Receptors and Upstream Components

The Hippo pathway is regulated by extracellular signals such as cell-cell contact, mechanical stress, and soluble growth factors, which are sensed through the following key upstream elements:

1. *Cell-Surface Proteins and Adherens Junctions*:
   - *Fat Cadherins (e.g., Fat4)*: Atypical cadherins that act as important upstream regulators of the Hippo pathway.
   - *Dachsous (Ds)*: Another cadherin that interacts with fat proteins to regulate signaling.
2. *G-Protein Coupled Receptors (GPCRs)*: GPCRs play a role in modulating Hippo signaling through their effects on cytoskeletal dynamics and mechanical tension.
3. *Integrins and Focal Adhesion Components*: These transmembrane proteins sense extracellular matrix signals and can modulate Hippo signaling by influencing the mechanical environment of cells.
4. *Growth Factor Receptors*:
   - Growth factor receptors like EGFR, VEGFR, and others indirectly influence Hippo signaling through pathways like PI3K/Akt and MAPK that can cross-talk with Hippo components.

The Core Hippo Pathway

The pathway itself involves a kinase cascade:

1. *MST1/2 (Mammalian Ste20-like kinases)*: Activated by upstream signals and phosphorylates:
2. *LATS1/2 (Large Tumor Suppressor kinases)*: These in turn phosphorylate and inhibit:
3. *YAP/TAZ (Yes-associated protein and WWTR1 transcription co-activator)*: When YAP/TAZ are phosphorylated, they are retained in the cytoplasm and

degraded. When unphosphorylated, they translocate to the nucleus to interact with TEAD1-4 transcription factor to promote transcription of genes involved in growth and proliferation.

Dysregulation of both mTORC1 and HIPPO pathways is commonly implicated in cancer, where hyperactivation of YAP/TAZ or mTOR leads to uncontrolled cell growth and survival [58] (Fig. 2.14).

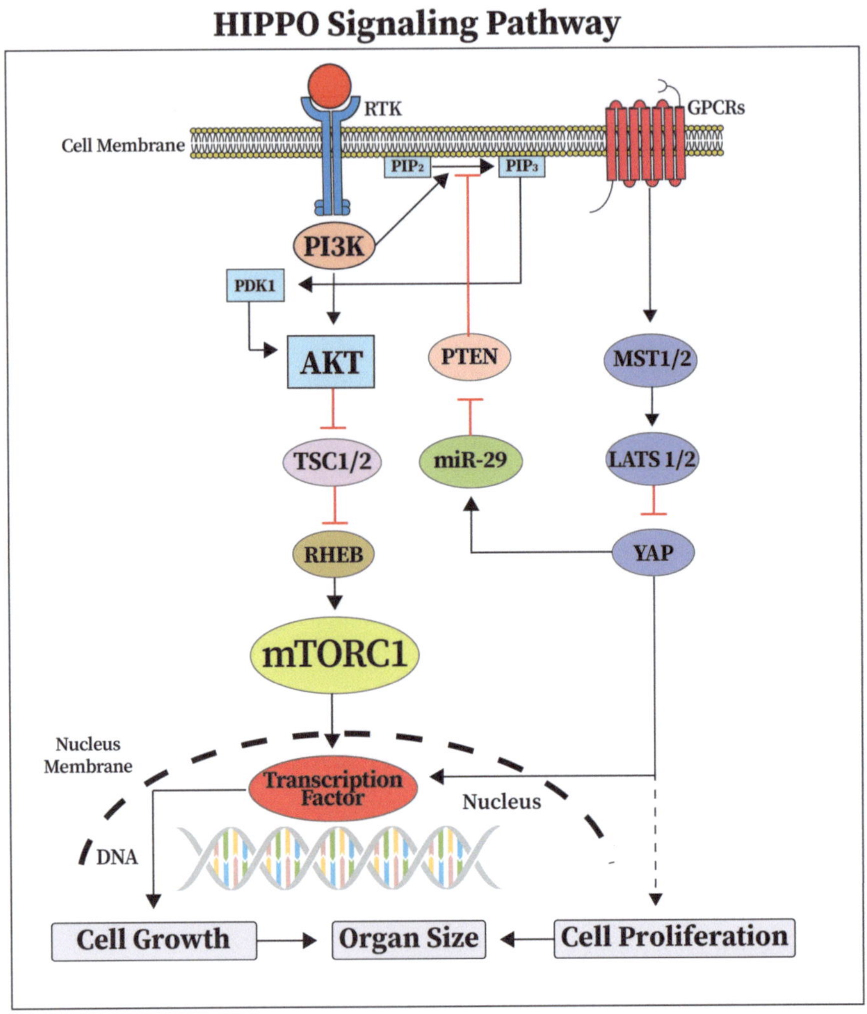

Fig. 2.14 The HIPPO pathway regulates organ size by integrating extracellular signals like cell-cell contact, mechanical stress, and growth factors. It involves receptor tyrosine kinases (RTKs) and GPCRs, which interact with pathways like mTORC1. Core kinases MST1/2 and LATS1/2 phosphorylate YAP, preventing their nuclear activity and controlling cell proliferation and apoptosis

Other Modulators of mTORC1

There are other factors that influence mTORC1 and as the result modulate the cellular function. mTORC1 is significantly modulated by both *calorie restriction (CR)* and *exercise*, two interventions known to promote metabolic health and longevity. These interventions influence mTORC1 activity primarily through changes in nutrient availability, energy balance, and cellular stress signals.

1. *Calorie Restriction (CR)* and mTORC1: Refers to a sustained reduction in caloric intake without malnutrition. It reduces mTORC1 activity through several mechanisms:

   (a) *Reduced Amino Acids and Nutrients*

   - mTORC1 is directly activated by amino acids, particularly *leucine* and other branched-chain amino acids (BCAAs), which promote mTORC1 localization to lysosomes for activation.
   - CR decreases circulating amino acids and glucose levels, leading to reduced mTORC1 activation.

   (b) *AMPK Activation*

   - CR reduces ATP levels and increases AMP:ATP ratio, activating *AMPK*.
   - AMPK phosphorylates and activates *TSC2*, which inhibits *Rheb*, a GTPase required for mTORC1 activation. This suppression reduces mTORC1 signaling.
   - AMPK also phosphorylates *Raptor*, an essential mTORC1 component, further inhibiting mTORC1.

   (c) *SIRT1 and NAD+ Levels*

   - CR increases *NAD+* levels and activates *SIRT1*, a deacetylase that can regulate downstream effectors of mTORC1, contributing to its suppression.

   (d) *Enhanced Autophagy*

   - Decreased mTORC1 activity during CR facilitates *autophagy*, a critical cellular process for clearing damaged organelles and maintaining cellular homeostasis (Fig. 2.15).

2. *Exercise* and mTORC1: Modulates mTORC1 in a context-dependent manner, balancing its roles in muscle adaptation and metabolic stress responses

   (a) *Exercise-Induced AMPK Activation*

   - Prolonged or intense exercise reduces ATP levels, activating AMPK. Similar to CR, AMPK inhibits mTORC1 via TSC2 and Raptor phosphorylation, promoting autophagy and energy homeostasis.

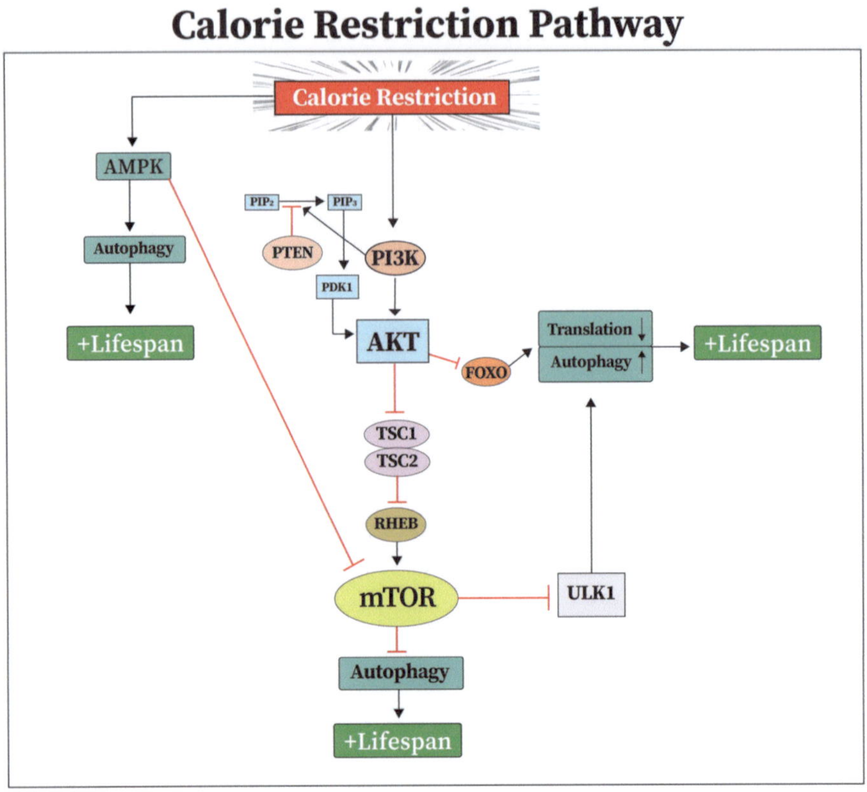

Fig. 2.15 Calorie restriction inhibits mTOR activity by reducing nutrient and growth factor availability, leading to decreased protein synthesis and cell growth. This activation of AMPK, a cellular energy sensor, further suppresses mTORC1, which enhances autophagy. Together, these effects support cellular maintenance, stress resistance, and longevity

- AMPK activation during exercise also enhances glucose uptake and fatty acid oxidation, creating an environment unfavorable for mTORC1 activity.

(b) *Mechanical Stimuli and Muscle Growth*

- Resistance exercise temporarily activates mTORC1 in *skeletal muscle* to stimulate *protein synthesis* and muscle hypertrophy via downstream effectors like *S6K1* and *4E-BP1.*
- However, this activation is tightly regulated, and endurance exercise or energy stress conditions can suppress mTORC1 via AMPK or REDD1 (regulated in development and DNA damage responses 1).

(c) *Nutrient and Hormonal Factors*

- Exercise depletes glycogen and reduces circulating insulin levels, both of which suppress mTORC1.

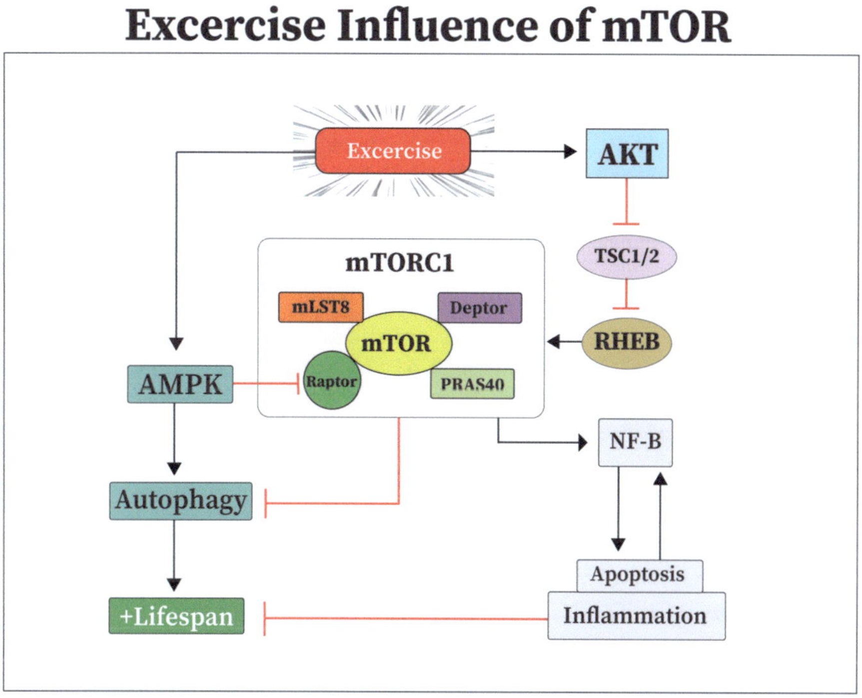

Fig. 2.16 AMPK, in response to energy depletion during exercise, inhibits mTORC1 to promote autophagy and energy conservation. Conversely, AKT can activate mTORC1, particularly in muscle cells, to stimulate protein synthesis and muscle growth

- Exercise-induced increases in *adiponectin* and *myokines* (e.g., irisin) further inhibit mTORC1 indirectly (Fig. 2.16).

Integrated Effects of CR and Exercise on mTORC1: When combined, calorie restriction and exercise synergistically modulate mTORC1 activity:

- *Acute Inhibition*: Both reduce mTORC1 signaling during periods of nutrient deprivation or energy stress, promoting autophagy, mitochondrial biogenesis, and stress resistance.
- *Adaptive Responses*: During recovery, moderate mTORC1 reactivation can support protein synthesis and repair processes, especially in muscle tissue after resistance exercise.

mTORC2 (Mechanistic Target of Rapamycin Complex 2)

mTORC2 is a critical protein complex involved in regulating cell survival, cytoskeletal organization, and lipid metabolism. Unlike mTORC1, mTORC2 is generally insensitive to rapamycin and includes distinct subunits such as RICTOR and mSIN1 alongside mTOR and mLST8. It plays a vital role in activating AKT by phosphorylating it at Ser473, a step essential for full activation of AKT. mTORC2's activity influences cellular processes like proliferation and migration, and it is increasingly recognized for its role in diseases like cancer and metabolic disorders [40].

mTORC1 and mTORC2 are integral components of cellular signaling pathways that adjust cellular growth, survival, and metabolism based on environmental inputs. mTORC1 is primarily activated by nutrients and growth factors to promote anabolism and inhibit autophagy, while mTORC2 responds to growth factors to regulate survival and organization. The activity of these complexes is modulated by various feedback and regulatory mechanisms, ensuring that cell growth and function are finely tuned in response to changing environmental and cellular conditions. Understanding these pathways is crucial for developing therapeutic strategies in diseases where mTOR signaling is dysregulated, such as cancer, metabolic disorders, and age-related diseases.

The regulatory dynamics of the mTORC2 pathway, particularly in the context of insulin/PI3K signaling and its interplay with mTORC1.

Mechanisms of mTORC2 Activation

mTORC2 is part of the larger mTOR signaling pathway and specifically responsible for the phosphorylation of AKT at S473.

mTORC2 is exclusively Regulated by Growth Factors and Unlike mTORC1, mTORC2 is activated exclusively by growth factor signaling mediated through RTK/PI3K but is less responsive to nutrients.

mTORC2 is crucial for regulating cell survival, metabolism, and cytoskeletal organization. It activates AGC family kinases, including AKT, SGK, and PKC, which are vital for these processes (Fig. 2.17).

mTORC2 Receptors

Insulin Receptor Substrate (IRS): IRS proteins are adaptor molecules that can link RTKs, especially the insulin receptor, to the PI3K-AKT signaling pathway. Upon phosphorylation by RTKs, IRS proteins provide docking sites for the SH2 domains of the p85 subunit of PI3K, facilitating PI3K activation.

mTORC2 and Cellular Localization

mTORC2 phosphorylation by Akt occurs on the endoplasmic reticulum (ER). This localization influences mTORC2 activity or downstream signaling and changes in response to different stimuli.

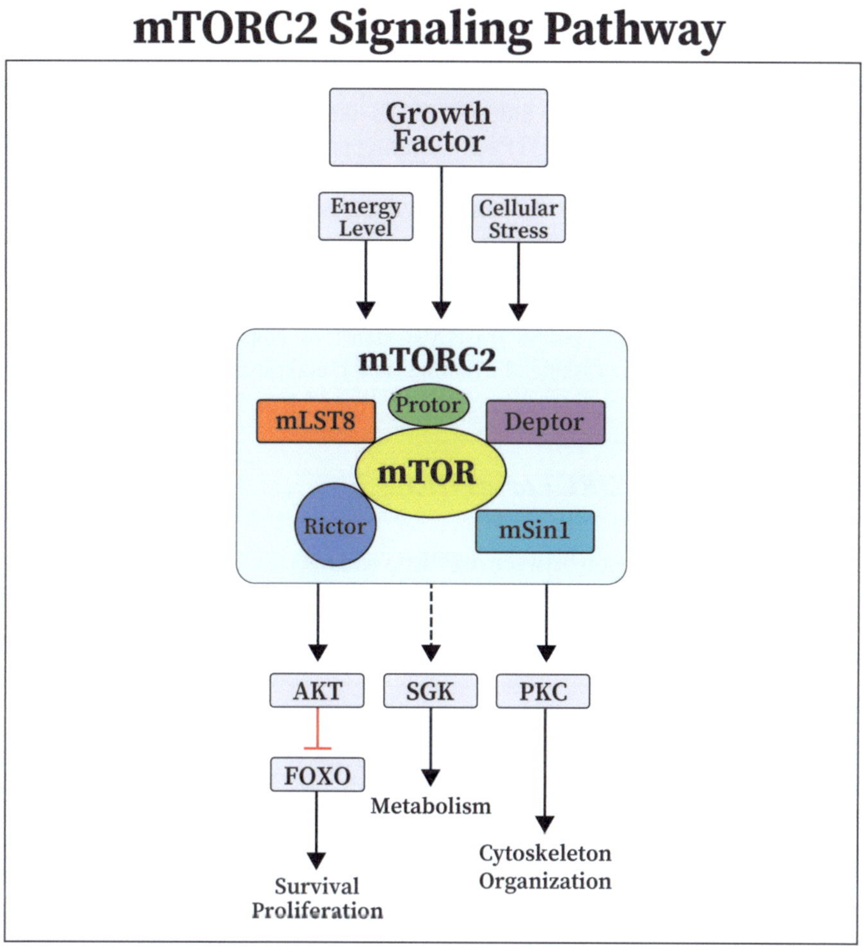

Fig. 2.17 mTORC2 signaling involves growth factors as the primary upstream regulators, activating the pathway through receptor tyrosine kinases. Downstream, mTORC2 phosphorylates and activates AKT, which drives various cellular functions, including cell survival, metabolism, and cytoskeletal organization

Rictor and GAP-Like Activity

- mTORC2 includes Rictor (rapamycin-insensitive companion of mTOR), which has been implicated in interacting with small GTPases, particularly those of the Rho family (e.g., Rac1, Cdc42, and RhoA).
- While Rictor does not act as a traditional GAP (GTPase-activating protein), it modulates the activity of small GTPases by influencing their activation state. This can resemble GAP-like behavior in certain contexts, such as cytoskeletal organization and cell migration.

TSC1/TSC2 in mTORC2 Regulation

mTORC2 indirectly regulates GTPase signaling by phosphorylating downstream targets, such as AKT which can influence GAPs like TSC2 (tuberous sclerosis complex 2). TSC2 acts as a GAP (GTPase-activating protein) for Rheb, a critical small GTPase in mTORC1 activation.

TSC1/TSC2 complex may promote mTORC2 activity independent of its GAP function. While mTORC2 itself does not have intrinsic GAP enzymatic activity, its components, particularly Rictor, are involved in modulating small GTPase signaling. This modulation may mimic GAP-like effects by altering the balance of GTP-bound (active) and GDP-bound (inactive) states of small GTPases, impacting cellular processes like cytoskeletal dynamics and metabolism.

Feedback from mTORC1 to mTORC2

The negative feedback loop between mTORC1 and mTORC2 is crucial as mTORC1 inhibits insulin/PI3K signaling (e.g., through IRS-1 degradation), which maintains cellular homeostasis

Regulation by mTORC2 and AGC Kinases

mTORC2 and its downstream AGC family kinases, particularly Akt (Protein Kinase B) and SGK1 (serum- and glucocorticoid-induced kinase 1), also play roles in modulating autophagy, both through transcription-dependent and -independent processes. mTORC2 activates Akt and SGK1, which can phosphorylate and inhibit components of the autophagy machinery, as well as transcription factors that promote autophagy and lysosomal biogenesis [5].

FoxO Transcription Factors

The cytoplasmic retention of Forkhead box O (FoxO) transcription factors by Akt and SGK1 also limits autophagic degradation. FoxO factors are crucial for the transcription of genes involved in various stages of autophagy and lysosomal function. When Akt and SGK1 are activated by mTORC2, they phosphorylate FoxO factors, leading to their retention in the cytoplasm and preventing them from activating autophagy-related genes.

The mTORC2 Signaling Network: Targets and Cross-Talks

1. *mTORC2 and AKT Activation*
   - *Full Activation of AKT*: mTORC2 phosphorylates AKT at Ser473, a step crucial for its full activation. This positions AKT both upstream (via mTORC1 regulation) and downstream of mTOR complexes.
   - *Phosphorylation of PKC Isoforms*: Includes PKCθ, which is critical for the activation of NF-κB in T cells, linking mTORC2 to the regulation of gene expression and T cell activation.
   - *Activation of SGK1*: Further influences T cell function by regulating ion transport and growth.

Feedback and Inter-Complex Regulation [40]

- *Feedback Inhibition*: mTORC1 activation leads to feedback inhibition mechanisms that impact both RTK/PI3K/AKT signaling and mTORC2:
  - *Inhibition of IRS*: mTORC1 activation results in the phosphorylation and subsequent inhibition of Insulin Receptor Substrate (IRS), dampening PI3K/AKT signaling.
  - *Activation of GRB10*: GRB10 is another protein that is activated by mTORC1 and acts to inhibit insulin and other growth factor signaling pathways, further reducing PI3K/AKT activity.

S6K-Mediated Inhibition S6 Kinase (S6K), a downstream effector of mTORC1, not only inhibits IRS but also negatively regulates mTORC2 through inhibitory phosphorylation, creating a complex interplay between the mTOR complexes and other signaling pathways [51].

Summary of mTORC2 Role in Cell

- *Upstream Signals*: Mainly Growth factors (PI3K), nutrients, and stress may also affect mTORC2.
- *Downstream Effects*: Activation of AKT, PKC, SGK1, and cytoskeletal remodeling, leading to enhanced cell survival, metabolism, and migration.
- *mTORC2 and T-Cell Fate*: The Sin1/mTORC2 complex plays a crucial role in $CD8^+$ T cell fate by influencing their differentiation into effector, memory, or exhausted states. mTORC2, through metabolic and survival pathway regulation,

enhances memory T cell generation while mTOR signaling overall is vital for T cell memory development, including tissue-resident memory cells. Additionally, mTOR activity contributes to T cell exhaustion during chronic infections or cancer, affecting the balance between progenitor and terminally exhausted T cells [36].

PI3K/AKT Pathways in Viral Infections

The *PI3K/AKT pathway* is often hijacked by viruses to promote their replication and survival. It facilitates viral entry, replication, and immune evasion by enhancing cell survival, suppressing apoptosis, and modulating host immune responses. We only use following examples as the list can be very large [50].

1. *Herpes Simplex Virus 1 (HSV-1)*
2. *Human Immunosuppression Virus (HIV)*
3. *Influenza Virus*
4. *human papillomavirus (HPV)*
5. *SARS-CoV-2 (Covid 19)* (Fig. 2.11)

Herpes Simplex Virus 1 (HSV-1) It is indeed a complex virus, and its ability to manipulate host cell signaling pathways is key to its successful infection and replication. HSV-1 encodes its own serine/threonine kinase, known as Us3, which plays a critical role in counteracting apoptosis by mimicking the activity of the host cell's Akt pathway. This allows the virus to prevent premature cell death, ensuring that it can replicate efficiently before the immune response clears the infection [29].

Early in HSV-1 infection, apoptosis is blocked in an Akt-dependent manner. Akt is a serine/threonine kinase that promotes cell survival and growth by inhibiting apoptotic pathways. By activating Akt signaling, HSV-1 ensures that the host cell does not undergo apoptosis too early, which would prevent the virus from completing its replication cycle.

As the infection progresses, HSV-1 accumulates sufficient levels of its Us3 protein kinase. Us3 has been shown to act similarly to Akt by phosphorylating various substrates that are involved in blocking apoptosis, thereby continuing to inhibit programmed cell death even after the initial Akt signaling fades.

This dual strategy by HSV-1—an initial reliance on the host's Akt signaling followed by its own kinase Us3— exemplifies how viruses can evolve redundancies to ensure successful replication, particularly by manipulating critical survival pathways such as those involving apoptosis.

Human Immunosuppression Virus (HIV) Upon exposure to HIV-1, the virus rapidly initiates signaling events within host T-cells, leading to significant changes in the phosphorylation landscape. Within one minute of HIV-1 exposure, over 200 phosphorylation sites in T-cells are modified, which impacts a range of cellular processes. This rapid and extensive modification suggests that HIV-1 manipulates the host cell's signaling machinery from the very outset of infection [27].

PI3K/Akt pathway plays a crucial role in cell survival, metabolism, and growth. HIV-1's ability to activate the PI3K/Akt pathway supports several essential aspects of viral replication:

1. *Cell Survival*: Activation of Akt promotes anti-apoptotic signals, helping to protect the infected T-cells from undergoing programmed cell death, which could otherwise hinder viral replication.
2. *Cellular Metabolism*: Akt signaling enhances glucose uptake and cellular metabolism, providing the energy and resources needed for efficient viral replication.
3. *Cytoskeletal Reorganization*: Phosphorylation events downstream of the PI3K/Akt pathway may also alter the host cell's cytoskeleton, facilitating the transport of HIV-1 to the nucleus and supporting viral entry and integration.

By manipulating these pathways, HIV-1 creates a favorable environment for its replication while simultaneously avoiding premature cell death, which is crucial for the successful establishment of infection. The virus's ability to rapidly induce such changes highlights its efficiency in hijacking host cell machinery to support its lifecycle.

Influenza virus The interplay between influenza virus and the PI3K/Akt/mTOR signaling pathway is critical for viral replication and host-pathogen interactions. The virus manipulates these pathways to create a favorable environment for its life cycle, while drugs like rapamycin, an mTOR inhibitor, can modulate these effects [28]

1. Influenza Virus and PI3K/Akt Pathway

   - The PI3K/Akt pathway is a key regulator of cellular processes like survival, metabolism, and growth. During influenza virus infection, the virus activates the PI3K/Akt pathway early in its lifecycle to promote its own replication. This pathway supports the survival of infected cells and aids in viral protein synthesis.

     • Influenza virus engages PI3K/Akt to block apoptosis in infected cells, which ensures that the host cells do not die prematurely, allowing the virus time to replicate and assemble its viral progeny. For example, viral proteins such as **NS1** can activate the PI3K/Akt pathway, thus promoting cell survival and enhancing viral replication.

2. mTOR Pathway in Influenza Virus Infection

   - The mTOR pathway is a downstream effector of the PI3K/Akt signaling axis and plays a crucial role in protein synthesis, cell growth, and metabolism. For influenza virus, the mTOR pathway is important for driving the translation of viral proteins. By activating the mTOR pathway, influenza virus ensures that the infected cell's machinery prioritizes viral protein production over normal cellular functions.

- mTORC1, a key complex in the mTOR pathway, regulates translation by controlling the activity of S6K1 and 4E-BP1, which are involved in mRNA translation. The influenza virus utilizes this mechanism to boost the translation of its own mRNAs, thereby enhancing viral replication.

Human Papilloma Virus (HPV) A virus known for causing cervical and other types of cancers engages the PI3K/Akt/mTOR pathway to enhance its replication, evade host immune responses, and drive oncogenesis. Understanding this interaction is crucial because targeting these pathways with drugs like rapamycin, an mTOR inhibitor, offers potential therapeutic strategies [2].

HPV and the PI3K/Akt Pathway

- HPV manipulates the *PI3K/Akt signaling pathway* early in infection. This pathway plays a critical role in regulating cellular processes such as cell survival, growth, and metabolism, all of which can support viral replication and persistence.
- HPV proteins, particularly *E6* and *E7*, directly or indirectly activate the PI3K/Akt pathway. By activating *Akt*, these viral proteins promote cell survival and block apoptotic mechanisms, thus preventing the premature death of infected cells. This pro-survival signaling ensures that the host cells remain viable long enough for the virus to complete its replication cycle.
- Activation of the PI3K/Akt pathway also promotes cell proliferation, which is key for the virus as it requires dividing cells to replicate its DNA and produce new virions.

mTOR Pathway in HPV Infection

- The *mTOR pathway* is a downstream effector of PI3K/Akt and is heavily exploited by HPV to support viral replication and oncogenesis. *mTORC1*, the primary complex in this pathway, regulates protein synthesis and cell growth, which the virus leverages for its replication.
- By activating mTORC1, HPV ensures that the host cell's protein synthesis machinery is focused on producing viral proteins. The *E6* and *E7 oncoproteins* are known to interact with components of the mTOR pathway, directly or indirectly, leading to increased viral protein translation and cell growth.
- The activation of mTOR also contributes to the maintenance of the *immortalized state* of HPV-infected cells, allowing the virus to persist in host tissues. This persistent activation is linked to HPV-driven carcinogenesis, as mTOR promotes the proliferation and survival of cells that accumulate mutations.

HPV and Oncogenesis

- Chronic activation of the *PI3K/Akt/mTOR pathway* by HPV oncoproteins is strongly associated with the progression to cancer. The E6 and E7 oncoproteins inactivate *tumor suppressor genes* such as *p53* and *Rb*, leading to unchecked cell proliferation and survival.
- The persistent activation of the mTOR pathway, through PI3K/Akt signaling, drives the growth of HPV-infected cells, leading to *cervical intraepithelial neo-*

plasia (CIN), which can progress to cervical cancer or other HPV-associated cancers.

SARS-CoV-2 (Covid 19)

The interaction between SARS-CoV-2, the virus responsible for COVID-19, and the PI3K/Akt/mTOR pathway is an area of active research. Like many viruses, SARS-CoV-2 hijacks host cell signaling pathways to facilitate its replication and evade immune responses. The PI3K/Akt/mTOR pathway plays a critical role in cell growth, survival, metabolism, and immune regulation, all of which are important for viral replication. Drugs like rapamycin, an mTOR inhibitor, have shown potential in modulating this pathway during SARS-CoV-2 infection and are being explored for therapeutic use in COVID-19 [12].

SARS-CoV-2 and PI3K/Akt Pathway

- *PI3K/Akt signaling* is a key regulatory pathway for cellular growth, metabolism, and survival. During SARS-CoV-2 infection, the virus is thought to activate the *PI3K/Akt pathway* to enhance viral replication and survival of the infected cells.
- *SARS-CoV-2 proteins*, such as *Nsp6* and *Nsp7*, may interact with components of the PI3K/Akt pathway to promote anti-apoptotic signaling. By keeping host cells alive longer, the virus ensures that it has sufficient time to replicate and assemble new virions.
- Activation of the PI3K/Akt pathway also increases cellular metabolism, providing the energy and resources necessary for the production of viral proteins and genomic material.

mTOR Pathway in SARS-CoV-2 Infection

- The *mTOR (mechanistic target of rapamycin) pathway* is a downstream effector of the PI3K/Akt signaling axis and plays a crucial role in cellular protein synthesis, metabolism, and immune regulation. mTORC1 is especially important for regulating cap-dependent translation, which the virus relies on for the synthesis of its own proteins.
- By activating the mTORC1 complex, SARS-CoV-2 ensures that the host cell's protein synthesis machinery is focused on producing viral proteins. This helps the virus propagate efficiently.
- *mTOR also regulates immune responses*: Dysregulated mTOR signaling can impact both the innate and adaptive immune responses, leading to either a failure to control the virus or excessive inflammation (such as the cytokine storm observed in severe COVID-19 cases).
- Additionally, mTOR inhibition has been associated with autophagy induction, a process that can degrade viral particles, although viruses like SARS-CoV-2 may have evolved mechanisms to evade or exploit autophagy for their own benefit.

PI3K-AKT Signaling Pathway Relationship with Oncogenesis

The *PI3K-AKT signaling pathway* is indeed central to many cellular processes, and its dysregulation is a hallmark of numerous cancers [20]. Here's a concise breakdown of the key points you've provided, enriched with additional context:

1. *Role in Cell Function and Oncogenesis*:
   - The PI3K-AKT pathway regulates critical cellular processes, including growth, survival, and proliferation.
   - Overactivation contributes to oncogenesis by driving uncontrolled cell proliferation and evasion of apoptosis.
2. *PI3K Mutations in Cancer*:
   - PI3K is often mutated in cancers, particularly in the PIK3CA gene, encoding the catalytic subunit p110α.
   - Mutations lead to persistent pathway activation, bypassing normal regulatory mechanisms like RTK signaling.
3. *Types of PIK3CA Mutations*:
   - Gene copy number abnormalities and point mutations are the most common alterations. Approximately 80% of the point mutations in PIK3CA gene.
   - Hotspot Mutations:
     - Mutations at E542K and E545K occur in the helical domain.
     - The H1047R mutation occurs in the kinase domain.
   - These mutations induce constitutive PI3K activation, independent of upstream RTK inputs.

Therapeutic Potential of mTOR Inhibition (Rapamycin)

Rapamycin, an mTOR inhibitor, is widely used in various fields [33]:

- *Transplantation*: Suppresses immune responses to prevent organ rejection.
- *Aging*: Modulates PI3K/AKT/mTOR to extend lifespan and improve health span.
- *Neurology*: Investigated for neuroprotection in diseases linked to mTOR dysregulation.
- *Antiviral effects*: Rapamycin's ability to suppress mTORC1 activity and induce autophagy provides a mechanism to reduce viral replication. By inhibiting the translation of viral proteins, rapamycin could decrease the viral load in infected individuals.
- *Anti-cancer effects*: Targets dysregulated PI3K/AKT/mTOR signaling to inhibit tumor growth. Rapamycin is being studied as a potential therapeutic in HPV-associated cancers. By targeting the mTOR pathway, rapamycin could limit the

growth of cancerous or pre-cancerous cells driven by HPV oncogenes. Additionally, rapamycin's anti-proliferative effects may slow tumor progression.
- *Immune modulation*: Rapamycin also modulates immune responses, which could be beneficial in the context of some viral infection.

Signaling Pathways of mTORC3 and mTORC4

The signaling pathways of mTORC3 and mTORC4 are under investigation at present and was discussed in the previous chapter of this book. The summary is presented below.

mTORC3 is recently discovered and less characterized compared to mTORC1 and mTORC2. According to Harwood [19]

- mTORC3 is described as a rapamycin-insensitive complex of mTOR.
- It phosphorylates key downstream targets such as 4E-BP1, P70S6K, and AKT, but operates independently of Raptor (mTORC1-specific) or Rictor (mTORC2-specific).
- Its formation is independent of ETV7's transcriptional activity, hinting at a unique and non-canonical signaling role for ETV7.

mTORC4, as described by He, is an emerging mTOR complex with a critical role in tumorigenesis and anticancer drug resistance [20].

Key functions include:

- Composed of mTOR, mLST8, DNA-PKcs, and mEAK7.
- Regulating the DNA damage response (DDR).
- Influencing the physiology of cancer stem cells (CSCs).

Bibliography

1. Afinanisa. AMPK localization: a key to differential energy regulation. Int J Mol Sci. 2021; https://doi.org/10.3390/ijms222010921.
2. Aguayo. PI3K/AKT/mTOR signaling pathway in HPV-Driven head and neck carcinogenesis: therapeutic implications. Biology. 2023; https://doi.org/10.3390/biology12050672.
3. Annunziata. The IGF system. Acta Diabetologica. 2010; https://doi.org/10.1007/s00592-010-0227-z.
4. Artimovič. The ability of microRNAs to regulate the immune response in ischemia/reperfusion inflammatory pathways. Genes Immun. 2024; https://doi.org/10.1038/s41435-024-00283-6.
5. Ballesteros-Álvarez. mTORC2: the other mTOR in autophagy regulation. Aging Cell. 2021; https://doi.org/10.1111/acel.13431.
6. Bayly-Jones. Structure of the human TSC: WIPI3 lysosomal recruitment complex. Science. 2024; https://doi.org/10.1126/sciadv.adr5807.
7. Choudhury. Polyploidy and mTOR signaling: a possible molecular link. Cell Commun Signal. 2024; https://doi.org/10.1186/s12964-024-01526-9.

8. Zeng C-M. Frizzled receptors as potential therapeutic targets in human cancers. Int J Mol Sci. 2018; https://doi.org/10.3390/ijms19051543.
9. He D. Gut stem cell aging is driven by mTORC1 via a p38 MAPK-p53 pathway. Nat Commun. 2020; https://doi.org/10.1038/s41467-019-13911-x.
10. Hwang D. YAP promotes global mRNA translation to fuel oncogenic growth despite starvation. Exp Mol Med. 2024; https://doi.org/10.1038/s12276-024-01316-w.
11. Davoody. mTOR signaling and Alzheimer's disease: what we know and where we are? CNS Neurosci Ther. 2023; https://doi.org/10.1111/cns.14463.
12. Dhawan. Regulatory T Cells (Tregs) and COVID-19: unveiling the mechanisms, and therapeutic potentialities with a special focus on long COVID. Vaccines. 2023; https://doi.org/10.3390/vaccines11030699.
13. Dostert. The TNF family of ligands and receptors: communication modules in the immune system and beyond. Physiol Rev. 2018; https://doi.org/10.1152/physrev.00045.2017.
14. Giguere. Canonical signaling and nuclear activity of mTOR—a teamwork effort to regulate metabolism and cell growth. FEBS J. 2016; https://doi.org/10.1111/febs.14384.
15. Glaviano. PI3K/AKT/mTOR signaling transduction pathway and targeted therapies in cancer. Mol Cancer. 2023; https://doi.org/10.1186/s12943-023-01827-6.
16. Gungor. The bright and the dark side of TGF-β signaling in hepatocellular carcinoma: mechanisms, dysregulation, and therapeutic implications. Cancers. 2022; https://doi.org/10.3390/cancers14040940.
17. Hao X-D. Longevity factor FOXO3a: a potential therapeutic target for age-related ocular diseases. Life Sci. 2024; https://doi.org/10.1016/j.lfs.2024.122769.
18. Hartung. The dual role of the TSC complex in cancer. Cell Host Microbe. 2024; https://doi.org/10.1016/j.molmed.2024.10.009.
19. Harwood. ETV7 is an essential component of a rapamycin-insensitive mTOR complex in cancer. Sci Adv. 2018; https://doi.org/10.1126/sciadv.aar3938.
20. He. Targeting PI3K/Akt signal transduction for cancer therapy. Signal Transduct Target Ther. 2021; https://doi.org/10.1038/s41392-021-00828-5.
21. Hua H. Targeting Akt in cancer for precision therapy. J Hematol Oncol. 2021; https://doi.org/10.1186/s13045-021-01137-8.
22. Hubert. Glucose deprivation impairs hypoxia-inducible factor-1α synthesis. Hypertens Res. 2024; https://doi.org/10.1007/s12672-024-01484-1.
23. Yu J. Components of the JNK–MAPK pathway play distinct roles in hepatocellular carcinoma. J Cancer Res Clin Oncol. 2023; https://doi.org/10.1007/s00432-023-05473-9.
24. Kasowanjete. A review of photobiomodulation on PI3K/AKT/mTOR in wound healing. J Photochem Photobiol. 2024; https://doi.org/10.1016/j.jpap.2023.100215.
25. Kazyken. Unexpected roles for AMPK in the suppression of autophagy and the reactivation of MTORC1 signaling during prolonged amino acid deprivation. Autophagy. 2024; https://doi.org/10.1080/15548627.2024.2355074.
26. Kilanowska. cAMP-dependent signaling and ovarian cancer. Cells. 2022; https://doi.org/10.3390/cells11233835.
27. Klute. Friends and foes: the ambivalent role of autophagy in HIV-1 infection. Viruses. 2024; https://doi.org/10.3390/v16040500.
28. Guo L. MicroRNA-4485 ameliorates severe influenza pneumonia via inhibition of the STAT3/PI3K/AKT signaling pathway. Oncol Lett. 2020; https://doi.org/10.3892/ol.2020.12078.
29. Xu L. The host cells suppress the proliferation of pseudorabies virus by regulating the PI3K/Akt/mTOR pathway. ASM J/Microbiol Spectr. 2024; https://doi.org/10.1128/spectrum.01351-24.
30. Zheng L. Recent advances in understanding amino acid sensing mechanisms that regulate mTORC1. Int J Mol Sci. 2016; https://doi.org/10.3390/ijms17101636.
31. Lama-Sherpa. Regulation of mTORC1 by the Rag GTPases. Biochem Soc Trans. 2023; https://doi.org/10.1042/BST20210038.
32. Lemmon. Cell signaling by receptor-tyrosine kinases. Cell. 2010; https://doi.org/10.1016/j.cell.2010.06.011.

33. Martin-Bocanegra. Involvement of mTOR signaling in physiopathology and its potential therapeutic interventions. Redox Exp Med. 2024; https://doi.org/10.1530/REM-23-0024.
34. Moon. MAPK/ERK signaling pathway in hepatocellular carcinoma. Cancers. 2021; https://doi.org/10.3390/cancers13123026.
35. Omolekan. PI3K/AKT/mTOR signaling network in human health and diseases. Cells. 2024; https://doi.org/10.3390/cells13171500.
36. Ouyang. Metabolic regulation of T cell development by Sin1–mTORC2 is mediated by pyruvate kinase M2. J Mol Cell Biol. 2018; https://doi.org/10.1093/jmcb/mjy065.
37. Panwar. Multifaceted role of mTOR (mammalian target of rapamycin) signaling pathway in human health and disease. Nature. 2023; https://doi.org/10.1038/s41392-023-01608-z.
38. Li Q. Targeting the PI3K/AKT/mTOR and RAF/MEK/ERK pathways for cancer therapy. Mol Biomed. 2022; https://doi.org/10.1186/s43556-022-00110-2.
39. Xie Q. The significance of lipid metabolism reprogramming of tumor-associated macrophages in hepatocellular carcinoma. Cancer Immunol Immunother. 2024; https://doi.org/10.1007/s00262-024-03748-9.
40. Ragupathi. The mTORC2 signaling network: targets and cross-talks. Biochem J. 2024; https://doi.org/10.1042/BCJ20220325.
41. Ramaiah. mTOR inhibition and p53 activation, microRNAs: the possible therapy against pandemic COVID-19. Gene Rep. 2020;20 https://doi.org/10.1016/j.genrep.2020.100765.
42. Raychaudhuri. JAK-STAT signaling and beyond in the pathogenesis of spondyloarthritis and their clinical significance. Curr Rheumatol Rep. 2024; https://doi.org/10.1007/s11926-024-01144-x.
43. Zhang S. Regulation of mTORC1 by amino acids in mammalian cells: a general picture of recent advances. Anim Nutr. 2021; https://doi.org/10.1016/j.aninu.2021.05.003.
44. Sambri. Ragopathies and the rising influence of RagGTPases on human diseases. Nat Commun. 2024; https://doi.org/10.1038/s41467-024-50034-4.
45. Santos. FOXO family isoforms. Cell Death & Disease. 2023; https://doi.org/10.1038/s41419-023-06177-1.
46. Shaw. The insulin receptor substrate (IRS) proteins. Cell Cycle. 2011; https://doi.org/10.4161/cc.10.11.15824.
47. Shorning. The PI3K-AKT-mTOR pathway and prostate cancer: at the crossroads of AR, MAPK, and WNT signaling. Int J Mol Sci. 2020; https://doi.org/10.3390/ijms21124507.
48. Taher. The role of the interleukin (IL)-6/IL-6 receptor axis in cancer. Biochem Soc Trans. 2018; https://doi.org/10.1042/BST20180136.
49. Tzavlaki. TGF-β Signaling. Biomolecules. 2020; https://doi.org/10.3390/biom10030487.
50. Volety. Mitigating viral invasion: mTORC2's role in neuroprotection and immunity. In: Stress: immunology and inflammation; 2024. p. 173–82. https://doi.org/10.1016/B978-0-12-817558-3.00008-1.
51. Wenxiang. Regulation of mTORC2 signaling. Genes. 2020; https://doi.org/10.3390/genes11091045.
52. Lee YJ. Exploring the key signaling pathways and ncRNAs in colorectal cancer. Int J Mol Sci. 2024; https://doi.org/10.3390/ijms25084548.
53. Wang Y. Targeting mTOR signaling pathways in multiple myeloma: biology and implication for therapy. Cell Commun Signal. 2024; https://doi.org/10.1186/s12964-024-01699-3.
54. Zhang Y. FoxO family members in cancer. Cancer Biol Ther. 2011; https://doi.org/10.4161/cbt.12.4.15954.
55. Yodhaanjali. Signaling and transduction mechanism of phospholipase C and isoforms in different cell types. In: Phospholipases in physiology and pathology, vol. 2; 2023. p. 199–210. https://doi.org/10.1016/B978-0-323-95696-3.00007-7.
56. Chia ZJ. Transforming growth factor-β receptors: versatile mechanisms of ligand activation. Acta Pharmacol Sin. 2024; https://doi.org/10.1038/s41401-024-01235-6.
57. Zhang Z. PI3K/Akt and HIF-1 signaling pathway in hypoxia-ischemia. Mol Med Rep. 2018; https://doi.org/10.3892/mmr.2018.9375.

58. Zhomg Z. The hippo signaling pathway in development and regeneration. Cell Rep. 2024; https://doi.org/10.1016/j.celrep.2024.113926.
59. Zhao. Nuclear mTOR signaling orchestrates transcriptional programs underlying cellular growth and metabolism. Cells. 2024; https://doi.org/10.3390/cells13090781.
60. Zwakenberg. mTORC1 restricts TFE3 activity by auto-regulating its presence on lysosomes. Mol Cell. 2024; https://doi.org/10.1016/j.molcel.2024.10.009.

Chapter 3
mTOR Effect on Eye Embryology

Contents

K. T. Moazed, *mTOR Signaling in Ophthalmology*,
https://doi.org/10.1007/978-3-032-05044-1_3

Abstract During embryonic eye development, mTOR signaling integrates metabolic, growth, and differentiation cues from PI3K/AKT, Wnt/β-catenin, Notch, and HIF-1α/VEGF, and other pathways, to ensure proper retinal progenitor proliferation, RPE formation, neurogenesis, and vascular development. Disruptions in these interactions can result in congenital ocular malformations such as microphthalmia, coloboma, retinal dysplasia, and optic nerve hypoplasia. Understanding these mechanisms provides insights into early-onset retinal diseases and potential therapeutic targets for congenital eye disorders.

Discussions

The development of the eye relies on the intricate interplay of many signaling pathways, which coordinate cellular proliferation, differentiation, and structural organization. Disruptions in any of these pathways can lead to congenital ocular anomalies, underscoring their significance in both developmental biology and disease pathogenesis.

Here we discuss how mTOR signaling facilitates the development of the eye from the earliest stages of embryogenesis. This chapter sets the stage for understanding the pathological conditions that are associated with its dysregulation.

Brief review of the embryology of the eye is necessary to understand the process of mTOR signaling.

Embryology of the Eye: An Overview

The development of the vertebrate eye begins early in embryogenesis and involves a series of coordinated morphogenetic events that shape its distinct structures.

1. Formation of the Optic Vesicles (3rd–4th Week)
    - The *eye primordium* appears as a thickening in the anterior neural plate.
    - Lateral outpouchings from the *diencephalon* of the neural tube form the *optic vesicles*.
    - The optic vesicles grow outward toward the surface ectoderm.
2. Lens Placode and Optic Cup Formation (4th–5th Week)
    - The optic vesicles induce the *surface ectoderm* to thicken, forming the *lens placode*.

- The lens placode invaginates, forming the *lens pit* and eventually pinches off as the *lens vesicle*.
- The optic vesicle also invaginates, folding into a *bilayered optic cup*.
  - The *inner layer* becomes the *neural retina*.
  - The *outer layer* forms the *retinal pigment epithelium (RPE)*.

3. Differentiation of Eye Structures (6th–8th Week)
   - The *lens vesicle* matures into the *lens*, with the posterior cells elongating into *lens fibers*.
   - The *optic stalk* extends and eventually forms the *optic nerve*.
   - The *cornea and anterior chamber* develop from the overlying ectoderm and surrounding mesenchyme.
   - The *iris and ciliary body* differentiate from the anterior optic cup.
4. Growth and Maturation (2nd–3rd Trimester)
   - The retina matures, with photoreceptors, ganglion cells, and supporting glial cells differentiating.
   - The vitreous *body* forms within the eye, providing structural support.
   - The extraocular muscles and eyelids develop.

By birth, the basic structure of the eye is complete, though postnatal growth and refinement (e.g., emmetropization) continue to optimize vision.

Molecular Pathways Involved in Embryology of the Eye

The *eye field* represents the earliest stage of vertebrate eye specification, setting the foundation for subsequent eye morphogenesis.

The *eye field* is a region in the anterior neuroectoderm of the developing embryo that gives rise to the eyes. It emerges during early *gastrulation* (critical phase in embryonic development where the single-layered blastula reorganizes into a three-layered structure; ectoderm, mesoderm, and endoderm, called the gastrula) and is marked by the expression of key transcription factors collectively known as the eye field transcription factors (EFTFs).

Influential Features of the Eye Field

- Located in the anterior neural plate.
- Contains progenitor cells that later divide into bilateral optic vesicles.
- Controlled by *EFTFs*, including *Pax6, Rx, Six3, Lhx2, and Otx2*, which regulate eye specification and development.

- Initially a single field, but later splits into two symmetrical optic vesicles under the influence of *Sonic Hedgehog (Shh)* signaling.

Signaling Pathways Involved

- *Pax6*: Master regulator of eye development.
- *Rx & Six3*: Essential for eye field formation and retinal progenitor proliferation.
- *Shh*: Splits the single eye field into two, preventing cyclopia (failure of eye separation).

The optical geometry and refractive state of the eye are shaped during embryonic and postnatal development, with genetics playing a dominant role in the embryonic phase, while both genetic and environmental factors influence postnatal eye growth through emmetropization. This process ensures that the posterior eye segment grows in proportion to the anterior segment's optical power, allowing images to focus precisely on the retina for clear vision. A mismatch in this balance results in hyperopia (if the eye is too short) or myopia (if the eye is too long). Visual input plays a crucial role, as optical defocus-driven feedback regulates posterior segment growth-hyperopic defocus (caused by negative lenses) accelerates eye elongation, leading to myopia, while myopic defocus (caused by positive lenses) slows growth, resulting in hyperopia [22].

Highlights of Vertebrate Eye Development and Key Signaling Pathways

Eye development in vertebrates is a highly regulated process involving coordinated morphogenetic movements and signaling pathways that establish distinct ocular structures. These signaling networks ensure the precise formation of ocular structures essential for vision (Table 3.1).

Brief Key Molecular Pathways in Different Stages of Eye Development

1. *Formation of the Optic Vesicles and Lens Induction*
    - The *optic vesicles* emerge as outpouchings of the neural tube (Fig. 3.1a–c).
    - The *presumptive lens epithelium (PLE)* invaginates, forming the *lens pits (LP)*.
    - *BMPs* from the surface ectoderm and PLE promote *neural retina development*.

Table 3.1 The table outlines key signaling pathways (e.g., Shh, FGF, Wnt, BMP) that orchestrate eye development by regulating stages like optic cup formation, retinal patterning, and lens induction, with molecules such as β-catenin and Pax6 coordinating spatial-temporal processes

Molecular pathways in eye development			
#	Pathway	Key molecules	Role in eye development
1	Wnt Signaling	WNT1, WNT3a, β-catenin	Regulates early eye field specification, optic cup formation, and retinal differentiation.
2	Sonic Hedgehog (Shh) Signaling	SHH, PTCH, GLI	Plays a role in the patterning of the optic vesicle and separation of eye fields.
3	Notch Signaling	NOTCH1, DLL1, JAGGED1	Controls cell fate decisions in the retina and regulates progenitor cell maintenance.
4	Retinoic Acid (RA) Pathway	RA, RAR, RXR	Essential for retinal progenitor proliferation and differentiation, photoreceptor development.
5	Bone Morphogenetic Protein (BMP) Signaling	BMP4, BMP7, SMADs	Involved in lens induction, retinal patterning, and optic cup morphogenesis.
6	Fibroblast Growth Factor (FGF) Signaling	FGF1, FGF2, FGFR	Promotes lens fiber differentiation, retinal neurogenesis, and optic cup formation.
7	Transforming Growth Factor β (TGF-β)	TGF-β2, SMADs	Regulates epithelial-mesenchymal transition (EMT) during eye development.
8	mTOR Signaling	PI3K, AKT, TSC1/TSC2 RHEB	Influences retinal progenitor cell proliferation, differentiation, and metabolism.
9	Hippo Signaling	MST1/2, LATS1/2, YAP/TAZ, TEAD1-4	Regulates retinal cell proliferation, differentiation, and apoptosis.
10	MAPK Signaling	RAS, RAF, MEK, ERK	Regulates retinal progenitor proliferation, differentiation, lens development, optic cup morphogenesis, and neuronal survival, ensuring proper eye formation and function.
11	PAX6 Pathway	PAX6, SOX2, OPTX2	Master regulator of eye development; mutations cause aniridia.
12	Ephrin-Eph	Ephrin-A/B, Eph receptors	Retinal ganglion cell axon guidance and topographic mapping.

Defects in these pathways disrupt critical events like choroid fissure closure or axon guidance, leading to congenital eye disorders such as coloboma or retinal miswiring

- *TGFβ* from the *periocular mesenchyme (POM)* activates *WNT/β-catenin signaling*, which *suppresses Pax6* expression in the *non-lens surface ectoderm*, preventing lens differentiation outside the *lens placode*.
- *In the lens placode, Pax6 inhibits WNT/β-catenin signaling*, initiating lens formation.

2. *Lens Vesicle Formation and Retinal Differentiation*

- The closure of the *lens pits* leads to the formation of the *lens vesicles (LV)*, which give rise to the *lens (LS)*.
- The *optic vesicles (OV)* differentiate into:

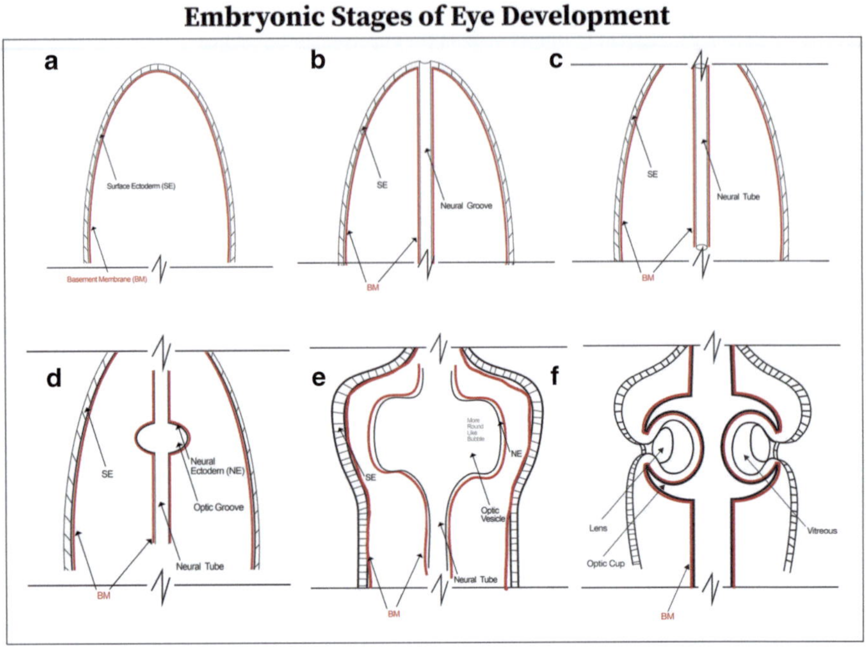

Fig. 3.1 Schematic representation of embryonic stages of eye develoment. (*a*) formation of surface ectoderm and the location of the basement membrane around 3rd week of gestation, (*b*) formation of the neural groove between 3rd and 4th week of gestation and location of basement membrane (BM), (*c*) closure of the neural groove and formation of the neural tube at 4th week of gestation and related position of the basement membrane (BM) adjacent to surface ectoderm (SE), (*d*) formation of the optic vesicle from neural tube by the 5th week of gestation and the location of the basement membrane (BM), (*e*) enlargement of the optic vesicle and its movement towards the surface ectoderm and the location of the basement membrane (BM), (*f*) formation of the optic cup by invagination of the optic vesicle and penetration of the surface ectoderm inside the optic cup to form the lens vesicle by the 12th week of gestation and the location of the basement membrane (BM)

  - The *retinal pigment epithelium (RPE)*
  - The *neural retina (NR) (*Fig. 3.1d–f)

- *WNT signaling from the surface ectoderm activates Otx2 and Mitf*, which drive *RPE differentiation* (Fig. 3.2).

3. *Lens and Retinal Maturation*

   - The *FGF signaling* from the retina and *vitreous (VT)* promotes lens fiber differentiation.
   - The *lens vesicle* fully matures into the *lens (LS)*, supporting light focusing and vision (Fig. 3.3).

Later Stages of Embryonic Eye Development

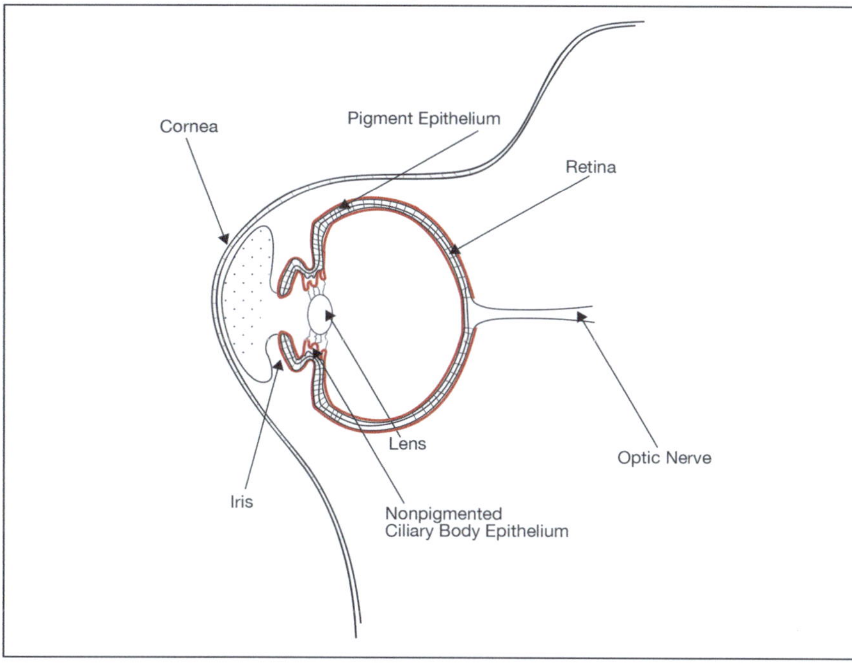

Fig. 3.2 By 20th week of gestation, the Iris and anterior chamber are formed. The tip of the invaginated optic cup forms the pupil and the 2 layers of the invaginated optic cup forms the posterior pigment epithelium of the iris and retina with the location of the basement membrane (BM) on either side

Major Signaling Pathways in Eye Development

- *BMPs* → Promote neural retina differentiation.
- *TGFβ/WNT-β-catenin* → Regulates Pax6 expression, controlling lens fate.
- *WNT signaling (Otx2, Mitf)* → Essential for RPE formation.
- *FGF* → Drives lens fiber differentiation.

Detailed Key Signaling Pathways in Eye Development

Eye development is orchestrated by a highly coordinated network of signaling pathways that regulate cellular proliferation, differentiation, and tissue organization. Among these, mTOR, FGF, Wnt, Hedgehog, and BMP pathways are the most influential players, each contributing to distinct aspects of ocular formation and function.

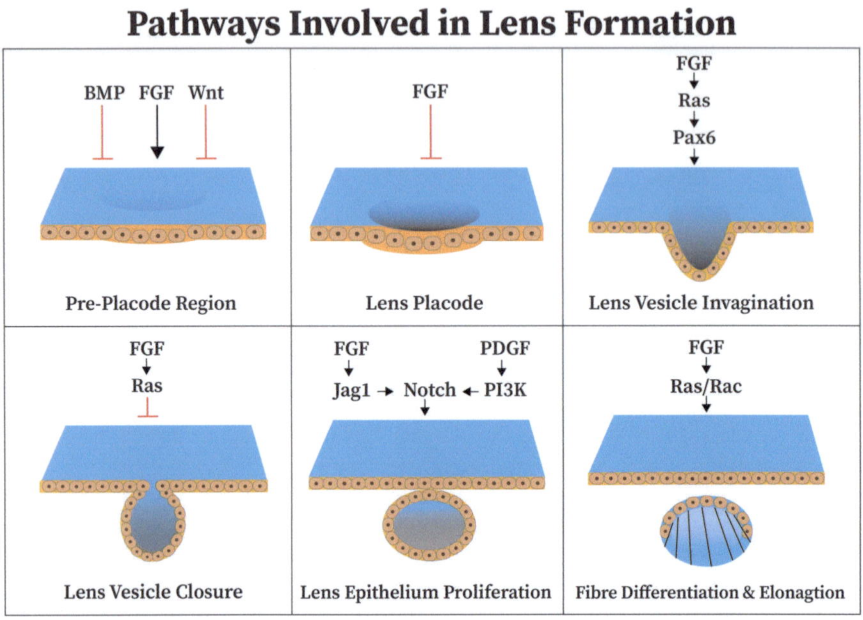

Fig. 3.3 Lens formation is a complex process that occurs during embryonic development and is regulated by a network of signaling pathways, transcription factors, and molecular interactions. The illustrations above depict the different stages of lens development, highlighting the key pathways involved. Activators are represented by black arrows, while inhibitors are shown with red crossbars, indicating their respective roles in regulating this process

mTOR Signaling (mTORC1 & mTORC2)

Role in Eye Development

- mTORC1 (via Raptor) regulates metabolic activity, protein synthesis, and progenitor cell proliferation during early retinal neurogenesis.
- Conditional deletion of Raptor in retinal progenitor cells leads to decreased proliferation, increased apoptosis, and aberrant lamination.
- mTORC2 (via Rictor) contributes to cytoskeletal organization and RGC axon guidance at the optic chiasm.
- Works in tandem with Akt signaling to regulate photoreceptor survival and retinal angiogenesis.

Defects Associated with mTOR Dysregulation

- mTORC1 inhibition results in thin retinas, loss of retinal stratification, and impaired visual processing.
- Overactive mTOR signaling is linked to retinal dystrophies, LCA (Leber congenital amaurosis), and tuberous sclerosis complex (TSC)-associated eye abnormalities.

mTOR Signaling in Early Ocular Development: Interactions with Transcription Factors and Signaling Pathways

Eye development originates from the anterior neural plate during late gastrulation, with the visual field emerging from the forebrain. This complex process is orchestrated by many transcription factors, for example, Rx, Pax6, Six3, and Optx2, which work in conjunction with various signaling pathways, including bone morphogenetic protein (BMP), Nodal, and Wnt/β-catenin. The mTOR pathway integrates these signals, ensuring proper cellular growth, metabolism, and differentiation during the early stages of ocular morphogenesis.

The key pathways that play a crucial role in eye development are outlined below

Fibroblast Growth Factor (FGF) Signaling

Role in Eye Development

- Essential for lens induction, retinal progenitor cell proliferation, and optic vesicle patterning [9].
- Regulates differentiation of lens fiber cells, with FGF gradients influencing epithelial cell proliferation (low FGF) and lens fiber elongation (high FGF).
- FGF1, FGF2, and FGF9 secreted from the developing lens and retina drive retinal differentiation and patterning.
- Works in coordination with MAPK and PI3K-AKT pathways to promote survival of retinal ganglion cells (RGCs).

Defects Associated with FGF Dysregulation

- FGF mutations can lead to lens defects, cataracts, microphthalmia, and retinal dysplasia.
- Disruptions in FGF signaling impair corneal and optic nerve development.

Key Roles of FGF Signaling in Eye Embryology

Fibroblast growth factor (FGF) signaling plays a crucial role in eye embryology, influencing various aspects of ocular development, including the formation of the lens, retina, cornea, and optic nerve. The FGF family, consisting of 23 ligands and 4 canonical receptors (FGFR1–FGFR4), interacts with heparan sulfate proteoglycans (HSPGs) to regulate cell proliferation, differentiation, survival, and tissue patterning during eye development [14].

1. Lens Induction and Development
    - FGF signaling is essential for lens placode formation and differentiation.
    - FGF ligands secreted from the retina and periocular mesenchyme induce lens fiber cell differentiation.
    - Gradients of FGF activity regulate lens epithelial cell proliferation (low FGF) and fiber cell elongation and differentiation (high FGF), primarily through FGFR1 and FGFR2.
    - Activation of the Ras-MAPK pathway promotes lens fiber differentiation.
2. Retina Development
    - FGFs are crucial for optic vesicle patterning and retinal progenitor cell proliferation.
    - FGF9 and FGF15 are important for early retina formation by maintaining the retinal progenitor pool.
    - FGFs secreted from the lens (e.g., FGF1, FGF2, FGF9*)* regulate differentiation of the neural retina and retinal pigment epithelium (RPE).
    - FGF signaling interacts with Sonic Hedgehog (Shh) and Wnt pathways to control retinal ganglion cell (RGC) development.
3. Corneal Development
    - FGFs, particularly FGF7 and FGF10, are involved in corneal epithelium proliferation and stromal development.
    - FGF10 mutations lead to congenital disorders such as lacrimo-auriculo-dento-digital (LADD) syndrome, affecting ocular structures.
    - FGF-mediated epithelial-mesenchymal interactions regulate corneal stromal and endothelial differentiation.
4. Optic Nerve and Glial Cell Development
    - FGF signaling supports the survival and differentiation of oligodendrocytes and astrocytes in the optic nerve.
    - FGF2 *and FGF9* promote optic nerve head morphogenesis and axonal guidance.
5. Ocular Vasculature Formation
    - FGF signaling regulates angiogenesis in the developing eye, particularly in retinal vascular development.
    - FGF2 is a key angiogenic factor that interacts with VEGF to promote retinal vascularization.

Clinical Relevance

A. Disruptions in FGF signaling are associated with congenital eye disorders such as microphthalmia, anophthalmia, cataracts, and coloboma.
B. FGFR mutations contribute to syndromic craniofacial and ocular abnormalities, such as Pfeiffer syndrome and Apert syndrome.

Wnt/β-Catenin Signaling in Eye Embryology

The Wnt/β-catenin pathway is a key regulator of eye development, influencing eye field specification, optic cup formation, retinal differentiation, and corneal development. Proper spatial and temporal regulation of Wnt signaling is essential, as both excessive and deficient Wnt activity can lead to congenital ocular disorders [7].

Role of Wnt/β-Catenin in Eye Development

A. Eye Field Specification and Optic Vesicle Formation

- Wnt signaling is repressed in the anterior neural plate to allow Pax6, Rx, and Six3 expression, which define the eye field.
- Overactive Wnt signaling in early stages disrupts eye formation, leading to anophthalmia or cyclopia.

B. Optic Cup and Retinal Differentiation

- Wnt/β-catenin promotes dorsal retinal identity, while low Wnt signaling is necessary for ventral retinal structures.
- Regulates retinal progenitor cell (RPC) proliferation and differentiation into retinal ganglion cells (RGCs), photoreceptors, and Müller glia.
- Maintains retinal pigmented epithelium (RPE) fate; excessive Wnt activity can convert RPE into neural retina.

C. Lens and Corneal Development

- Wnt inhibition is required for lens induction; excessive Wnt signaling leads to failure in lens placode formation.
- Corneal epithelial stratification and stem cell maintenance rely on Wnt/β--catenin activity.

Wnt Dysregulation and Ocular Disorders

- Anophthalmia & Microphthalmia: Wnt overactivation disrupts early eye field specification.
- Coloboma: Wnt misregulation affects optic fissure closure.
- Retinal Dystrophies: Wnt pathway mutations alter photoreceptor and RGC survival.
- Glaucoma: Wnt dysfunction impacts trabecular meshwork and aqueous humor drainage.
- Corneal Dystrophies: Imbalanced Wnt activity affects corneal transparency and repair.3. Therapeutic Implications
- Wnt modulators (e.g., inhibitors for hyperactivation, activators for retinal repair) are potential treatments for retinal degeneration and corneal diseases.
- Stem cell therapy: Wnt/β-catenin is being explored for RGC regeneration and optic nerve repair.

Role in Eye Development (R.[10])

- Regulates the formation of the optic cup, RPE (retinal pigment epithelium), and corneal epithelial maintenance.
- Wnt2b and Wnt3a play a role in maintaining retinal progenitor cells and promoting optic nerve head development.
- Essential for retinal vascularization, working with VEGF (vascular endothelial growth factor) to guide angiogenesis.

Defects Associated with Wnt Dysregulation

- Mutations in Wnt pathway components cause coloboma, anophthalmia, and defective corneal wound healing.
- Aberrant Wnt signaling is implicated in congenital glaucoma and retinal degenerative diseases.

Sonic Hedgehog (Shh) Signaling Pathway

Sonic Hedgehog (Shh) is a critical morphogen that plays a key role in embryonic development, tissue regeneration, and stem cell maintenance. It is part of the Hedgehog (Hh) signaling pathway, which also includes Indian Hedgehog (Ihh) and Desert Hedgehog (Dhh). Shh signaling is essential for the regulation of cell proliferation, differentiation, and survival, particularly in the development of the central nervous system, limbs, and eyes [2].

Role in Eye Development

- Drives optic stalk formation, retinal cell fate specification, and axonal guidance of retinal ganglion cells.
- Sonic Hedgehog (Shh) secreted from the ventral forebrain and retina helps regulate the dorsoventral patterning of the eye.
- Promotes proliferation of retinal progenitor cells and ciliary body development.

Defects Associated with Hedgehog Dysregulation

- Shh mutations result in holoprosencephaly, optic nerve hypoplasia, and midline fusion defects.
- Impaired Shh signaling leads to microphthalmia and RGC loss.

Shh Pathway Components and Mechanism

1. Shh Ligand Production and Secretion
    - Shh is synthesized as a precursor protein that undergoes autocatalytic cleavage and lipid modification (palmitoylation and cholesterol attachment), which are necessary for its full activity.
    - The mature, lipid-modified Shh ligand is secreted and can act in a paracrine or autocrine manner.
2. Shh Binding to Patched (Ptch1)
    - In the absence of Shh, the receptor Patched-1 (Ptch1) inhibits Smoothened (Smo), a key transmembrane protein.
    - Shh binding to Ptch1 relieves this inhibition, allowing Smo to become active.
3. Activation of Gli Transcription Factors
    - Active Smo initiates a signaling cascade leading to the activation of Gli transcription factors (Gli1, Gli2, Gli3).
    - Gli proteins translocate to the nucleus and regulate the transcription of Hedgehog target genes, which control cell fate, proliferation, and survival.

4. Regulatory Feedback Mechanisms
   - The pathway is tightly regulated by various feedback loops, including negative feedback via Ptch1 upregulation and positive feedback through Gli1 activation.

Shh in Development and Disease

1. Role in Embryonic Development
   - Neural Tube Patterning: Shh is crucial for dorsoventral patterning of the neural tube and the formation of the floor plate.
   - Limb Development: Governs anterior-posterior limb patterning via the Zone of Polarizing Activity (ZPA).
   - Ocular Development: Essential for optic cup and retinal differentiation.
2. Shh in Ocular Health and Disease
   - Retinal Development: Regulates differentiation of retinal progenitor cells.
   - Ocular Malformations: Mutations in Shh can result in holoprosencephaly, microphthalmia, and coloboma.
   - Glaucoma and Retinal Degeneration: Dysregulation of Shh has been implicated in neurodegenerative diseases of the eye.
3. Shh in Cancer
   - Aberrant activation of the Shh pathway is linked to various cancers, including medulloblastoma, basal cell carcinoma, and glioblastoma.
   - Shh signaling promotes tumorigenesis by driving proliferation, stemness, and survival of cancer cells.
4. Therapeutic Targeting of Shh
   - Hedgehog pathway inhibitors such as Vismodegib and Sonidegib are used in the treatment of Hedgehog-dependent cancers.
   - Potential applications in ocular diseases, regenerative medicine, and neuroprotection

Shh and Its Crosstalk with mTOR

- *mTOR-Shh Interactions*: Studies suggest that mTOR signaling intersects with Shh in regulating stem cell maintenance and cancer progression.
- *Autophagy and Growth Regulation*: Shh signaling influences autophagy and cell survival pathways that involve mTORC1.

Bone Morphogenetic Protein (BMP) Signaling

Role in Eye Development

- BMPs, particularly BMP4 and BMP7, are required for optic vesicle invagination and retinal patterning.
- Interacts with Noggin (BMP antagonist) to balance proliferation and differentiation in the developing neural retina.
- Important for lens development, where BMP signaling helps specify the lens placode.

Defects Associated with BMP Dysregulation

- BMP deficiencies lead to optic nerve colobomas, aniridia, and defective RPE formation.
- BMP mutations are linked to congenital cataracts and defective lens formation.

Bone Morphogenetic Proteins (BMPs) in Eye Development

Bone Morphogenetic Proteins (BMPs) are a subgroup of the Transforming Growth Factor-Beta (TGF-β) superfamily and play a crucial role in embryonic development, including the formation and differentiation of the eye. BMP signaling is indispensable for multiple stages of eye development, from early optic vesicle formation to the differentiation of the retina, lens, and cornea. Given its broad influence, BMPs represent potential therapeutic targets for congenital and degenerative eye diseases [3].

They regulate various stages of eye development, including optic vesicle patterning, lens induction, retinal differentiation, and corneal morphogenesis.

BMP is a subset of the TGF-β superfamily, regulates eye morphogenesis, lens induction, retinal differentiation, and corneal development through Smad1/5/8 phosphorylation and non-Smad pathways. BMPs are categorized based on sequence homology and function:

Group 1: Prototypical BMPs (Involved in Bone, Cartilage, and Eye Development)

- BMP2, BMP4 → Optic vesicle, lens, and retinal development
- BMP5, BMP6, BMP7 → Corneal differentiation, lens fiber formation
- BMP8a, BMP8b → Less studied in ocular biology

Group 2: GDF Subfamily (Growth and Differentiation Factors)

- GDF5, GDF6, GDF7 → Retina, neural crest, and scleral development

Group 3: Divergent BMPs (Act in Morphogenesis and Neurogenesis)

- BMP9, BMP10 → Retinal vascularization and angiogenesis

BMPs in Early Eye Development

BMP signaling is essential for the initial specification of the eye field in the anterior neural plate. It works in coordination with Sonic Hedgehog (Shh), Fibroblast Growth Factors (FGFs), and Wnt signaling to define the boundaries of the optic vesicle and optic cup.

- BMP4 and BMP7 are highly expressed in the developing optic vesicle and are necessary for proper optic vesicle morphogenesis.
- BMP signaling suppresses neural crest invasion into the optic vesicle, allowing it to properly invaginate and form the optic cup.

Corneal and Ocular Surface Development

BMP signaling contributes to the development of the corneal epithelium, stroma, and endothelium.

- BMP4 and BMP7 are required for corneal epithelial differentiation.
- BMP6 is involved in corneal stromal development.
- BMP signaling interacts with TGF-β pathways to regulate corneal transparency and wound healing.

Lens Induction and Differentiation

BMP signaling plays a key role in lens placode formation and its subsequent differentiation into the lens.

- BMP4 and BMP7 are expressed in the surface ectoderm and the optic vesicle, driving lens induction.
- BMP signaling in conjunction with FGF stimulates Pax6 expression, a master regulator of lens development.
- Knockout models of BMP4 or BMP7 result in failure of lens induction, leading to anophthalmia or severe ocular malformations.

Retinal Development and Patterning

BMP signaling regulates proliferation, differentiation, and survival of retinal progenitor cells.

- BMP4 and BMP2 are expressed in the retinal pigmented epithelium (RPE) and promote its differentiation.
- BMP signaling helps specify dorsoventral polarity in the retina.
- BMP-mediated Smad1/5/8 phosphorylation influences retinal ganglion cell (RGC) differentiation.
- Inhibition of BMP signaling in the retina leads to microphthalmia, coloboma, and disorganized retinal layers.

BMP Dysregulation and Ocular Diseases

Disruptions in BMP signaling are associated with several ocular diseases:

- Congenital Anophthalmia and Microphthalmia: BMP mutations or misregulation cause defects in optic vesicle morphogenesis.
- Congenital Cataracts: Defective BMP signaling can impair lens fiber differentiation.
- Retinal Degeneration: BMP4 mutations have been implicated in retinal cell survival deficits.
- Glaucoma: BMP pathway alterations affect trabecular meshwork function, leading to dysregulated intraocular pressure.
- Corneal Dystrophies: BMP dysfunction contributes to improper corneal epithelial maintenance.

Nodal Pathway in Eye Embryology

The Nodal signaling pathway, a member of the TGF-β superfamily, is essential for early eye development, particularly in eye field specification, dorsoventral patterning, and optic cup morphogenesis [5].

Key Roles in Eye Development

1. Eye Field Specification

    - Nodal signaling helps establish the eye field in the anterior neural plate by regulating Pax6, Rx, and Six3—key transcription factors for eye formation.

- Loss of Nodal signaling results in anophthalmia or microphthalmia due to failure in optic vesicle formation.

2. Optic Cup and Retinal Development
   - Nodal regulates the balance between neural retina (NR) and retinal pigmented epithelium (RPE) differentiation.
   - It controls dorsoventral patterning of the optic vesicle, influencing optic fissure closure—defects can lead to coloboma.

3. Lens and Corneal Development
   - Nodal signaling interacts with BMP and FGF pathways to regulate lens placode induction.
   - It also plays a role in corneal epithelial morphogenesis and transparency.

Clinical Implications

- Nodal pathway dysregulation is linked to congenital eye malformations, including anophthalmia, microphthalmia, and coloboma.
- Mutations in Nodal pathway genes (e.g., NODAL, FOXH1, Lefty1/2) contribute to ocular and craniofacial syndromes.

  Establishment of the Eye Field: Role of mTOR in Eye Field Specification

- The eye field is specified in the developing forebrain by a coordinated network of transcription factors:
  - Rx (Retina and anterior neural fold homeobox): Essential for retinal progenitor cell (RPC) formation and optic vesicle development.
  - Pax6 (Paired box 6): A key master regulator of eye development, required for the formation of the optic vesicle and lens placode.
  - Six3 (Sine oculis homeobox 3): Suppresses Wnt signaling to allow proper anterior forebrain and eye field formation.
  - Optx2 (Orthodenticle homeobox 2, also known as Otx2): Critical for RPE and neural retina formation.

mTORC1 and Eye Field Proliferation

- mTORC1 is activated by PI3K/AKT signaling in response to growth factors such as FGF (Fibroblast Growth Factor), promoting cell proliferation and metabolic support for the expansion of the eye field.
- mTORC1 integrates BMP, Nodal, and Wnt signaling cues to modulate the balance between self-renewal and differentiation of the eye field progenitor cells.

Dysregulation and Developmental Defects

- Hyperactivation of mTORC1 can lead to abnormal expansion of retinal progenitor cells (RPCs), resulting in ocular overgrowth (megalophthalmia) or ectopic eye formation.
- Loss of mTOR function can cause microphthalmia (small eyes) or anophthalmia (absence of eyes) due to reduced progenitor proliferation and metabolic insufficiency.

Optic Vesicle Formation and Patterning: Role of mTOR in Morphogenesis

After the establishment of the eye field, the neuroepithelium invaginates to form the optic vesicles, which later give rise to the optic cup (retina and RPE) and the optic stalk (future optic nerve). Eye field specification occurs prior to optic vesicle formation, during the neural plate stage. This process is marked by the activation of eye field-specific transcription factors (EFTFs), including *Rax, Pax6, Six3, Lhx2,* and *Six6.*

Studies in *Xenopus* have demonstrated that inhibiting FGF signaling before *Lhx2* expression leads to a reduced population of eye field cells. FGF signaling is crucial for the induction—but not the maintenance—of the eye field.

Wnt/β-Catenin and mTOR Crosstalk in Optic Vesicle Development

- Wnt signaling inhibition in the anterior forebrain is essential for the emergence of the eye field.
- mTORC1 activation is required for optic vesicle expansion, promoting neural progenitor proliferation.
- Wnt/mTOR interactions regulate RPE vs. neural retina fate specification:
  - High Wnt/mTOR activity → promotes RPE differentiation.
  - Low Wnt/mTOR activity → promotes neural retina development.

Pax6 and Six3 in Lens Induction: mTOR's Role in Cellular Differentiation

- Pax6 and Six3 regulate the formation of the lens placode, which thickens to form the lens vesicle.
- mTORC1 activation by growth factors such as IGF-1 supports lens epithelial proliferation and early differentiation.

- Inhibition of mTOR disrupts lens fiber differentiation, leading to congenital aphakia (absence of a lens) or lens dysgenesis.

mTOR and Retinal Progenitor Maintenance: Integration with Notch and HIF-1α

Once the optic vesicle develops into the optic cup, the neural retina and RPE undergo further differentiation.

mTOR and Notch Signaling in Retinal Progenitor Cell (RPC) Maintenance

- Notch signaling is crucial for maintaining RPCs in a proliferative state.
- mTORC1 enhances metabolic activity and protein synthesis, ensuring RPCs remain viable for extended neurogenesis.
- Disruptions in Notch-mTOR balance can lead to retinal malformations, such as:
  - Excess mTOR activity → premature differentiation → depletion of progenitors → retinal hypoplasia.
  - Reduced mTOR activity → delayed differentiation → optic nerve coloboma.

mTORC1 and HIF-1α in Retinal Vasculogenesis

- In the hypoxic embryonic environment, HIF-1α is stabilized by mTORC1, promoting VEGF secretion for early retinal vascular development.
- mTORC1-HIF-1α signaling is critical for choroidal and retinal vascularization.
- Defective mTOR signaling results in ocular ischemia and optic nerve hypoplasia.

Final Stages of Embryonic Eye Development: mTOR in RPE Maturation and Optic Nerve Formation

- RPE Development:
  - mTORC1 interacts with Wnt signaling to guide RPE maturation, pigmentation, and metabolic function.

- Defective mTOR activity results in RPE hypoplasia, affecting photoreceptor survival.

- Optic Nerve Development:
  - mTORC1 regulates axonal growth and myelination of retinal ganglion cells (RGCs) through PI3K/AKT signaling.
  - Disruptions in mTOR signaling lead to optic nerve hypoplasia or atrophy, affecting visual transmission to the brain.

Role of mTOR in Eye Embryological Development [12]

1. Corneal Morphogenesis:
   - mTOR modulates the migration and proliferation of corneal epithelial cells, contributing to corneal morphogenesis and transparency.
2. Iris and Ciliary Body Development:
   - mTOR signaling supports the differentiation and structural development of the iris and ciliary body, which are critical for aqueous humor production and pupil function.
3. Lens Development:
   - Cell Proliferation: mTOR regulates the proliferation of lens epithelial cells by controlling the G1/S phase transition of the cell cycle.
   - Differentiation: It promotes the differentiation of lens epithelial cells into lens fiber cells, a process that requires high metabolic activity and protein synthesis, both of which are mTOR-regulated.
4. Retinal Development:
   - Neurogenesis: mTOR influences retinal progenitor cell proliferation and differentiation. It ensures the proper formation of retinal neurons and glial cells.
   - Angiogenesis: mTOR is involved in the formation of retinal vasculature by regulating vascular endothelial growth factor (VEGF) signaling.
   - Photoreceptor Development: The high metabolic demands of photoreceptor cells during their differentiation and maturation depend on mTOR-driven anabolic processes.
5. Optic Nerve Formation:
   - mTOR plays a role in axonal growth and myelination of retinal ganglion cells (RGCs), contributing to the proper formation and function of the optic nerve.

6. Regulation of Metabolism:
    - mTOR integrates signals from nutrients, growth factors, and oxygen availability to ensure energy homeostasis during the highly dynamic process of eye organogenesis.

Pathological Implications of Dysregulated mTOR in Eye Development

- Congenital Ocular Disorders: Aberrant mTOR signaling can lead to structural malformations, such as anophthalmia or microphthalmia.
- Lens Opacities: Dysregulated mTOR in lens epithelial cells may contribute to congenital cataract formation.
- Retinal Dysplasia: Overactivation of mTOR is implicated in abnormal retinal layer formation and neurodevelopmental defects.
- Vascular Anomalies: mTOR dysregulation can result in improper retinal vascularization, leading to ischemic conditions or retinal neovascularization.

Therapeutic Considerations

- Understanding mTOR's role in eye embryology highlights potential therapeutic strategies for preventing or managing congenital eye disorders.
- mTOR inhibitors, like rapamycin, may have applications in modulating overactive mTOR signaling during embryological development, but their use would require careful timing and dosing to avoid adverse effects on normal growth processes.

mTOR Complex-Specific Roles in Eye Development

The inner retina expresses high levels of mTORC1 and mTORC2 [13]

mTORC1 (mTOR Complex 1)

- Primary Functions:
    - Promotes protein synthesis, cell growth, and metabolic regulation by phosphorylating key targets such as S6 kinase (S6K) and 4E-BP1.

  - Regulates cellular energy balance by integrating signals from nutrients, growth factors, and oxygen levels.
- Specific Effects on Ocular Development:
  - Lens Fiber Differentiation: mTORC1 facilitates the high rates of protein synthesis needed for lens fiber elongation and transparency.
  - Retinal Development:
    - Photoreceptor Layer Formation: mTORC1 controls the high energy demands and protein production during the differentiation of photoreceptors.
    - Synaptic Connections: Supports synaptic development between retinal neurons by driving lipid and protein synthesis.
  - Angiogenesis: mTORC1 mediates VEGF expression in endothelial cells, ensuring proper vascularization of the retina.
- Animal Model Insights:
  - Mouse Models:
    - Conditional deletion of Raptor (a key component of mTORC1) in retinal progenitors leads to microphthalmia, underdeveloped retinal layers, and apoptosis.
    - Overactive mTORC1 causes retinal dysplasia due to excessive cell proliferation and disrupted differentiation.
  - Zebrafish Studies:
    - mTORC1 hyperactivation disturbs retinal lamination, underscoring its role in retinal layer stratification [24].

mTORC2 (mTOR Complex 2)

- Primary Functions:
  - Regulates the actin cytoskeleton, cell survival, and metabolism via downstream targets such as AKT (Ser473), SGK1, and PKCα.
- Specific Effects on Ocular Development:
  - Iris and Corneal Formation:
    - Regulates cell polarity in the epithelium of the developing cornea and iris.
  - Cell Polarity and Migration:
    - mTORC2 governs cytoskeletal dynamics required for proper migration of lens epithelial cells and retinal progenitors.

- Retinal Ganglion Cell (RGC) Axonal Growth:
    - Promotes the extension and guidance of RGC axons, contributing to the formation of the optic nerve.

- Animal Model Insights:
  - Mouse Models:
    - Rictor (mTORC2 component) deletion disrupts RGC survival, leading to optic nerve malformations.
    - Aberrant mTORC2 activity impacts lens epithelial cell polarity, causing defects in lens curvature and transparency.
  - Drosophila Studies:
    - mTORC2 dysfunction impairs eye disc development, reducing size and disrupting normal ommatidial patterns.

mTOR Pathway Interactions with Other Signaling Networks in Eye Development

1. PI3K/AKT Pathway:
   - Critical upstream regulator of both mTORC1 and mTORC2.
   - Enhances RGC axon guidance and photoreceptor survival by promoting cell survival and metabolic activity.
2. Wnt/β-Catenin Pathway:
   - Intersects with mTOR signaling during retinal neurogenesis and RPE (retinal pigment epithelium) differentiation.
   - Wnt-driven mTOR activation supports retinal progenitor cell fate determination.
3. Notch Signaling:
   - Works with mTORC1 in controlling the timing of retinal progenitor differentiation, ensuring proper layer formation.
4. HIF-1α and VEGF Pathways:
   - mTORC1 regulates HIF-1α expression under hypoxic conditions during embryogenesis, promoting VEGF-mediated vascular development.

Impact of Dysregulated mTOR Complexes in Animal Models

mTORC1 Hyperactivation

- Retinal Dysplasia: Overactivation leads to excessive proliferation of progenitors without differentiation.
- Lens Opacities: Results in abnormal protein aggregation and structural disorganization.

mTORC1 Inhibition

- Growth Arrest: Reduced retinal size and failure of lens fiber elongation due to insufficient protein synthesis.
- Cell Death: Leads to apoptosis of progenitor cells and photoreceptors.

mTORC2 Dysregulation

- Defective Optic Nerve Formation: Impaired RGC axon extension in Rictor-null models.
- Cytoskeletal Abnormalities: Disrupted epithelial integrity and morphogenesis in the cornea and lens.

Emerging Research and Applications

- Dual mTORC Modulators:
  - Fine-tuning both mTORC1 and mTORC2 activity may offer therapeutic potential for treating congenital disorders like microphthalmia and anophthalmia.
- mTOR Inhibitors in Model Systems:
  - Low-dose rapamycin has shown promise in rescuing hyperactivation phenotypes, but timing is crucial to avoid stunting development.

mTOR Pathway Interactions with Other Signaling Networks in Embryonic Eye Development

During embryogenesis, the mTOR pathway serves as a central regulator of cellular growth, metabolism, and differentiation in the developing eye. It integrates signals from multiple pathways to guide the formation of distinct ocular structures, including the retina, retinal pigment epithelium (RPE), and vasculature. Below is an elaboration of its interactions with key signaling networks in embryonic eye development [1].

1. PI3K/AKT Pathway: Essential for Retinal Progenitor Expansion and Survival [11]

   - Regulation of Retinal Ganglion Cell (RGC) Differentiation:
     During early embryonic eye development, the PI3K/AKT/mTOR axis promotes the survival and differentiation of retinal ganglion cells (RGCs), which are the first neuronal cells to form in the retina. mTORC1 enhances neurite outgrowth and axon guidance, ensuring proper connectivity between the retina and the brain.
   - Neural Retinal Progenitor (NRPC) Maintenance and Expansion:
     mTORC1, activated downstream of PI3K/AKT, supports proliferation and metabolic demands of NRPCs, ensuring a sufficient pool of progenitors before differentiation. Loss of mTOR activity during early embryogenesis leads to microphthalmia (small eye syndrome) due to reduced NRPC proliferation [8].
   - Photoreceptor Survival:
     PI3K/AKT/mTOR signaling is essential for cone and rod photoreceptor progenitor survival, protecting them from apoptosis during early eye development.

2. Wnt/β-Catenin Pathway: Coordination of Retinal Neurogenesis and RPE Development

   - Regulation of Retinal Lineage Specification [4]:
     During early embryonic stages, the Wnt/β-catenin pathway activates mTORC1 to regulate the self-renewal and differentiation of retinal progenitor cells (RPCs) into various neuronal lineages, including photoreceptors and interneurons.
   - Retinal Pigment Epithelium (RPE) Formation:
     The RPE, which originates from the optic vesicle, requires Wnt signaling for differentiation. Wnt-driven mTOR activation is necessary for pigmentation, metabolism, and maturation of the RPE, ensuring the proper support of photoreceptors later in development.
   - Defects in Wnt-mTOR Interactions:
     If Wnt/mTOR signaling is disrupted in the embryo, it can result in coloboma (failure of optic fissure closure) and defective RPE differentiation, leading to early retinal degeneration.

3. Notch Signaling: Timing of Retinal Differentiation and Layer Formation
   The balance between *transactivation* and *cis-inhibition* ensures precise spatial and temporal control of Notch activity, which is critical for tissue homeostasis, development, and differentiation (D.[6]).

   - *Transactivation* occurs when a Notch receptor interacts with a ligand (e.g., Delta-like or Jagged) presented by an adjacent cell. This interaction leads to proteolytic cleavage of Notch and the release of its intracellular domain (NICD), which translocates to the nucleus to regulate gene transcription.
   - *Cis-inhibition* happens when Notch receptors and ligands co-expressed in the same cell bind to each other, preventing receptor activation by ligands from neighboring cells. This mechanism effectively fine-tunes Notch activity and prevents excessive signaling.
     The interplay between these two mechanisms allows for intricate control of cell fate decisions, particularly in *lateral inhibition*, boundary formation, and *stem cell niche maintenance*. Disruptions in this balance are implicated in numerous pathologies, including *developmental disorders, cancer, and degenerative diseases*.
   - Maintenance of Progenitor Pools:
     In the embryonic retina, Notch signaling inhibits premature differentiation, ensuring a balance between progenitor expansion and differentiation. Notch-mTORC1 crosstalk helps coordinate the timing of retinal cell fate determination.
   - Formation of Retinal Cell Layers:
     The retina develops through a highly organized sequence of neurogenesis, where Notch ensures that progenitors remain in a proliferative state until the appropriate time for differentiation. mTORC1 integrates metabolic and growth cues to regulate this transition.
   - Developmental Disorders Associated with Dysregulation:
     If Notch or mTOR activity is abnormally high, RPCs fail to differentiate properly, leading to hyperproliferation and disorganized retinal layering, seen in congenital retinal dysplasia. Conversely, reduced mTOR activity can cause retinal hypoplasia.
4. HIF-1α and VEGF Pathways: Retinal Vascularization and Oxygen Regulation

   - Hypoxia-Driven Retinal Vasculogenesis [19]:
     During early embryogenesis, the developing eye exists in a relatively hypoxic environment. mTORC1 regulates hypoxia-inducible factor 1-alpha (HIF-1α), which promotes the formation of the hyaloid and choroidal vasculature through vascular endothelial growth factor (VEGF) signaling [21].
   - Formation of the Primary Ocular Vasculature:
     VEGF secretion, controlled by mTORC1, ensures proper choroidal and retinal capillary development, supplying nutrients to the growing retina.
   - Failure of mTOR-HIF-1α-VEGF Regulation:

- Overactivation leads to abnormal vascular proliferation, contributing to congenital disorders like persistent fetal vasculature (PFV).
- Insufficient activity can cause optic nerve hypoplasia (ONH) and ischemic retinal damage.

mTOR signaling plays a crucial role in neural stem cell (NSC) proliferation and differentiation, particularly examining the effects of rapamycin (Rapa)-mediated inhibition of the mTOR pathway. The role of NSC is highly relevant to neurodevelopmental disorders such as epilepsy and autism spectrum disorders (ASDs).

mTOR in NSC Regulation

- The mTOR pathway controls NSC self-renewal, proliferation, and lineage specification.
- mTORC1 (via S6K1/eIF4E) promotes NSC proliferation and differentiation into neurons, while mTORC2 influences cytoskeletal organization and migration.
- Disruptions in mTOR signaling are implicated in tuberous sclerosis complex (TSC), focal cortical dysplasia, epilepsy, and ASD [20].

Tuberous Sclerosis Complex (TSC)

TCS, as a prototypical mTORopathy, highlights its molecular pathogenesis and clinical variability. TSC effectively highlights its genetic basis, inheritance pattern, and incidence (A.[15]).

Here are a few key points that could be expanded or refined for clarity and completeness:

1. Genetic Basis and mTOR Hyperactivation
   - TSC1 (Hamartin) and TSC2 (Tuberin) form a complex that inhibits Rheb, a small GTPase that activates mTORC1.
   - Pathogenic variants in TSC1 or TSC2 disrupt this inhibition, leading to hyperactive mTORC1 signaling, which drives uncontrolled cell growth and tumor formation.
   - TSC2 mutations are generally associated with more severe phenotypes than TSC1 mutations.
2. Inheritance and Mosaicism
   - Autosomal dominant inheritance accounts for ~30% of cases, often with variable expressivity.
   - De novo mutations and mosaicism account for ~70% of cases, explaining sporadic presentations.

- Mosaicism leads to variable disease severity, as the mutation may not be present in all cells.

3. Epidemiology
   - The incidence of TSC is estimated to range between 1 in 5800 and 1 in 13,520 live births.
   - The prevalence in the general population is estimated to be 1 in 20,000 to 1 in 50,000 individuals, depending on diagnostic criteria and access to genetic testing.
   - Genotype-phenotype correlation: TSC2 mutations tend to result in more widespread and severe manifestations, including earlier-onset epilepsy and intellectual disability.

Key Aspects to Consider

1. Molecular Pathogenesis of TSC and mTOR Dysregulation
   - TSC1 (Hamartin) and TSC2 (Tuberin) form a GTPase-activating protein (GAP) complex that inhibits Rheb, a key activator of mTORC1.
   - Loss-of-function mutations in TSC1 or TSC2 lead to hyperactive mTORC1 signaling, causing uncontrolled cell proliferation, metabolic dysregulation, and neuronal hyperexcitability.
   - TSC2 Mutations & Disease Severity:
     - TSC2 has GAP activity, making mutations in its catalytic domain particularly pathogenic.
     - Missense mutations may retain partial function, while truncating mutations result in more severe phenotypes.
2. Genotype-Phenotype Correlation
   - TSC2 mutations generally cause a more severe phenotype than TSC1 mutations.
   - Variants in non-coding regions or less essential exons may modulate expressivity and lead to milder presentations.
   - Mosaicism and second-hit mutations influence tumor burden and neurological manifestations.
   - Penetrance is nearly complete, but expressivity varies widely, even within families, leading to variability in seizure onset, cognitive impairment, and autism spectrum disorder (ASD) risk.
3. Neurological Implications of mTOR Hyperactivation in TSC
   - Cortical Tubers: Developmental malformations leading to epilepsy.
   - Subependymal Giant Cell Astrocytoma (SEGAs): Benign brain tumors requiring mTOR-targeted therapy.

- Epilepsy & Autism: TSC is a leading cause of infantile spasms, with a high incidence of ASD (40–50%).
- Dysregulated Synaptic Plasticity: Excess mTORC1 activity impairs neuronal connectivity and cortical network balance.

PTEN (Phosphatase and Tensin Homolog)

It is a key regulator of ocular development and homeostasis, and its dysregulation leads to diverse congenital and acquired eye diseases, including retinal dystrophies, glaucoma, optic nerve pathologies, and ocular tumors. Understanding PTEN-related mechanisms provides therapeutic targets for treating PTEN-associated ocular disorders.

PTEN is a tumor suppressor gene that regulates cell growth, proliferation, and survival by antagonizing the PI3K-Akt-mTOR pathway. In ocular development, PTEN plays a crucial role in retinal, lens, and optic nerve formation, and its dysregulation is implicated in various congenital and acquired eye diseases.

PTEN in Eye Development (Embryology)

PTEN is critical for early eye field specification, progenitor proliferation, and differentiation in various ocular structures [23]:

A. Retinal Development

- PTEN regulates retinal progenitor cell (RPC) proliferation and differentiation.
- Conditional PTEN knockout (KO) models show retinal hyperplasia and disorganized retinal layers, leading to dysfunctional vision.
- Balances retinal ganglion cell (RGC) survival by inhibiting excessive Akt signaling.
- PTEN deficiency can result in retinal vascular abnormalities, contributing to persistent fetal vasculature (PFV).

B. Lens Development

- PTEN controls lens epithelial cell proliferation and prevents abnormal lens fiber differentiation.
- Loss of PTEN leads to lens epithelial hyperplasia, cataract formation, and disrupted lens transparency.
- PI3K-Akt-mTOR overactivation in PTEN-deficient lenses causes aberrant epithelial-mesenchymal transition (EMT).

C. Optic Nerve and Cornea Development

- PTEN regulates axon growth and myelination in the optic nerve by modulating Akt/mTOR signaling.
- PTEN mutations or deletions lead to optic nerve gliomas, megalencephaly, and retinal ganglion cell (RGC) dysfunction.
- In corneal development, PTEN influences epithelial stratification and wound healing, impacting corneal transparency and homeostasis.

PTEN-Related Ocular Pathologies

PTEN mutations or loss-of-function variants are associated with both congenital and acquired eye diseases.

A. PTEN Hamartoma Tumor Syndrome (PHTS) & Ocular Manifestations

- Cowden Syndrome (CS): A PTEN-related disorder with ocular findings such as conjunctival hamartomas, papillomas, and strabismus.
- Bannayan-Riley-Ruvalcaba Syndrome (BRRS): Associated with hypertelorism, retinal vascular anomalies, and megalencephaly.

B. PTEN Loss and Retinal Diseases

- PTEN loss in retinal cells leads to retinal hypertrophy, RGC loss, and retinal vascular malformations.
- Linked to retinal dystrophies, macular edema, and proliferative vitreoretinopathy (PVR).
- Plays a role in age-related macular degeneration (AMD) and diabetic retinopathy (DR) via PI3K-Akt-mediated vascular dysfunction.

C. PTEN and Glaucoma

- PTEN loss contributes to glaucoma pathogenesis by promoting retinal ganglion cell apoptosis and increasing trabecular meshwork fibrosis.
- PTEN deficiency enhances susceptibility to optic nerve damage in normal-tension glaucoma (NTG) and primary open-angle glaucoma (POAG).

D. PTEN and Ocular Tumors

- Uveal Melanoma: PTEN mutations are frequently found in aggressive, metastatic cases with PI3K-Akt-mTOR overactivation.
- Retinoblastoma: PTEN loss cooperates with RB1 mutations to drive tumor progression.
- Gliomas of the Optic Nerve: PTEN deletion leads to neurofibromatosis-associated gliomas, linked to NF1 mutations.

Therapeutic Implications

- mTOR Inhibitors (Rapamycin, Everolimus): Target PTEN-deficient ocular tumors and retinal diseases.
- PI3K Inhibitors (Buparlisib, Alpelisib): Potential treatments for uveal melanoma and retinal vascular diseases.
- Gene Therapy: PTEN re-expression strategies for retinal neuroprotection and optic nerve regeneration.

mTORC1 Gene Deletion

Disruption of eye development has been demonstrated through Rptor gene deletion, whereby loss of mTORC1 signaling in retinal progenitor cells results in impaired retinal lamination and defective embryologic organization of the eye [18].

Conditional deletion of Rptor gene in retinal progenitor cells leads to decreased proliferation and increased apoptosis during embryogenesis. These developmental deficits preceded structural abnormalities in adult retinas, most notably the fusion of the outer and inner nuclear layers and the absence of an outer plexiform layer.

Despite Rptor ablation, ganglion cell axons exhibit normal segregation at the optic chiasm, with both contralateral and ipsilateral projections showing overlapping termination patterns within several retinorecipient nuclei. Together, these defects in retinal structure and visual pathway organization contributes to impaired visually mediated behaviors.

During embryonic eye development, mTOR signaling integrates key transcription factors (Rx, Pax6, Six3, Optx2) with major pathways (BMP, Nodal, Wnt, Notch, and HIF-1α/VEGF) to orchestrate:

1. Eye field specification in the anterior neural plate.
2. Optic vesicle formation and retinal progenitor expansion.
3. Proliferation, differentiation, and vascularization of the retina and RPE.
4. Formation of the lens and optic nerve.

Disruptions in these interactions can result in congenital ocular anomalies such as microphthalmia, coloboma, RPE hypoplasia, retinal dysplasia, and optic nerve malformations. Understanding the role of mTOR in these processes offers potential therapeutic targets for congenital and developmental eye disorders.

mTOR (mechanistic Target of Rapamycin) plays a significant role in ocular embryological development, as it is integral to regulating cell growth, proliferation, differentiation, and metabolism. These processes are critical during the development of the eye, which requires precise spatial and temporal coordination of signaling pathways.

Role of MAPK Signaling in Eye Development

The mitogen-activated protein kinase (MAPK) signaling pathway plays a crucial role in eye development, regulating processes such as progenitor cell proliferation, differentiation, apoptosis, and tissue patterning. The MAPK cascade transmits extracellular signals via RAF-MEK-ERK, JNK, and p38 kinases, influencing various stages of ocular development [16].

Key Functions of MAPK in Eye Development

1. Regulation of Retinal Progenitor Cells
   - MAPK/ERK signaling is critical for retinal progenitor cell proliferation and survival.
   - Activation of ERK1/2 supports the expansion of progenitor pools and prevents premature differentiation.
   - ERK inhibition leads to reduced proliferation and increased apoptosis in retinal progenitor cells.
2. Lens Development and Differentiation
   - MAPK signaling contributes to lens induction, fiber cell differentiation, and lens epithelial cell survival.
   - FGF-mediated MAPK activation is essential for lens fiber differentiation.
   - Disruption of MAPK pathways results in defective lens development and cataract formation.
3. Optic Cup and Retinal Patterning
   - ERK1/2 activation in the developing optic cup influences dorsal-ventral patterning and cell fate determination.
   - Defects in MAPK signaling lead to abnormal optic cup morphogenesis, potentially contributing to conditions like microphthalmia.
4. Photoreceptor and RPE (Retinal Pigment Epithelium) Development
   - MAPK regulates retinal cell fate decisions, particularly in photoreceptor and retinal pigment epithelium (RPE) differentiation.
   - MAPK activation through growth factors (e.g., IGF-1, EGF, FGF) supports photoreceptor survival and maturation.
5. Axon Guidance and Optic Nerve Development
   - MAPK signaling modulates retinal ganglion cell (RGC) survival and axon guidance toward the optic chiasm.
   - ERK and JNK pathways help regulate neuronal growth cone dynamics and synaptic connectivity.

6. Regulation of Apoptosis and Neuroprotection
   - MAPK signaling protects against oxidative stress and apoptosis in developing retinal cells.
   - Dysregulation can lead to retinal degeneration and congenital ocular anomalies.

Clinical Relevance

- MAPK mutations are linked to congenital eye disorders such as coloboma, anophthalmia, and microphthalmia.
- Dysregulation of MAPK contributes to retinopathy of prematurity (ROP), glaucoma, and retinal dystrophies.
- MAPK-targeting therapies (e.g., MEK inhibitors) are being explored for treating ocular malignancies like uveal melanoma.

Ephrin-Eph Signaling

It plays a crucial role in eye development, particularly in the formation of the retina and the establishment of retinotopic maps, which ensure proper spatial organization of neural connections [17].

Key functions include:

1. Retinal Axon Guidance: Ephrins and Eph receptors guide retinal ganglion cell (RGC) axons to their correct targets in the brain, such as the optic tectum (in non-mammals) or superior colliculus (in mammals), through repulsive or attractive cues.
2. Retinotopic Mapping: They help create precise spatial maps by regulating the ordered projection of RGCs from the retina to the brain, ensuring that neighboring retinal cells connect to neighboring target cells.
3. Boundary Formation: Ephrin-Eph interactions establish boundaries between different regions of the eye, such as the dorsal and ventral retina, critical for proper visual processing.
4. Cell Sorting and Patterning: They contribute to the organization and differentiation of retinal cells during development.

Dysregulation of Ephrin-Eph signaling can lead to visual system defects, such as misrouted axons or improper retinotopic maps, highlighting its importance in eye development.

Bibliography

1. Albano. Repurposing development genes for axonal regeneration following injury: examining the roles of Wnt signaling. Front Cell Dev Biol. 2024; https://doi.org/10.3389/fcell.2024.1417928.
2. Azuma. Sonic hedgehog determines early retinal development and adjusts eyeball architecture. Int J Mol Sci. 2025; https://doi.org/10.3390/ijms26020496.
3. Callan. TGF-β Signaling pathways in the development of diabetic retinopathy. Int J Mol Sci. 2024; https://doi.org/10.3390/ijms25053052.
4. Campos. Non-canonical Wnt pathway expression in the developing mouse and human retina. Exp Eye Res. 2024;244 https://doi.org/10.1016/j.exer.2024.109947.
5. Casey. Eye morphogenesis in vertebrates. Annu Rev Vis Sci. 2023; https://doi.org/10.1146/annurev-vision-100720-111125.
6. Chen D. A model of notch signalling control of angiogenesis: evidence of a role for notch ligand heterodimerization. PLoS Comput Biol. 2025; https://doi.org/10.1371/journal.pcbi.1012825.
7. Diacou. Cell fate decisions, transcription factors and signaling during early retinal development. Prog Retin Eye Res. 2022;91 https://doi.org/10.1016/j.preteyeres.2022.101093.
8. Durate-Silva. Chemical signaling in the developing avian retina: focus on cyclic AMP and AKT-dependent pathways. Front Cell Dev Biol. 2022; https://doi.org/10.3389/fcell.2022.1058925.
9. Edirisinghe. Pathology and therapeutic significance of fibroblast growth factors. Targets. 2025; https://doi.org/10.3390/targets3010005.
10. Guo R. Roles of Wnt signaling pathway and ROR2 receptor in embryonic development: an update review article. Epi Insights. 2022; https://doi.org/10.1177/25168657211064232.
11. Kalous. A role of PI3K/Akt Signaling in oocyte maturation and early embryo development. Cells. 2023; https://doi.org/10.3390/cells12141830.
12. Karami. Signaling pathway regulators in preimplantation embryos. J Mol Histol. 2024; https://doi.org/10.1007/s10735-024-10338-7.
13. Losiewicz. mTORC1 and mTORC2 expression in inner retinal neurons and glial cells. Exp Eye Res. 2020,197 https://doi.org/10.1016/j.exer.2020.108131.
14. Makrides. Jack of all trades, master of each: the diversity of fibroblast growth factor signalling in eye development. Open Biol. The Royal Scociety Publishing. 2022; https://doi.org/10.1098/rsob.210265.
15. Man A. The genetics of tuberous sclerosis complex and related mTORopathies: current understanding and future directions. Genes. 2024; https://doi.org/10.3390/genes15030332.
16. Moustardas. MAPK pathways in ocular pathophysiology: potential therapeutic drugs and challenges. Cells. 2023; https://doi.org/10.3390/cells12040617.
17. Murcia-Belmante. EphA4 mediates ephrinB1-dependent adhesion in retinal ganglion cells. J Neurosci. 2025; https://doi.org/10.1523/JNEUROSCI.0043-24.2024.
18. Nord. Reduced mTORC1-signaling in progenitor cells leads to retinal lamination deficits. Dev Dyn. 2024; https://doi.org/10.1002/dvdy.707.
19. Plastino. MicroRNAs and the HIF/VEGF axis in ocular neovascular diseases. Acta Ophthalmol. 2021; https://doi.org/10.1111/aos.14845.
20. Romanyuk. mTOR pathway inhibition alters proliferation as well as differentiation of neural stem cells. Front Cell Neurosci. 2024; https://doi.org/10.3389/fncel.2024.1298182.
21. Shaw. VEGF signaling: role in angiogenesis and beyond. Biochim Biophys Acta. 2024;1879(2) https://doi.org/10.1016/j.bbcan.2024.189079.
22. Summers. Functional integration of eye tissues and refractive eye development: mechanisms and pathways. Exp Eye Res. 2021;209 https://doi.org/10.1016/j.exer.2021.108693.

23. Touahri. Pten regulates endocytic trafficking of cell adhesion and Wnt signaling molecules to pattern the retina. Cell Rep. 2024; https://doi.org/10.1016/j.celrep.2024.114005.
24. Zibetti. Deciphering the retinal epigenome during development, disease and reprogramming: advancements, challenges and perspectives. Cells. 2022; https://doi.org/10.3390/cells11050806.

Chapter 4
mTOR Effect on Conjunctiva

Contents

Abstract The mTOR pathway has significant effects on the conjunctiva, influencing its development, homeostasis, and response to various pathological conditions. The conjunctiva, being a dynamic tissue with roles in ocular surface protection, immune surveillance, and tear production, is influenced by mTOR signaling. The mTOR pathway is a central regulator of conjunctival homeostasis and pathological conditions, influencing epithelial repair, fibroblast proliferation, angiogenesis, immune modulation, and tumor growth. Targeting mTOR presents therapeutic potential in conditions such as dry eye syndrome, pterygium, fibrosis, malignancies, and thyroid-associated ophthalmopathy (TAO), offering new avenues for intervention in ocular surfaces and orbital diseases.

K. T. Moazed, *mTOR Signaling in Ophthalmology*,
https://doi.org/10.1007/978-3-032-05044-1_4

Discussion

The mechanistic target of rapamycin (mTOR) is a key regulator of conjunctival hemostasis, orchestrating a complex interplay of cellular and molecular processes that maintain vascular stability, fibroblast activity, epithelial integrity, and immune homeostasis. Through its regulation of angiogenesis, fibroblast proliferation, and epithelial repair, mTOR plays a critical role in sustaining conjunctival homeostasis and facilitating effective responses to injury.

In vascular stability, mTOR modulates endothelial cell function and angiogenesis, ensuring proper blood supply and oxygenation to the conjunctival tissue. Its role in fibroblast activity is equally significant, as it governs fibroblast proliferation, extracellular matrix production, and tissue remodeling, all of which are crucial for wound healing and maintaining the conjunctival structure.

Epithelial integrity is another fundamental aspect influenced by mTOR, as it regulates epithelial cell proliferation, differentiation, and barrier function, thereby preventing excessive tissue damage and promoting regeneration. Additionally, mTOR has a key role in immune regulation, balancing pro-inflammatory and anti-inflammatory responses in the conjunctiva. This function is particularly relevant in conditions such as conjunctival fibrosis, dry eye syndrome, and other ocular surface disorders, where dysregulated inflammation contributes to disease progression.

Given its multifaceted role in conjunctival repair and inflammation, targeted modulation of mTOR signaling presents a potential therapeutic strategy for various ocular surface diseases. Inhibiting or fine-tuning mTOR activity could help mitigate pathological fibrosis, excessive angiogenesis, or chronic inflammation, offering novel approaches for managing conjunctival disorders.

Key Roles of mTOR in Conjunctival Hemostasis

mTOR in Conjunctival Hemostasis

- Hemostasis in the conjunctiva is essential for maintaining tissue integrity, vascular stability, and immune homeostasis. mTOR (mechanistic target of rapamycin), a key regulator of cell growth and metabolism, plays a significant role in multiple roles [15].

Goblet Cell Maintenance

- mTOR supports the production and secretion of mucins by goblet cells.
- This activity is crucial for maintaining the tear film and protecting the ocular surface.

Immune Modulation

- mTOR regulates immune cell activity and cytokine production, controlling inflammation in conjunctiva, particularly T-cell activation and macrophage responses, contributing to immune surveillance and inflammation.
- Controlling and preventing excessive immune activation. Disruptions in mTOR signaling contribute to pathological conditions of the conjunctiva.
- Other mTOR-related conditions include dry eye disease, pterygium, conjunctival fibrosis, malignancies, and thyroid-associated ophthalmopathy (TAO).

Regulation of Angiogenesis and Vascular Integrity

- mTOR, particularly mTORC1, controls endothelial cell proliferation and migration, essential for maintaining vascular homeostasis in the conjunctiva.
- Activation of mTOR enhances VEGF (vascular endothelial growth factor) signaling, promoting new blood vessel formation, which is critical for maintaining conjunctival microcirculation and conjunctival repair after injury.
- Excessive mTOR activation may lead to pathological angiogenesis, contributing to conditions such as pterygium or conjunctival hyperemia.

Fibroblast Proliferation and Wound Healing

- mTOR regulates conjunctival fibroblast proliferation and differentiation, influencing extracellular matrix (ECM) remodeling.
- After injury, mTOR signaling supports conjunctival healing by driving fibroblast activation and collagen deposition.
- However, dysregulated mTOR activity may promote fibrotic responses, leading to excessive scarring or conditions like conjunctival fibrosis.

Epithelial Repair and Barrier Function

- The conjunctival epithelium relies on mTOR for cell survival, proliferation, and migration.
- mTORC1 activation supports epithelial cell growth and repair, ensuring the restoration of the ocular surface following injury or inflammation.
- Inhibiting mTOR (e.g., with rapamycin) can slow epithelial proliferation, which may be beneficial in conditions involving hyperproliferative disorders, but could delay wound healing in cases of trauma.

Inflammatory Regulation and Immune Modulation

- mTOR is a key modulator of immune responses in the conjunctiva.
- It influences macrophage polarization and cytokine production, affecting inflammation and immune-mediated conjunctival diseases.
- Inhibiting mTOR can suppress inflammatory responses, which is useful for conditions like allergic conjunctivitis or autoimmune ocular surface diseases.

Pathological Implications of Dysregulated mTOR in the Conjunctiva Diseases

Here, we explore the role of mTOR in some of the conjunctiva's most common conditions, highlighting its regulatory influence on cellular processes such as proliferation, inflammation, fibrosis, and angiogenesis. The mechanistic target of rapamycin (mTOR) signaling pathway plays a crucial role in maintaining conjunctival homeostasis, and its dysregulation has been implicated in various pathological conditions. These include:

1. Dry eye syndrome (DES)
2. Allergic conjunctivitis
3. Pterygium
4. Conjunctival fibrosis
5. Conjunctival pemphigoid
6. Conjunctival malignancies
7. Thyroid-associated ophthalmopathy (TAO) (Fig. 4.1)

mTOR in Dry Eye Syndrome (DES)

mTOR influences epithelial cell survival, mucin production, and autophagy, all of which are crucial for tear film stability. Dysregulated mTOR signaling has been linked to increased oxidative stress and inflammation, exacerbating ocular surface damage in DES.

Dysregulated mTOR signaling in goblet cells can reduce mucin production, exacerbating dry eye symptoms. Hyperactivation of mTOR in immune cells can promote chronic inflammation in the conjunctiva (Fig. 4.2).

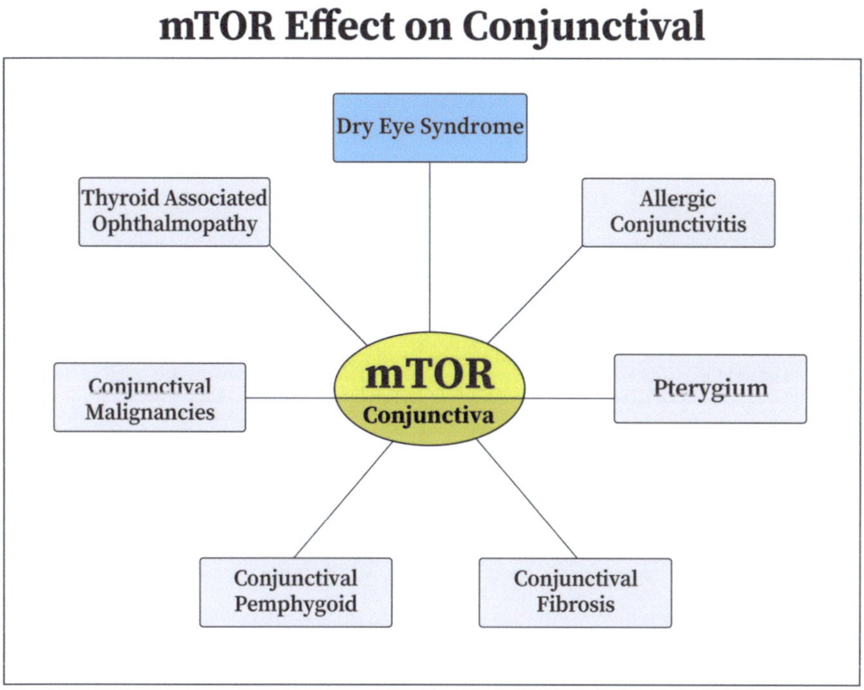

Fig. 4.1 The image above represents the direct effect of mTOR on various pathological conditions of conjunctiva

Pathophysiology Highlights

- Dry eye disease involves chronic inflammation, epithelial damage, and tear film instability.
- Dysregulated mTOR signaling can impair conjunctival goblet cell function, reducing mucin production and exacerbating tear film dysfunction.
- Hyperactive mTOR in immune cells enhances pro-inflammatory cytokine release (e.g., IL-6 and TNF-α), worsening ocular surface inflammation.

Dry eye disease involves ocular surface inflammation, tear film instability, and reduced mucin production. mTOR is a key regulator in these processes.

mTOR's Role in DED Pathogenesis

1. *Goblet Cell Dysfunction:*
    - mTORC1 activity is essential for goblet cell proliferation and mucin (e.g., MUC5AC) production.

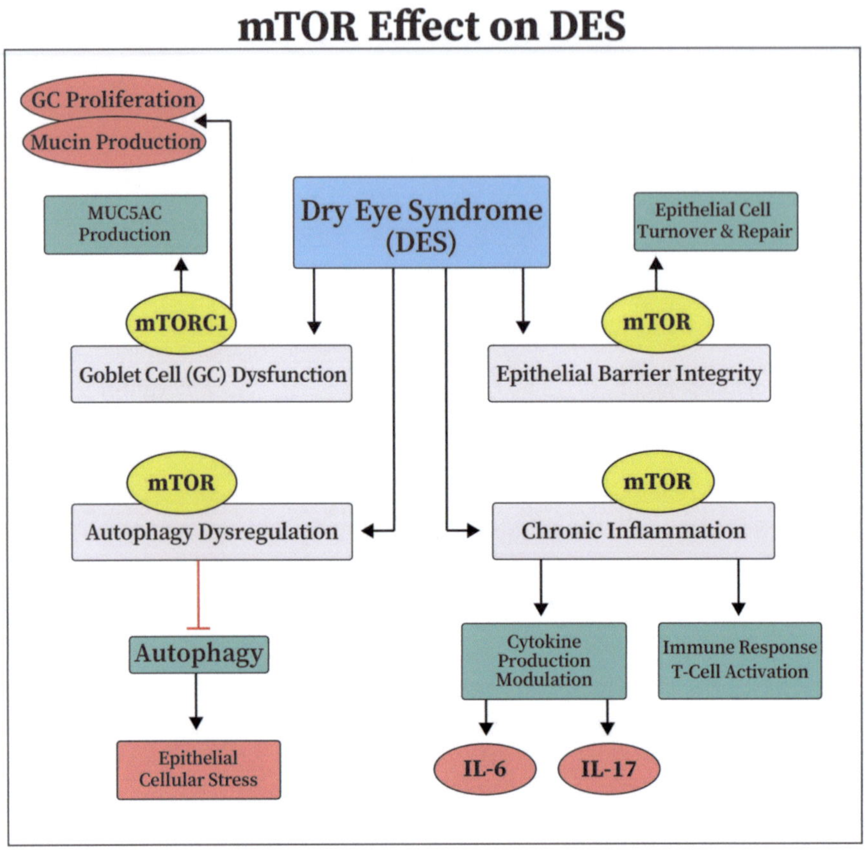

Fig. 4.2 The image above represents the mTOR effect on different aspects of dry eye syndome

- In chronic dry eye, mTORC1 dysregulation leads to impaired goblet cell differentiation and reduced mucin secretion, worsening tear film instability.

2. *Epithelial Barrier Integrity:*

   - mTOR regulates epithelial cell turnover and repair. Hyperactivation may cause excessive proliferation, while reduced mTOR activity compromises epithelial regeneration.

3. *Chronic Inflammation:*

   - mTOR influences immune responses by modulating cytokine production (e.g., IL-6 and IL-17) and T-cell activation.
   - Overactive mTORC1 amplifies inflammatory pathways in conjunctival epithelial cells and immune cells, perpetuating DED symptoms.

4. *Autophagy Dysregulation:*
   - mTOR suppresses autophagy under hyperactivated conditions, leading to cellular stress in the conjunctiva and corneal epithelium.

Therapeutic Implications for DED

1. *mTOR Inhibitors:*
   - Low-dose *rapamycin* or topical mTOR modulators could restore goblet cell function and suppress inflammation.
   - Targeting mTORC1 might balance epithelial cell turnover and improve mucin production.
2. *Anti-inflammatory Strategies:*
   - Therapies targeting mTOR-regulated cytokines (e.g., IL-6 inhibitors) could mitigate chronic inflammation in DED.

mTOR Role in Allergic Conjunctivitis

In allergic inflammation, mTOR modulates immune cell activation and cytokine production. Inhibition of mTOR has been shown to attenuate mast cell degranulation and reduce pro-inflammatory cytokines, suggesting a potential role in controlling chronic allergic conjunctivitis.

mTOR plays a key role in allergic conjunctivitis by enhancing Th2 immune responses, mast cell activation, vascular permeability, mucin secretion, and tissue remodeling. Targeting mTOR may provide a novel therapeutic approach to modulate allergic inflammation in the conjunctiva. mTOR modulates mast cell activity and inflammatory mediator release, which are central to allergic responses in the conjunctiva (Fig. 4.3).

The mechanistic target of rapamycin (mTOR) plays a significant role in allergic conjunctivitis (AC) by modulating immune responses, inflammation, and tissue remodeling in the conjunctiva. Its involvement can be summarized as follows:

1. Regulation of Immune Cells in Allergic Responses
   - mTOR regulates the activation and differentiation of T-helper 2 (Th2) cells, which are central to allergic responses.
   - Activation of the mTORC1 pathway promotes Th2-mediated cytokine release (IL-4, IL-5, and IL-13), leading to eosinophil recruitment and mast cell activation.
   - mTORC2 supports the survival and function of mast cells, which degranulate upon allergen exposure and release histamine, tryptase, and other mediators.

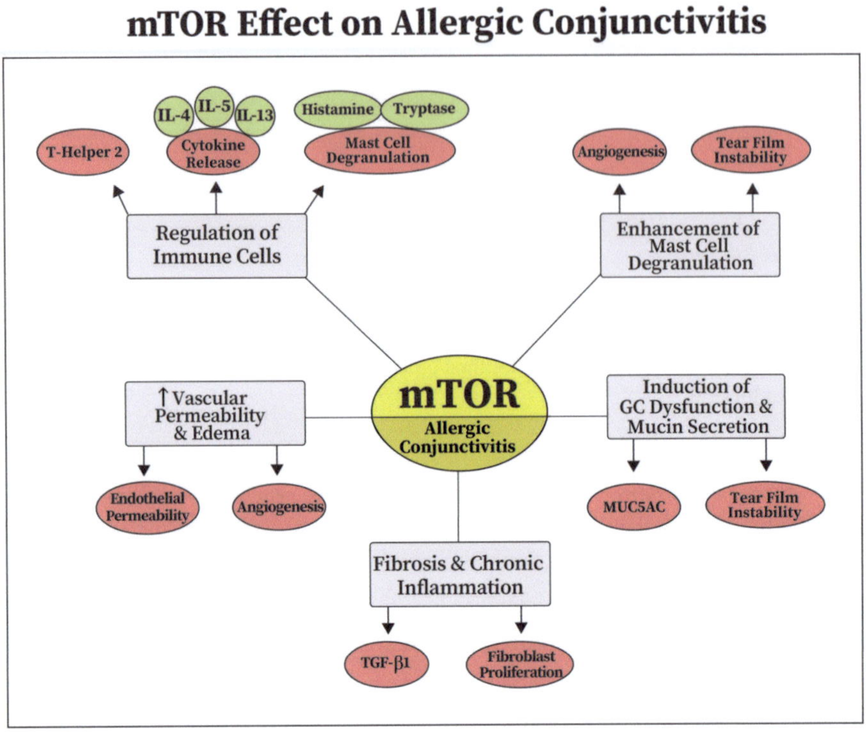

Fig. 4.3 The image above represents the direct effect of mTOR on various pathological conditions of conjunctiva

2. Enhancement of Mast Cell Degranulation
   - mTOR signaling modulates FcεRI (high-affinity IgE receptor) activation in mast cells, amplifying their degranulation response upon allergen exposure.
   - Inhibition of mTOR using rapamycin reduces histamine and inflammatory mediator release, dampening the allergic response.
3. Increased Vascular Permeability and Edema
   - mTORC1 activation in endothelial cells enhances vascular permeability, leading to conjunctival redness, swelling, and tear film instability.
   - It also promotes angiogenesis, contributing to chronic conjunctival changes in severe allergic conjunctivitis.
4. Induction of Goblet Cell Dysfunction and Mucin Secretion
   - mTOR influences the function of conjunctival goblet cells, which secrete mucin (MUC5AC) to maintain tear film stability.
   - Dysregulated mTOR signaling leads to excessive mucin production or depletion, worsening ocular surface irritation and contributing to the itchy, watery eyes seen in allergic conjunctivitis.

5. Fibrosis and Chronic Inflammation in Severe Forms
    - In chronic allergic conjunctivitis (e.g., vernal keratoconjunctivitis and atopic keratoconjunctivitis), persistent mTOR activation promotes fibroblast proliferation, extracellular matrix deposition, and conjunctival fibrosis.
    - TGF-β1-induced fibrosis is partially mediated through mTOR, linking allergic inflammation to conjunctival remodeling.

Potential Therapeutic Implications

- Rapamycin (mTOR inhibitor) has shown anti-inflammatory and anti-allergic effects by suppressing mast cell degranulation and Th2 cytokine production.
- Topical or systemic mTOR inhibitors could reduce allergic conjunctivitis severity, particularly in steroid-resistant cases.

mTOR Role in Pterygium

Pterygium is characterized by fibrovascular overgrowth extending onto the cornea, driven by UV-induced oxidative stress and chronic inflammation. Aberrant mTOR activation contributes to fibrovascular proliferation, epithelial–mesenchymal transition (EMT), and angiogenesis in pterygium development. Targeting mTOR has been proposed as a potential therapeutic approach to prevent recurrence after surgical excision (Fig. 4.4).

mTORC activation promotes fibroblast proliferation, angiogenesis, and ECM deposition, contributing to pterygium growth. VEGF upregulation via mTOR leads to increased vascularization, supporting pterygium progression. The functions of AMPK/mTOR signaling in TGF-β1-induced pterygium fibroblast proliferation and transdifferentiation have been well documented [3].

The AMPK/mTOR signaling pathway plays a regulatory role in TGF-β1-driven processes in human pterygium fibroblasts (HPFs), influencing both proliferation and transdifferentiation. While TGF-β1 activates mTOR to promote fibroblast growth, AMPK acts as a negative regulator. Modulating this pathway presents a potential strategy for therapeutic intervention in pterygium, possibly reducing its recurrence after surgical excision. Risk factors for pterygium and latest research progress on major pathogenesis of pterygium are discussed in the literature [5].

The long noncoding RNA FOXD2-AS1 (FOXD2 antisense RNA 1) is implicated in recurrent pterygium through an epigenetic and post-transcriptional regulatory mechanism involving H3K27 acetylation, VEGF-A expression, and miR-205-5p.

The epigenetic–post-transcriptional axis is crucial in pterygium recurrence and suggests FOXD2-AS1 and miR-205-5p as potential therapeutic targets [13].

H3K27 Acetylation-Induced Activation of FOXD2-AS1

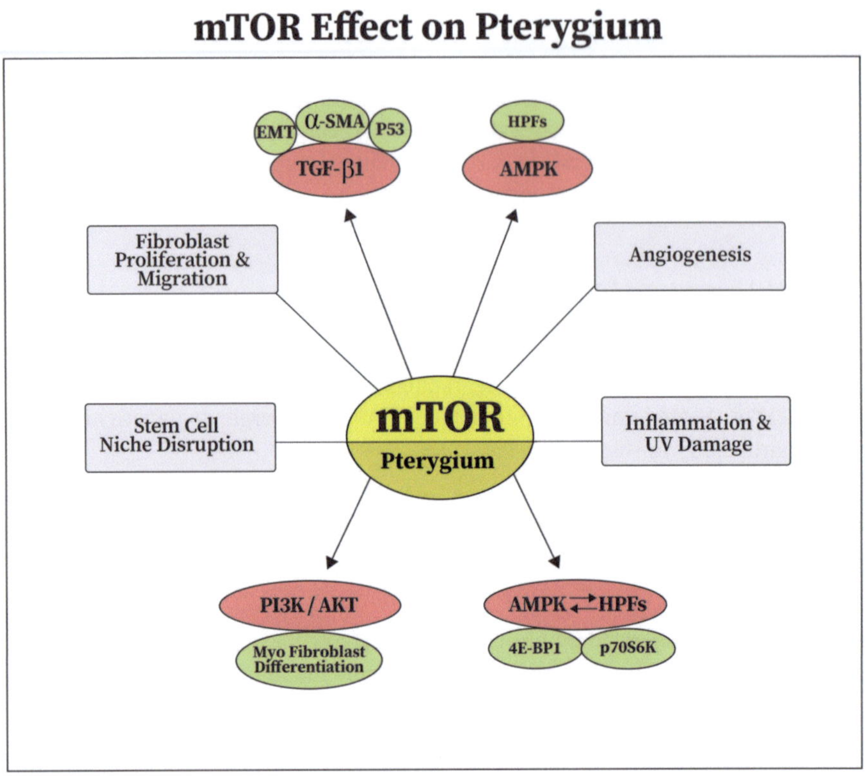

Fig. 4.4 The image above represents the direct effect of mTOR on various pathological conditions of conjunctiva

- Histone H3 lysine 27 acetylation (H3K27ac) is an epigenetic modification associated with active gene transcription.
- In recurrent pterygium, H3K27ac upregulates FOXD2-AS1, enhancing its transcription and function.

FOXD2-AS1 as a Competing Endogenous RNA (ceRNA)

- FOXD2-AS1 acts as a miRNA sponge, binding to miR-205-5p and preventing it from targeting its downstream mRNA.

Regulation of VEGF-A Expression

- miR-205-5p normally suppresses VEGF-A (vascular endothelial growth factor-A), which is a key player in angiogenesis and fibrosis.
- By sponging miR-205-5p, FOXD2-AS1 relieves repression on VEGF-A, leading to increased VEGF-A expression.

Impact on Recurrent Pterygium

- Enhanced VEGF-A expression promotes abnormal angiogenesis, fibrovascular proliferation, and recurrence of pterygium after surgical excision.
- This mechanism contributes to high recurrence rates due to excessive wound healing and fibrovascular tissue growth.

Key Mechanisms

1. *TGF-β1 as a Driver of Fibrosis and Transdifferentiation:*
   - TGF-β1 is a major pro-fibrotic cytokine that induces epithelial-to-mesenchymal transition (EMT) and fibroblast-to-myofibroblast transdifferentiation in HPFs.
   - It promotes increased expression of α-SMA (α-smooth muscle actin) and extracellular matrix (ECM) components, contributing to fibrosis and the progression of pterygium.
   - P53 and mTOR in TGF-β1-induced pterygium causes fibroblast proliferation and transdifferentiation [14].
2. *AMPK Activation as an Antagonist to mTOR:*
   - AMPK serves as an energy sensor and is activated in response to cellular stress or low ATP levels.
   - Activation of AMPK negatively regulates mTOR signaling, thereby inhibiting cell proliferation and metabolic activity.
   - In HPFs, AMPK activation may suppress TGF-β1-induced proliferation and differentiation, preventing excessive fibroblast activation.
3. *mTOR Pathway and TGF-β1-Induced Proliferation:*
   - The mechanistic target of rapamycin (mTOR) functions as a central regulator of cell growth and metabolism.
   - TGF-β1 activates mTOR via PI3K/Akt signaling, leading to enhanced fibroblast proliferation and myofibroblast differentiation.
   - This contributes to increased tissue remodeling and the growth of pterygial tissue.
4. *Crosstalk Between AMPK and mTOR in HPFs:*
   - AMPK activation inhibits mTORC1 activity, reducing the expression of downstream pro-growth effectors like p70S6K and 4E-BP1, thereby suppressing proliferation.
   - Conversely, TGF-β1-driven activation of mTOR may override AMPK-mediated suppression, promoting HPF proliferation and transdifferentiation.

5. *Potential Therapeutic Implications:*
   - Rapamycin (mTOR inhibitor) could reduce TGF-β1-induced proliferation in HPFs, slowing pterygium progression.
   - AMPK activators (e.g., metformin and AICAR) might counteract TGF-β1 effects by reducing mTOR signaling and suppressing fibroblast transdifferentiation.
   - Targeting the AMPK/mTOR axis could offer a novel approach for preventing fibrovascular tissue overgrowth in pterygium.

mTOR's Role in Pterygium Pathogenesis

1. *Fibroblast Proliferation and Migration:*
   - mTORC1 drives fibroblast proliferation and extracellular matrix (ECM) production in the conjunctiva, contributing to pterygium growth.
   - mTORC2 regulates cytoskeletal dynamics, enabling fibroblast migration and pterygium progression.
2. *Angiogenesis:*
   - mTOR promotes VEGF expression, driving neovascularization in pterygium tissues. VEGF-mediated vascularization is critical for lesion growth.
3. *Inflammation and UV Damage:*
   - mTOR amplifies inflammatory responses through cytokine production and oxidative stress pathways, particularly after UV-induced DNA damage.
   - Reduced autophagy due to mTOR hyperactivation exacerbates oxidative stress, leading to further tissue damage and fibrosis.
4. *Stem Cell Niche Disruption:*
   - Dysregulated mTOR affects the conjunctival stem cell niche, impairing epithelial repair and contributing to abnormal tissue proliferation.

Therapeutic Implications for Pterygium

1. *mTOR Inhibitors:*
   - Rapamycin and related drugs can suppress fibroblast proliferation, ECM deposition, and VEGF-driven angiogenesis.
   - Topical formulations of mTOR inhibitors are being investigated for limiting pterygium recurrence post-surgery.

2. *Anti-VEGF Therapy:*
   - Combining mTOR inhibitors with anti-VEGF agents could enhance efficacy in reducing vascularization and lesion growth.
3. *UV Protection:*
   - UV-induced mTOR activation highlights the importance of UV-blocking measures in preventing pterygium progression.

mTOR Role in Conjunctival Fibrosis (Ocular Cicatricial Diseases)

mTOR plays a central role in fibroblast proliferation and extracellular matrix (ECM) deposition, contributing to scarring in conjunctival fibrosis. In conditions such as ocular cicatricial pemphigoid, mTOR inhibition may help mitigate progressive conjunctival scarring.

Overactivation of mTOR, particularly mTORC1, leads to fibroblast proliferation and extracellular matrix deposition, contributing to conjunctival scarring in diseases such as ocular cicatricial pemphigoid or Stevens–Johnson's syndrome (Fig. 4.5).

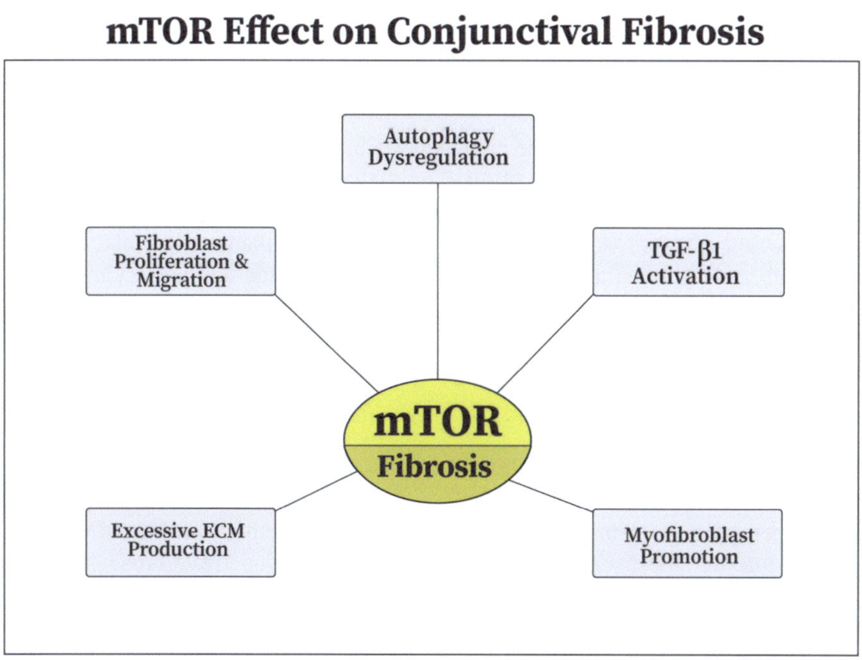

Fig. 4.5 The image above represents the direct effect of mTOR on various pathological pathways of inducing conjunctival fibrosis

mTOR in Conjunctival Fibrosis

- TGF-β1-induced fibroblast activation is mediated by mTORC1, promoting myofibroblast differentiation and excessive ECM production.
- Autophagy dysregulation due to mTOR hyperactivation contributes to fibrotic tissue remodeling.

Therapeutic Implications:

- Rapamycin and other mTOR inhibitors can reduce fibroblast proliferation and prevent excessive fibrosis.
- Targeting mTOR in conjunction with antifibrotic agents may enhance conjunctival healing while minimizing scarring.

Pathophysiology:

- Conjunctival fibrosis occurs in conditions like ocular cicatricial pemphigoid (OCP), Stevens–Johnson's syndrome (SJS), and postsurgical scarring (glaucoma filtering surgery).

mTOR Role in Conjunctival Pemphigoid

mTOR plays a critical role in the pathogenesis of ocular pemphigoid, contributing to fibroblast-driven conjunctival fibrosis, epithelial dysfunction, chronic inflammation, and pathological angiogenesis. Targeting the mTOR pathway may offer a novel therapeutic approach to reduce fibrosis, control inflammation, and improve epithelial healing, potentially delaying disease progression and preserving vision. There are studies on small molecules to inhibit the fibrotic response of conjunctival fibroblasts by regulating the checkpoint kinase 1/*P53* and *PI3K*/*AKT* pathways [4] (Fig. 4.6).

Role of mTOR in Ocular Pemphigoid

Ocular pemphigoid, primarily seen in mucous membrane pemphigoid (MMP), is a chronic autoimmune disease that leads to progressive conjunctival fibrosis, scarring, and blindness if left untreated. The mTOR (mechanistic target of rapamycin) pathway plays a crucial role in fibroblast activation, epithelial healing, immune modulation, and inflammation, all of which contribute to disease progression.

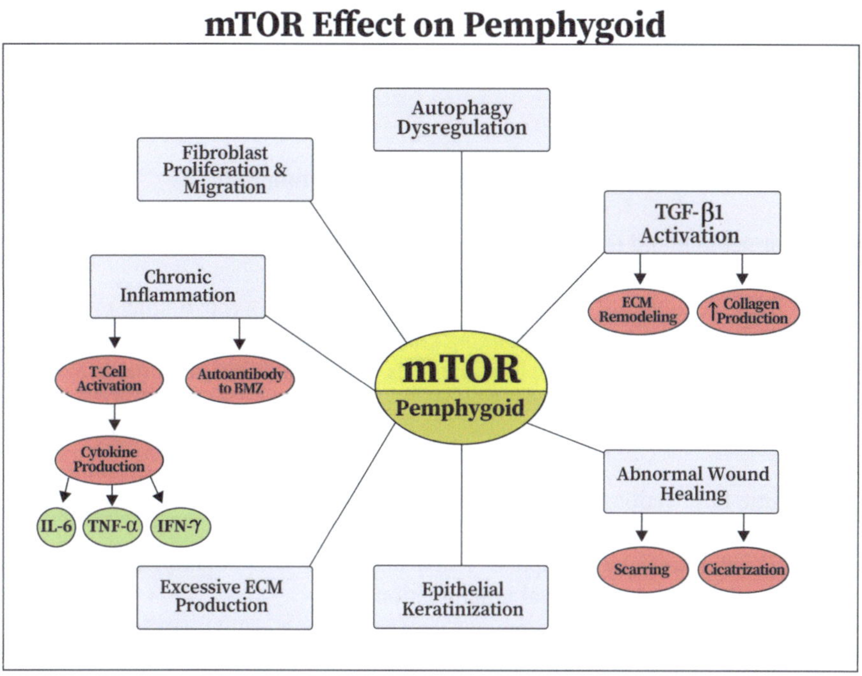

Fig. 4.6 The image above represents the direct effect of mTOR on multiple pathological pathways involved in the progression of conjunctival pemphigoid

mTOR in fibroblast activation and conjunctival fibrosis inhibition of mTOR differently modulates planar and subepithelial fibrogenesis in human conjunctival fibroblasts [12].

The hallmark of ocular pemphigoid is persistent conjunctival inflammation, leading to fibroblast activation and excessive extracellular matrix (ECM) deposition.

- mTORC1 signaling promotes fibroblast proliferation and differentiation into myofibroblasts, which contribute to subepithelial scarring and cicatrization.
- TGF-β1-mediated mTOR activation enhances collagen production and ECM remodeling, worsening conjunctival fibrosis.
- mTOR dysregulation impairs autophagy, which normally degrades excessive fibrotic tissue, exacerbating conjunctival scarring.

mTOR in Epithelial Damage and Wound Healing

- The conjunctival epithelium is progressively damaged in ocular pemphigoid, leading to poor wound healing and keratinization.
- mTORC1 regulates epithelial cell proliferation and migration, which are necessary for tissue repair.

- However, chronic mTOR activation may promote excessive epithelial proliferation and abnormal differentiation, worsening keratinization and ocular surface pathology.

mTOR in Immune Modulation and Chronic Inflammation

- Ocular pemphigoid is an autoimmune disease, with autoantibody-driven inflammation against the basement membrane zone (BMZ).
- mTORC1 regulates T-cell activation and inflammatory cytokine production (IL-6, TNF-α, and IFN-γ), sustaining chronic inflammation.
- Hyperactivation of mTOR in immune cells promotes a pro-inflammatory microenvironment, worsening tissue damage.

Therapeutic Implications

- mTOR inhibitors may suppress T-cell activation and inflammatory cytokine release, reducing conjunctival inflammation.
- Targeting mTOR alongside immunosuppressants (e.g., rituximab and corticosteroids) could enhance disease control.

mTOR in Angiogenesis and Conjunctival Vascular Changes

- mTORC1 upregulates VEGF (vascular endothelial growth factor), promoting abnormal conjunctival angiogenesis.
- Increased vascularization supports chronic inflammation and fibroblast activation, worsening disease progression.

Therapeutic Implications

- mTOR inhibition could reduce VEGF expression, limiting pathological angiogenesis.
- Combining anti-VEGF therapy (e.g., bevacizumab) with mTOR inhibitors may help control vascular changes in ocular pemphigoid.

mTOR. Role in Conjunctival Malignancies

mTOR is a key driver of cell cycle progression and survival in conjunctival malignancies. Hyperactivation of mTOR has been observed in these malignancies, making it a promising therapeutic target for pharmacologic intervention. mTOR is often implicated in conjunctival malignancies where increased mTORC1 activity drives cell proliferation and metabolic adaptation (Fig. 4.7).

mTOR plays a pivotal role in the pathogenesis of conjunctival malignancies by driving uncontrolled cell proliferation, survival, and angiogenesis. Its involvement in multiple oncogenic pathways makes it a promising target for therapeutic intervention. Further research is needed to optimize mTOR-targeted therapies in ocular oncology and to determine their efficacy in combination with existing treatments.

Aberrant activation of mTOR signaling has been implicated in the progression of various conjunctival neoplasms, including conjunctival squamous cell carcinoma (SCC), melanoma, lymphoma, and leiomyosarcoma.

mTOR in Conjunctival Squamous Cell Carcinoma (SCC)

mTOR is frequently hyperactivated in conjunctival SCC, a malignancy arising from the conjunctival epithelium. This activation promotes uncontrolled cell proliferation, resistance to apoptosis, and increased metabolic demands that drive tumor growth. Upstream oncogenic pathways, such as PI3K/AKT and EGFR signaling, contribute to mTOR dysregulation in SCC, further enhancing tumor aggressiveness. Additionally, mTOR activation supports epithelial-to-mesenchymal transition (EMT), which facilitates invasion and metastasis [6].

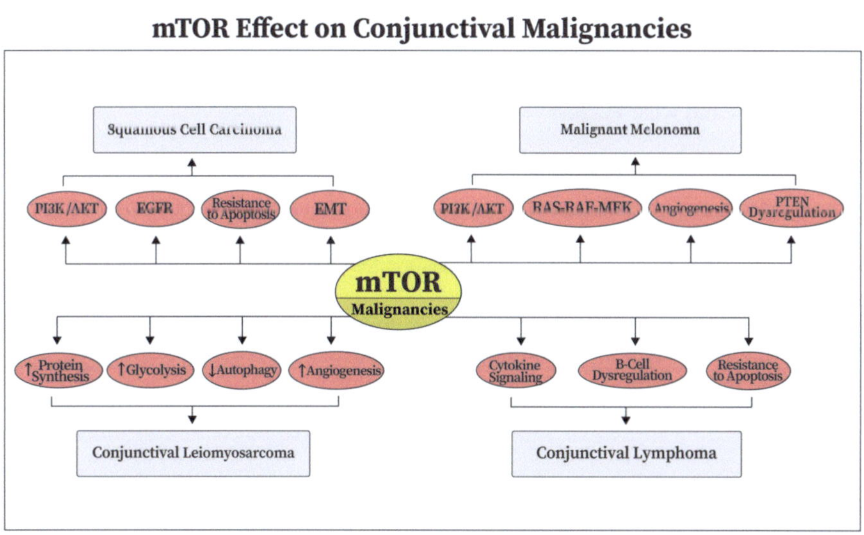

Fig. 4.7 The image above represents the direct effect of mTOR on various pathological pathways contributing to the development of malignancies in conjunctiva

mTOR in Conjunctival Melanoma

Conjunctival melanoma is a rare but aggressive malignancy with a high risk of local recurrence and distant metastases. mTOR signaling plays a crucial role in tumor progression, making it a potential therapeutic target. Further research is needed to optimize mTOR-targeted therapies and their integration with immunotherapy and targeted kinase inhibitors to improve outcomes in patients with this challenging ocular malignancy.

mTOR signaling plays a crucial role in conjunctival melanoma, a rare but aggressive malignancy with a high risk of recurrence and metastasis. In melanoma, mTOR regulates cell survival, invasion, and resistance to apoptosis by integrating signals from RAS-RAF-MEK and PI3K/AKT pathways. Overactive mTOR contributes to increased melanocyte proliferation and tumor progression. Moreover, mTOR-driven angiogenesis supports tumor vascularization, allowing melanoma cells to invade deeper tissues and metastasize [2].

Conjunctival melanoma (Co-M) is a rare but highly aggressive ocular surface malignancy that is frequently misdiagnosed or overlooked, leading to significant visual impairment, reduced quality of life, and a high risk of metastasis-related mortality. It occurs predominantly in fair-skinned populations, with an incidence of approximately 0.46 cases per 1,000,000 persons per year, accounting for 0.25% of all melanomas and 5% of ocular melanomas. Co-M is the second most common conjunctival malignancy after squamous cell carcinoma (SCC) and originates from basal melanocytes within the conjunctival epithelium.

Pathogenesis and Risk Factors

The majority (~70%) of conjunctival melanoma cases develop from conjunctival melanocytic intraepithelial neoplasia (C-MIN), also known as primary acquired melanosis (PAM) with atypia, while others arise from pre-existing conjunctival naevi or de novo. Key risk factors include:

- Ultraviolet (UV) radiation exposure, similar to cutaneous melanoma
- Genetic predisposition, including mutations in BRAF, NRAS, and KIT
- Chronic inflammation and environmental factors
- Light skin pigmentation, which is associated with increased susceptibility

mTOR Signaling in Conjunctival Melanoma

The mTOR pathway plays a critical role in the progression of Co-M by promoting tumor cell proliferation, invasion, metabolic adaptation, and resistance to apoptosis. mTOR activation in conjunctival melanoma is driven by the following:

- Oncogenic BRAF (BRAF V600E) and NRAS mutations, which hyperactivate the PI3K/AKT/mTOR axis

- Dysregulation of PTEN, a tumor suppressor that normally inhibits mTOR signaling
- Hypoxia-induced metabolic reprogramming, enhancing angiogenesis and tumor invasion

Clinical Features and Prognosis

Co-M often presents as a pigmented, vascularized, nodular, or diffuse lesion on the bulbar conjunctiva, with possible involvement of the fornix and palpebral conjunctiva [9]. The prognosis is influenced by:

- Tumor thickness and extent of local invasion
- Presence of ulceration and high mitotic activity
- Regional lymph node involvement (common in Co-M, unlike uveal melanoma)
- Genetic alterations, such as BRAF mutations, which influence therapeutic response

Therapeutic Implications: mTOR Inhibition in Conjunctival Melanoma

Given the role of mTOR in tumor progression, invasion, and metastasis, targeting this pathway has emerged as a promising approach in conjunctival melanoma treatment. mTOR inhibitors (rapamycin, everolimus, and temsirolimus) may have therapeutic benefits by:

- Reducing tumor cell proliferation and inducing apoptosis
- Suppressing angiogenesis, limiting metastatic spread
- Enhancing response to targeted therapies, such as BRAF and MEK inhibitors in BRAF-mutant melanomas

Additionally, immunotherapy (checkpoint inhibitors targeting PD-1/PD-L1) and targeted kinase inhibitors (BRAF/MEK inhibitors) are being explored in Co-M, with combination strategies involving mTOR inhibition showing potential for improving treatment outcomes.

mTOR in Conjunctival Lymphoma

Conjunctival lymphomas, including extranodal marginal zone B-cell lymphoma (MALT lymphoma), also exhibit mTOR dysregulation. The pathway contributes to enhanced lymphocyte proliferation and survival by modulating protein synthesis and metabolic activity. Given that mTOR is a downstream effector of B-cell receptor (BCR) and cytokine signaling, its upregulation promotes the expansion of malignant B-cell clones and resistance to apoptosis, which sustains lymphoma growth [10].

Conjunctival lymphoma is a low-grade B-cell malignancy with variable prognosis, ranging from localized disease to systemic involvement. The mTOR pathway plays a key role in B-cell proliferation and survival, making it a promising target for therapy. mTOR inhibitors, either alone or in combination with standard chemoimmunotherapy (e.g., rituximab), may improve treatment outcomes in refractory or aggressive cases. Further studies are needed to optimize targeted therapies in conjunctival lymphoma.

Conjunctival Lymphoma: Overview, Pathogenesis, and the Role of mTOR Signaling

Overview

Conjunctival lymphoma is a slow-growing, extranodal malignancy of the mucosa-associated lymphoid tissue (MALT) within the conjunctiva. It is part of the spectrum of ocular adnexal lymphomas (OALs) and is most commonly classified as extranodal marginal zone B-cell lymphoma (EMZL), although other subtypes such as diffuse large B-cell lymphoma (DLBCL) and follicular lymphoma can also occur. While often presenting as a painless, salmon-colored subconjunctival mass, conjunctival lymphoma can cause ocular discomfort, conjunctival chemosis, and visual disturbances in advanced cases.

The incidence of conjunctival lymphoma is relatively low, but early diagnosis is crucial, as it can either be localized or associated with systemic lymphoma. Prognosis depends on the histological subtype, extent of disease, and response to therapy.

Pathogenesis and Risk Factors

Conjunctival lymphomas arise from the dysregulated clonal expansion of B-cells within conjunctival lymphoid tissue. The precise cause remains unclear, but factors contributing to lymphomagenesis include:

- Chronic antigenic stimulation (e.g., chronic inflammation and infections such as *Chlamydia psittaci*)
- Dysregulation of B-cell receptor (BCR) signaling
- Genetic and epigenetic alterations (e.g., t(11;18) translocation and BCL2 overexpression)
- Deregulation of PI3K/AKT/mTOR signaling, leading to uncontrolled cell growth and survival

Approximately 5–20% of conjunctival lymphomas are associated with systemic lymphoma, emphasizing the importance of systemic evaluation upon diagnosis.

Role of mTOR in Conjunctival Lymphoma

The mTOR pathway plays a central role in B-cell proliferation, survival, metabolism, and drug resistance in lymphomas. Aberrant activation of PI3K/AKT/mTOR signaling in conjunctival lymphoma contributes to:

1. Enhanced B-cell survival by preventing apoptosis
2. Increased metabolic activity, supporting rapid cell growth
3. Lymphoma cell proliferation via downstream effectors (e.g., S6K1 and 4EBP1)
4. Drug resistance, particularly in aggressive or relapsed lymphomas

Mutations in PI3K, PTEN loss, and AKT activation frequently lead to uncontrolled mTOR signaling, making it an attractive target for therapy.

Clinical Features and Diagnosis

Symptoms

- Painless, slow-growing salmon-colored subconjunctival mass
- Unilateral or bilateral involvement
- Possible foreign body sensation or ocular discomfort
- Conjunctival swelling (chemosis)
- Blurred vision or diplopia (if orbital extension occurs)

Diagnosis

1. Slit-lamp examination to assess lesion characteristics
2. Histopathology and immunohistochemistry (IHC)
    - CD20+, CD79a + (B-cell markers)
    - CD5- and CD10- (to exclude other lymphomas)
    - BCL2 overexpression
3. Fluorescence in situ hybridization (FISH) or PCR for genetic aberrations
4. Systemic evaluation (CT/PET scan and bone marrow biopsy) to rule out systemic lymphoma

Therapeutic Implications: Targeting mTOR in Conjunctival Lymphoma

Given the role of mTOR in lymphoma progression, its inhibition has emerged as a promising therapeutic strategy. mTOR inhibitors (rapamycin/sirolimus, everolimus, and temsirolimus) have shown antilymphoma activity by:

- Inducing apoptosis in malignant B-cells
- Inhibiting cell cycle progression
- Enhancing response to monoclonal antibodies (e.g., rituximab)
- Reducing angiogenesis and metabolic reprogramming

Standard Treatment Approaches

- Radiotherapy (for localized disease)
- Systemic therapy (for advanced disease)
  - Rituximab (anti-CD20 monoclonal antibody)
  - Chemoimmunotherapy (e.g., CHOP regimen in aggressive cases)
  - Targeted PI3K/mTOR inhibitors for refractory/relapsed disease

mTOR in Leiomyosarcoma (LMS)

LMS is a malignant mesenchymal neoplasm with frequent local recurrences and distant metastases composed of cells showing smooth muscle differentiation. Leiomyosarcoma of the conjunctiva is a rare but aggressive malignancy with high recurrence and metastatic potential. The mTOR pathway plays a crucial role in tumor progression, making it a viable therapeutic target. Further research into mTOR inhibitors and combination therapies may improve outcomes in patients with this rare ocular malignancy. Leiomyosarcoma (LMS) of the conjunctiva is a rare but highly aggressive malignant mesenchymal neoplasm characterized by smooth muscle differentiation. It exhibits frequent local recurrences and a high potential for distant metastasis, posing significant therapeutic challenges [7].

Pathogenesis and Molecular Characteristics of LMS

LMS arises from smooth muscle cells, possibly from the vascular smooth muscle of conjunctival blood vessels. Histologically, it is composed of spindle-shaped cells with eosinophilic cytoplasm, elongated nuclei, and a high mitotic index, often accompanied by necrosis and pleomorphism. Immunohistochemical markers used for diagnosis include:

- Smooth muscle actin (SMA) and desmin, which confirm smooth muscle differentiation
- Ki-67, which indicates high proliferative activity
- Myosin heavy chain and caldesmon, which further support smooth muscle lineage

mTOR Signaling in Conjunctival Leiomyosarcoma

The mTOR pathway plays a significant role in cell proliferation, survival, and metabolism in LMS. Dysregulation of PI3K/AKT/mTOR signaling contributes to uncontrolled tumor growth, chemoresistance, and enhanced metastatic potential. Activation of mTOR promotes:

1. Increased protein synthesis (via S6K1 and 4EBP1)
2. Enhanced glycolysis and metabolic adaptation, fueling tumor progression
3. Suppression of autophagy, preventing the degradation of oncogenic proteins
4. Promotion of angiogenesis, increasing tumor vascularization and aggressiveness

Clinical Features and Prognosis

Patients with conjunctival LMS typically present with a slowly growing, painless mass that may cause surface ulceration or vascularization. Given its high recurrence rate and propensity for metastasis, early diagnosis and aggressive management are crucial. The prognosis depends on:

- Tumor size and location
- Histopathological grade
- Presence of necrosis and mitotic activity
- Degree of mTOR pathway activation

Pathophysiology of the Role of mTOR in Conjunctival Malignancies

- Conjunctival tumors, such as squamous cell carcinoma (SCC) and melanoma, exhibit aberrant mTOR activation, driving uncontrolled cell growth, survival, and angiogenesis.
- mTORC1 activation enhances protein synthesis (via p70S6K and 4E-BP1) and metabolic adaptation, supporting tumor progression.

Therapeutic Implications: Targeting mTOR in Conjunctival Leiomyosarcoma

Given the role of mTOR in LMS pathogenesis, its inhibition represents a promising therapeutic strategy. mTOR inhibitors (rapamycin, everolimus, and temsirolimus) have been explored in systemic leiomyosarcomas and may provide benefits in reducing tumor growth, inhibiting metastasis, and enhancing chemotherapy sensitivity in conjunctival LMS. Potential therapeutic approaches include:

- mTOR inhibitors alone to reduce tumor proliferation
- Combination therapy with PI3K/AKT inhibitors to overcome resistance
- Adjunctive radiotherapy or chemotherapy to target residual disease after surgical excision

mTOR Role in Thyroid-Associated Ophthalmopathy (TAO) and Thyroid Eye Disease (TED)

Thyroid-associated eye disease is an immune-mediated orbital disorder characterized by autoimmune activation, cytokine-induced inflammation, and orbital fibroblast remodeling. The interplay between TSHR, IGF-1R, immune cells, and pro-inflammatory mediators leads to fibrosis, fat expansion, and glycosaminoglycan accumulation, causing proptosis and orbital dysfunction. The mTOR pathway plays a key role in driving fibroblast proliferation and adipogenesis, making it a potential target for future TED therapies [1] (Fig. 4.8).

Pathogenesis of Thyroid Eye Disease (TED)

Thyroid eye disease (TED), also known as thyroid-associated orbitopathy (TAO), is an autoimmune inflammatory disorder affecting the orbit and periorbital tissues, primarily associated with Graves' disease. The pathogenesis involves a complex interplay of immune activation, fibroblast proliferation, adipogenesis, and extracellular matrix expansion, leading to orbital inflammation, fibrosis, and proptosis [8].

Key Pathogenic Mechanisms in TED

1. *Immune Dysregulation and Autoantigen Recognition*
    - TED is driven by autoantibodies against the thyroid-stimulating hormone receptor (TSHR) and insulin-like growth factor 1 receptor (IGF-1R).
    - Antigen-presenting cells (APCs) present autoantigens via major histocompatibility complex class II (MHC-II) molecules, initiating an autoimmune response.

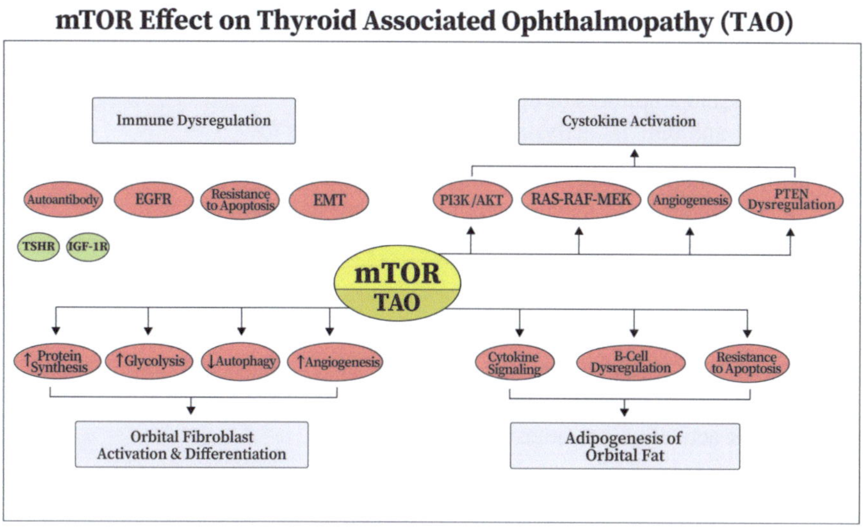

Fig. 4.8 The image above represents the direct effect of mTOR on various pathological pathways contributing to the development of malignancies in conjunctiva

- T-helper (Th1 and Th2) immune responses are triggered, leading to the secretion of inflammatory cytokines.

2. *Cytokine and Chemokine Activation*

- Pro-inflammatory cytokines play a major role in TED, promoting fibroblast activation, adipogenesis, and tissue remodeling.
- Key cytokines involved:
  - Interferon-gamma (IFN-γ): Enhances MHC-II expression, increasing antigen presentation.
  - Tumor necrosis factor-alpha (TNF-α): Induces fibroblast proliferation and cytokine release.
  - Interleukins (IL):
    - IL-1β and IL-6: Promote inflammation and orbital fibroblast differentiation.
    - IL-4 and IL-10: Modulate immune responses, with IL-4 driving fibroblast to adipocyte transformation.
  - Transforming growth factor-beta (TGF-β): Contributes to fibrosis and tissue remodeling.
  - Regulated on activation, normal T-cell-expressed and secreted (RANTES): Recruits T-cells and macrophages, amplifying inflammation.

3. *Orbital Fibroblast Activation and Differentiation*

   - Orbital fibroblasts are central to TED pathogenesis and serve as both immune targets and amplifiers of disease.
   - TSHR and IGF-1R activation on fibroblasts leads to:

     – ↑ Proliferation and extracellular matrix (ECM) deposition, causing fibrosis.
     – ↑ Adipogenesis, leading to orbital fat expansion and proptosis.
     – ↑ Glycosaminoglycan (GAG) production, particularly hyaluronic acid, causing edema and swelling.

4. *Role of mTOR Signaling in TED*

   - The mTOR pathway is hyperactivated in TED, influencing fibroblast proliferation, adipogenesis, and cytokine signaling.
   - mTOR activation promotes:

     – Orbital fibroblast proliferation, contributing to tissue remodeling.
     – Adipogenesis via AKT/mTOR signaling, leading to orbital fat expansion.
     – Increased inflammatory cytokine secretion, worsening the disease progression.

   - mTOR inhibitors (e.g., rapamycin and everolimus) have been proposed as potential therapeutic targets to mitigate fibroblast-driven tissue changes in TED.

Pathophysiology:
- Thyroid-associated orbitopathy (TAO) is an autoimmune orbital disorder associated with fibroblast proliferation, adipogenesis, and inflammation.
- mTORC1 regulates orbital fibroblast proliferation and differentiation, contributing to fibrosis and adipose tissue expansion.
- mTOR-driven VEGF upregulation exacerbates orbital congestion and edema (Fig. 4.9).

Therapeutic Implications:
- mTOR inhibitors may suppress fibroblast activation and adipogenesis, reducing orbital tissue remodeling.
- Combining mTOR inhibition with IGF-1 blockade may help control fibroblast-driven inflammation in TAO.

mTOR plays a critical role in TAO by promoting orbital fibroblast activation, adipogenesis, inflammation, and angiogenesis. Targeting mTOR could provide novel therapeutic strategies to reduce fibrosis, adipose tissue expansion, and immune-mediated damage in TAO.

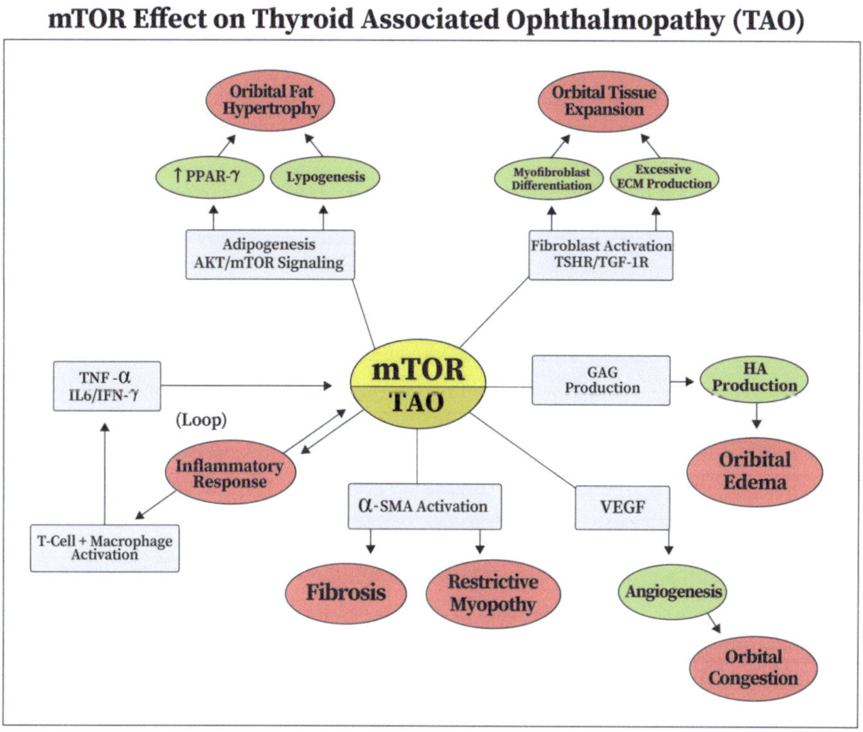

Fig. 4.9 The image above represents the intricate and multifactorial interaction between different signaling pathways, which in turn effect the complex outcome of orbital disease associated with TAO

Role of mTOR in Thyroid-Associated Ophthalmopathy (TAO)

Thyroid-associated ophthalmopathy (TAO) is an autoimmune condition primarily affecting the orbital and periorbital tissues, often associated with Graves' disease. The mTOR signaling pathway plays a crucial role in TAO by regulating fibroblast activation, adipogenesis, inflammation, and tissue remodeling, contributing to disease pathogenesis.

1. *Fibroblast Activation and Myofibroblast Differentiation*

   - Orbital fibroblasts (OFs) are central to TAO pathogenesis, differentiating into myofibroblasts and secreting excessive extracellular matrix components.
   - TGF-β1 and IGF-1 activate mTORC1, driving fibroblast proliferation, differentiation, and fibrosis, leading to orbital tissue expansion.
   - mTOR activation enhances α-SMA (alpha-smooth muscle actin) expression, promoting fibrosis and restrictive myopathy in TAO.

2. *Adipogenesis and Orbital Fat Expansion*
   - mTORC1 is a key regulator of adipogenesis in orbital fibroblasts.
   - Activation of PPAR-γ (peroxisome proliferator-activated receptor gamma) by mTORC1 enhances lipogenesis, leading to orbital fat hypertrophy, a hallmark of TAO.
   - Increased fat accumulation contributes to proptosis (exophthalmos) and orbital congestion.
3. *Inflammatory Response and Cytokine Production*
   - mTOR modulates immune cell function, particularly T-cells and macrophages, contributing to inflammation in TAO.
   - Pro-inflammatory cytokines such as TNF-α, IL-6, and IFN-γ activate mTOR signaling, sustaining orbital inflammation.
   - Inhibition of mTOR reduces fibroblast proliferation, cytokine release, and immune cell activation, highlighting its potential as a therapeutic target.
4. Angiogenesis and Orbital Tissue Remodeling
   - mTOR enhances VEGF (vascular endothelial growth factor) expression, promoting abnormal angiogenesis in orbital tissues.
   - Increased vascularization may exacerbate orbital congestion and edema in active TAO.

Potential Therapeutic Targeting of mTOR in TAO
- mTOR inhibitors (e.g., rapamycin and everolimus) may suppress fibroblast proliferation, adipogenesis, and inflammation in TAO.
- PPAR-γ agonists (e.g., pioglitazone) modulate adipogenesis and could complement mTOR-targeted therapies.
- Autophagy regulation via mTOR modulation could impact fibrosis and immune activation in TAO.

Infectious Conjunctivitis

The immune-regulatory function of mTOR impacts pathogen recognition and antimicrobial responses in conjunctival infections. Properly balanced mTOR signaling is essential for effective immune defense while preventing excessive inflammation and tissue damage [11] (Fig. 4.10).

Infectious conjunctivitis, whether bacterial or viral, involves an immune response that is regulated in part by mTOR signaling. mTOR influences innate immune responses, including pathogen recognition, cytokine release, and antimicrobial peptide production. While proper mTOR activation is essential for an effective immune defense, excessive activation can lead to prolonged inflammation and tissue damage. In viral conjunctivitis, such as that caused by adenovirus or herpes simplex virus, mTOR inhibition has been studied for its potential antiviral effects by

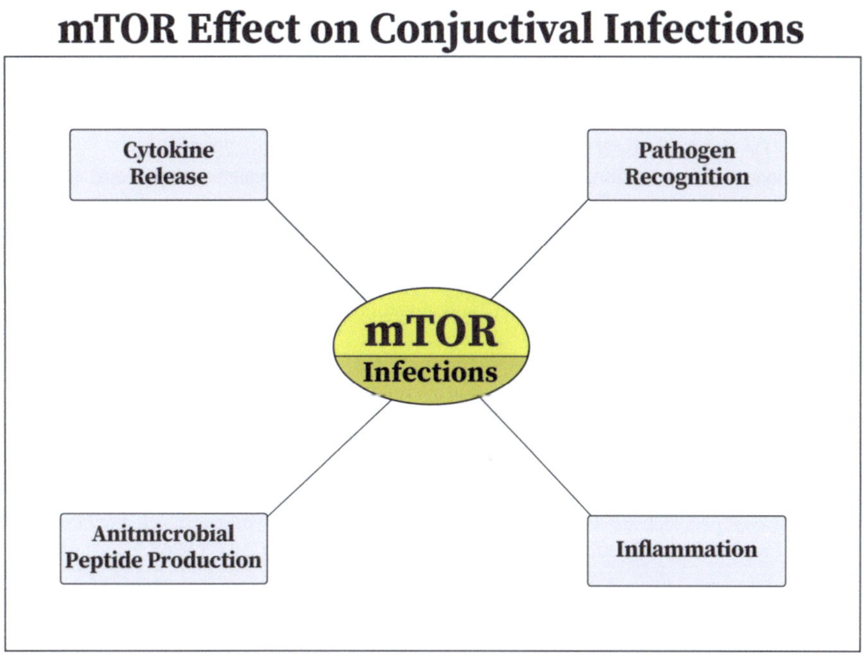

Fig. 4.10 The image above represents the direct effect of mTOR's role on various mechanisms of interactions with infectious pathogens

reducing viral replication and inflammation. However, the balance between immune activation and resolution must be carefully managed to avoid impairing the host defense.

Bibliography

1. Aoun. Orbital inflammation in thyroid eye disease: stress responses and their implications. Stress. 2024;4 https://doi.org/10.3390/stresses4010004.
2. Butt. Conjunctival melanoma: a clinical review and update. Cancer. 2024;16 https://doi.org/10.3390/cancers16183121.
3. Hua Y. Function of AMPK/mTOR signaling in TGF-β1-induced Pterygium fibroblast proliferation and transdifferentiation. 2025; https://doi.org/10.1080/02713683.2025.2470410.
4. Huang L. AZD6738 inhibits fibrotic response of conjunctival fibroblasts by regulating checkpoint kinase 1/P 53 and PI3K/AKT pathways. Front Pharmacol. 2022;13 https://doi.org/10.3389/fphar.2022.990401.
5. Ding P. Risk factors for pterygium: latest research progress on major pathogenesis. Experimental Eye Research. 2024;243 https://doi.org/10.1016/j.exer.2024.109900.
6. Sakai. Expression, intracellular localization, and mutation of EGFR in conjunctival squamous cell carcinoma and the association with prognosis and treatment. PLoS. 2020;15 https://doi.org/10.1371/journal.pone.0238120.

7. Santoro. Conjunctival leiomyosarcoma: a clinico-pathological study with in deep molecular characterization. Pathol Res Pract. 2024;255 https://doi.org/10.1016/j.prp.2024.155182.
8. Scarabosio. Thyroid eye disease: advancements in orbital and ocular pathology management. J Pers Med. 2024;14 https://doi.org/10.3390/jpm14070776.
9. Shields. Conjunctival melanoma: Insights into classification, outcomes, and biomarkers. Clinic Dermatol. 2024;42(1) https://doi.org/10.1016/j.clindermatol.2023.10.010.
10. Tanenbaum. Classification, diagnosis, and management of conjunctival lymphoma. Eye and Vision. 2019;6 https://doi.org/10.1186/s40662-019-0146-1.
11. Ye W. SGK1 mediates herpes simplex keratitis via the PI3K/SGK1/Wnt signaling pathways. Cell Signall. 2025;127 https://doi.org/10.1016/j.cellsig.2024.111566.
12. Watanabe. Inhibition of mTOR differently modulates planar and subepithelial fibrogenesis in human conjunctival fibroblasts. Arch Clin Exp Ophthalmol. 2024;263 https://doi.org/10.1007/s00417-024-06481-2.
13. Gao Y. Activation of LncRNA FOXD2-AS1 by H3K27 acetylation regulates VEGF-A expression by sponging miR-205-5p in recurrent pterygium. J Cell Mol Med. 2020;24 https://doi.org/10.1111/jcmm.16024.
14. Hua Y. Function of P53 and mammalian target of rapamycin in TGF-β1-induced pterygium fibroblast proliferation and transdifferentiation. Research Square. 2024; https://doi.org/10.21203/rs.3.rs-4777255/v1.
15. Li Z. Novel perspectives on the pharmacological treatment of thyroid-associated ophthalmopathy. Front Endocrinol. 2025;15 https://doi.org/10.3389/fendo.2024.1469268.

Chapter 5
mTOR Role in Cornea

Contents

Abstract The mechanistic target of rapamycin (mTOR) is a central regulator of cellular metabolism, growth, proliferation, and survival and plays a critical role in maintaining corneal health and function. In the corneal epithelium, mTOR signaling influences cell proliferation, wound healing, and barrier integrity. Within the stroma, it regulates keratocyte activation, extracellular matrix remodeling, and responses to injury or fibrosis. In the endothelium, mTOR supports cell survival and maintains pump function critical for corneal transparency. Dysregulation of mTOR signaling has been implicated in various corneal pathologies, including degenerations, infections, fibrosis, and dystrophies. Therapeutically, modulation of the mTOR pathway offers potential strategies for enhancing corneal regeneration, controlling scarring, and mitigating degenerative changes. Understanding the nuanced role of mTOR in the corneal layers provides valuable insights for the development of targeted interventions in corneal disease management.

K. T. Moazed, *mTOR Signaling in Ophthalmology*,
https://doi.org/10.1007/978-3-032-05044-1_5

Discussion

The mTOR pathway has a profound effect on the cornea, playing a crucial role in its development, maintenance, repair, and pathology. In this chapter, the detailed exploration of mTOR's impact on the cornea is studied, which is influenced by two major recycling pathways:

- Autophagy [15] which includes degradation and recycling of damaged organelles, proteins, and other cellular components
- Mitophagy [27] which includes selective degradation of damaged or dysfunctional mitochondria by autophagy, across corneal layers in both noninfectious and infectious corneal diseases, dystrophies, and degenerations

Effect of mTOR on Methylation in Cornea and Corneal Disease

mTOR influences DNA and histone methylation in the cornea by regulating enzymes involved in epigenetic modification. Dysregulated mTOR signaling may alter gene expression patterns linked to corneal development, wound healing, and disease progression. This has been discussed in a systematic review in a recent literature [28].

mTOR Role in Corneal Homeostasis

mTOR maintains corneal homeostasis by regulating cell proliferation, metabolism, autophagy, and response to stress, ensuring epithelial turnover, stromal integrity, and endothelial function.

1. Epithelial Turnover [13]
    - mTORC1 regulates the rapid turnover of corneal epithelial cells, ensuring repair and protection from environmental insults.
    - Dysregulation can lead to imbalances, with either delayed healing or hyperproliferative conditions.
2. Energy and Nutrient Sensing [16]
    - mTOR integrates signals from nutrients and growth factors to maintain corneal epithelial cell metabolism, critical for sustaining high turnover and repair rates.
3. Immune Surveillance [1]
    - mTOR regulates immune cell activity in the cornea, controlling inflammation and maintaining an immune-privileged environment.

mTOR's Role in Corneal Development

1. Cell Proliferation and Differentiation:
   - mTORC1 regulates the proliferation of corneal epithelial and stromal cells during embryogenesis.
   - mTORC2 contributes to cytoskeletal organization and polarity, critical for epithelial stratification and corneal curvature.
2. Limbal Stem Cell Function:
   - Limbal stem cells at the corneal periphery depend on mTOR signaling to maintain their metabolic activity and balance between quiescence and proliferation.
3. Corneal Transparency:
   - mTOR modulates the synthesis of collagen and proteoglycans in stromal keratocytes, ensuring proper extracellular matrix (ECM) organization required for corneal clarity.

Pathological Implications of Dysregulated mTOR in the Cornea

Dysregulation of mTOR in the cornea disrupts cellular homeostasis, leading to impaired wound healing, excessive fibrosis, reduced autophagy, and increased inflammation. This contributes to the pathogenesis of corneal degenerations, delayed wound healing, infections, dry eye syndrome, keratoconus, neovascularization, dystrophies, and ultimately compromising corneal transparency and function.

1. Wound Healing Delayed and Fibrosis: Insufficient mTORC1 activity impairs epithelial cell migration and proliferation, leading to chronic wounds. Overactive mTOR signaling in stromal keratocytes leads to excessive collagen deposition and scarring, reducing corneal transparency [12]. The verification is observed with the fact that rapamycin inhibits corneal inflammatory response and neovascularization in a mouse model of corneal alkali burn [7]. Aberrant mTOR activation may promote fibrotic responses, alter stromal remodeling, and contribute to chronic low-grade inflammation, all of which may worsen corneal opacity [10].
2. Infectious Keratitis: mTOR modulates immune responses during infections. Hyperactivation can amplify inflammation, causing collateral tissue damage [17].
3. Dry Eye Disease: mTOR dysregulation in corneal epithelial cells contributes to reduced barrier integrity and increased inflammation, worsening tear film instability exacerbating dry eye symptoms [2].

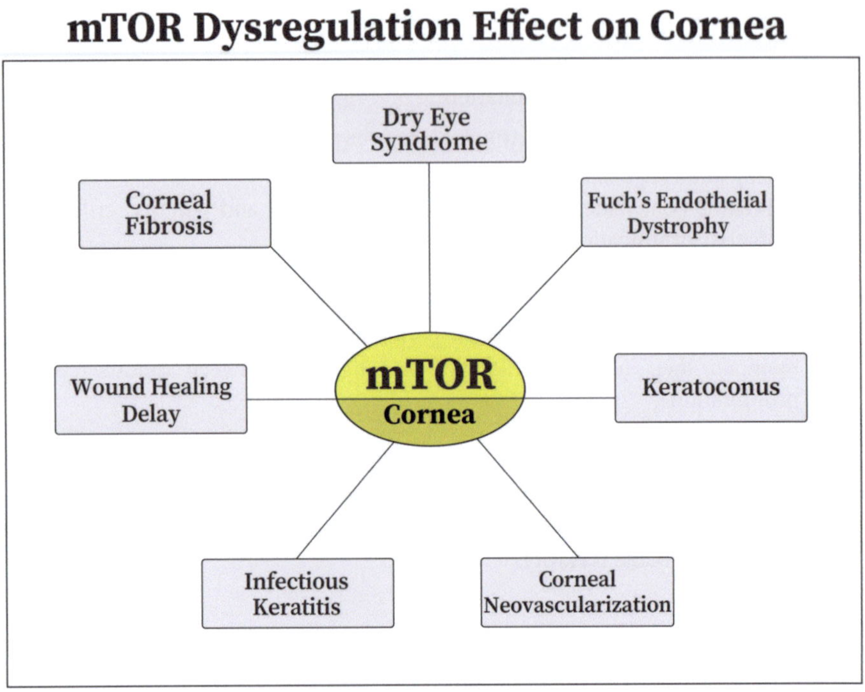

Fig. 5.1 The image above represents the various effects of mTOR dysregulation on the cornea

4. Keratoconus: Altered mTOR signaling affects ECM synthesis in stromal keratocytes, contributing to the thinning and biomechanical weakening of the cornea [4].
5. Corneal Neovascularization: mTOR, particularly mTORC1, promotes angiogenesis by upregulating VEGF expression in the cornea, a response observed in chronic inflammation or hypoxic conditions [25]. The insulin-like growth factor (IGF) promotes angiogenesis by stimulating endothelial cell proliferation, migration, and survival through activation of the PI3K/AKT/mTOR and MAPK pathways and by upregulating pro-angiogenic factors like VEGF [22].
6. Corneal Dystrophies: The mechanistic target of rapamycin (mTOR) signaling pathway plays a significant role in the pathogenesis of various corneal dystrophies, particularly those associated with GFBI (transforming growth factor beta-induced protein, also known as TGFBIp) mutations, such as granular corneal dystrophy (GCD). Mutations in the GFBI gene lead to abnormal protein folding and aggregation within the corneal stroma, forming deposits that impair corneal transparency (Fig. 5.1).

mTOR in Corneal Repair and Regeneration

1. Epithelial Wound Repair [5]
   - mTORC1 promotes epithelial migration and proliferation, critical for re-epithelialization of corneal wounds.
   - Autophagy, regulated by mTOR, contributes to cellular clearance during repair.
2. Stromal Regeneration [20]
   - mTOR modulates keratocyte activity, balancing collagen synthesis and degradation during stromal healing.
3. Endothelial Regeneration: [23]
   - mTOR promotes corneal endothelial regeneration by supporting cell survival, proliferation, and metabolic activity, but its overactivation may impair autophagy and lead to cellular stress or senescence.
4. Limbal Stem Cell Therapy [26]
   - mTOR signaling supports the expansion and differentiation of limbal stem cells in regenerative therapies for limbal stem cell deficiency.

Relationship Between mTOR and AMPK in the Human Cornea

The mechanistic target of rapamycin (mTOR) and AMP-activated protein kinase (AMPK) are two key signaling pathways that function antagonistically to regulate cellular energy balance, growth, and stress responses. In the human cornea, they play crucial roles in maintaining corneal homeostasis, wound healing, and protection against oxidative stress [21].

1. Antagonistic Energy Sensors
   - AMPK is activated in low-energy states (high AMP/ATP ratio), promoting catabolic processes to generate ATP (e.g., autophagy and fatty acid oxidation).
   - mTOR, particularly mTORC1, is activated in high-energy states and promotes anabolic processes (e.g., protein synthesis and cell proliferation).
2. Regulation of Autophagy
   - AMPK stimulates autophagy in the cornea by inhibiting mTORC1 through:
     - Phosphorylation of TSC2 (tuberous sclerosis complex 2), which inhibits Rheb and mTORC1.
     - Direct phosphorylation of Raptor, an essential component of mTORC1.

- This is critical in corneal epithelial cells during oxidative stress or nutrient deprivation, helping remove damaged organelles and proteins.

3. Wound Healing and Cell Proliferation

- During corneal epithelial injury, mTORC1 is transiently activated to promote cell migration and proliferation for wound closure.
- AMPK may be transiently suppressed during this early healing phase but is later reactivated to restore homeostasis and prevent excessive proliferation.

4. Oxidative Stress and Inflammation

- In conditions like dry eye disease or UV exposure, AMPK activation counters oxidative damage by enhancing mitochondrial biogenesis and antioxidant defense, while suppressing mTORC1-driven inflammation.
- mTORC1 activation under stress may exacerbate inflammation unless modulated by AMPK.

5. Corneal Endothelial and Stromal Cell Function

- Endothelial cells rely on AMPK for barrier integrity and antisenescent effects, while mTOR dysregulation can contribute to cellular senescence and dysfunction.
- In stromal keratocytes, mTOR activation can drive fibrosis or myofibroblast transition, while AMPK counters these effects via TGF-β signaling modulation.

mTOR Effect in Cornea: Layer-Specific Roles and Pathology (Fig. 5.2)

Corneal Epithelium [9]

The corneal epithelium is the outermost layer of the cornea, serving as a protective barrier against environmental insults while maintaining corneal transparency. It is composed of five to seven layers of nonkeratinized, stratified squamous epithelial cells, including basal cells, wing cells, and superficial cells. The basal cells are mitotically active and anchored to the basement membrane, giving rise to differentiated cells that migrate anteriorly and are eventually shed. Tight junctions among superficial cells preserve corneal hydration and prevent pathogen entry. Continuous regeneration from limbal stem cells is essential for maintaining epithelial integrity and function.

STAT3 and PI3K/AKT signaling pathways are pivotal regulators of the transdifferentiation of keratinocyte progenitor cells (KPCs) into corneal epithelial-like cells. Activation of STAT3 (signal transducer and activator of transcription 3) promotes cellular reprogramming by enhancing the expression of genes associated

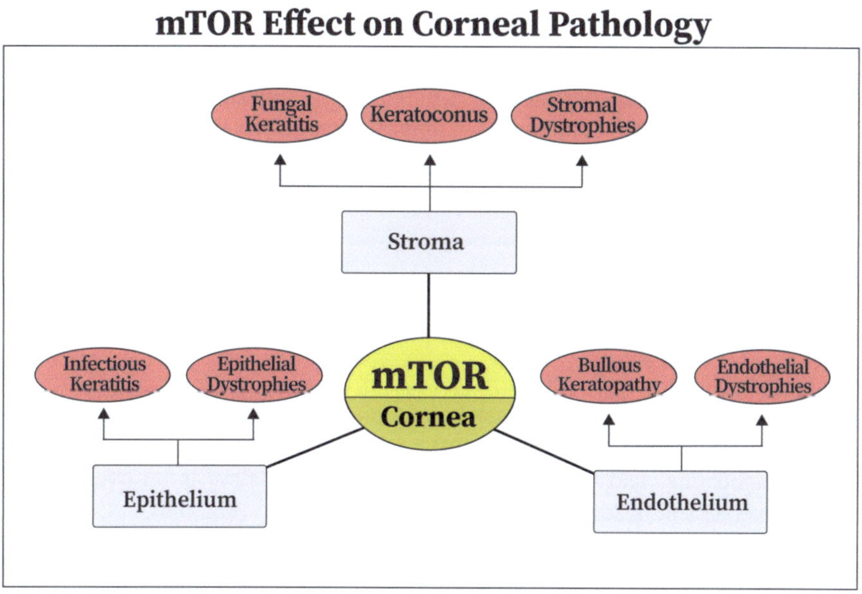

Fig. 5.2 The image above represents mTOR's layer-specific impact on pathological disorders of the epithelium, stroma, and endothelium

with epithelial identity and suppressing those linked to epidermal differentiation. Simultaneously, the PI3K/AKT pathway facilitates cell survival, proliferation, and cytoskeletal reorganization, creating a permissive intracellular environment for phenotypic transition ([11]).

Together, these pathways coordinate the shift in transcriptional programming, enabling KPCs to lose their native keratinocyte characteristics and acquire corneal epithelial-specific markers, such as KRT12. STAT3 predominantly governs transcriptional control, while PI3K/AKT ensures cellular plasticity, resistance to stress, and remodeling of adhesion and barrier properties necessary for successful corneal epithelial integration. Their synergistic activation is thus critical for achieving and maintaining stable transdifferentiation.

mTOR Role in Corneal Epithelial Degeneration (e.g., Exposure Keratitis)

The mechanistic target of rapamycin (mTOR) signaling pathway is increasingly recognized as a key modulator in corneal degenerative processes, including exposure keratitis. Exposure keratitis, resulting from incomplete eyelid closure (lagophthalmos), leads to persistent corneal epithelial injury, desiccation, inflammation, and stromal remodeling [24].

Infectious Keratitis (e.g., HSV and Bacterial)

In infectious keratitis, mTOR modulates immune responses and autophagy. Its dysregulation can exacerbate inflammation, impair pathogen clearance, and delay corneal healing. Upregulated autophagy acts as a host defense but may be hijacked by pathogens [3].

Role of mTOR in Corneal Epithelial Dystrophies

The mechanistic target of rapamycin (mTOR) is a central regulator of cell growth, protein synthesis, autophagy, and metabolism. Its dysregulation has been implicated in various corneal epithelial dystrophies through its influence on epithelial turnover, matrix remodeling, and stress response mechanisms. Below is an overview of mTOR involvement in several major epithelial dystrophies (Fig. 5.3).

1. Epithelial Basement Membrane Dystrophy (EBMD)
   - Pathogenesis: Characterized by abnormal production and organization of basement membrane and epithelial adhesion abnormalities.
   - mTOR involvement:
     - Overactive mTORC1 promotes excess synthesis of extracellular matrix proteins (e.g., laminins and collagens), contributing to redundant basement membrane formation.
     - Inhibits autophagy, leading to intracellular accumulation of debris.

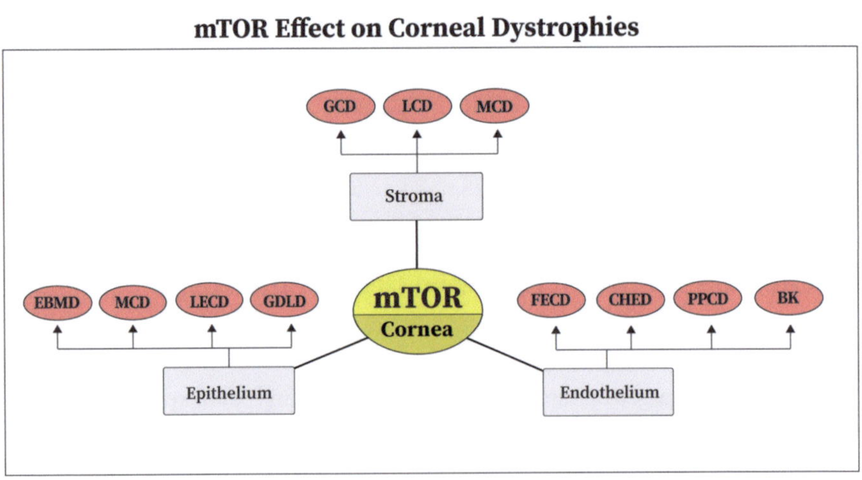

Fig. 5.3 The image above represents mTOR's layer-specific impact on corneal dystrophies across the epithelial, stromal, and endothelial disorders

- Impairs normal epithelial cell desquamation and promotes epithelial hyperplasia.

2. Messman's Corneal Dystrophy

   - Pathogenesis: Mutations in keratin genes (KRT3 and KRT12) lead to cytoskeletal fragility and intraepithelial cyst formation.
   - mTOR involvement:

     - Chronic endoplasmic reticulum (ER) stress from misfolded keratins may activate mTORC1, further suppressing autophagy.
     - mTOR dysregulation may prevent proper degradation of protein aggregates and exacerbate epithelial degeneration.

3. Lisch Epithelial Corneal Dystrophy

   - Pathogenesis: Characterized by whorled, feathery gray opacities due to vacuolated epithelial cells containing glycosaminoglycan-like material.
   - mTOR involvement (hypothetical):

     - mTOR may influence glycogen metabolism and epithelial vesicle trafficking.
     - Disrupted mTOR signaling could impair vacuole clearance and epithelial integrity.

4. Gelatinous Drop-Like Corneal Dystrophy (GDLD)

   - Pathogenesis: Caused by *TACSTD2* mutations leading to epithelial barrier dysfunction and subepithelial amyloid deposition.
   - mTOR involvement:

     - Chronic epithelial stress and inflammation may lead to mTORC1 activation.
     - Promotes proinflammatory cytokine production and fibrosis through NF-\u03baB signaling.
     - Suppresses autophagy, reducing clearance of amyloid precursors such as lactoferrin.

Therapeutic Implications

- mTOR inhibition (e.g., rapamycin):

  - May reduce excessive ECM production and normalize epithelial turnover in EBMD.
  - Enhances autophagy to clear cytoplasmic debris in Meesmann dystrophy.
  - Decreases inflammatory signaling and amyloid accumulation in GDLD.

- AMPK activation (e.g., metformin):

  - Provides cytoprotective effects by inhibiting mTORC1.
  - Promotes energy homeostasis and enhances epithelial resilience under stress.

Corneal Stroma [19]

The corneal stroma is the thickest layer of the cornea, comprising approximately 90% of its total thickness. It is primarily composed of regularly arranged collagen fibrils (mainly type I collagen) embedded in a highly hydrated extracellular matrix, which is critical for maintaining corneal transparency and mechanical strength. Keratocytes, the resident stromal cells, are sparsely distributed between the collagen lamellae and are responsible for synthesizing and remodeling the extracellular matrix. The precise organization of collagen fibers, uniform spacing, and relative avascularity of the stroma are essential for its optical clarity and refractive properties.

mTOR Role in Stromal Corneal Diseases

Infectious (e.g., fungal keratitis): Autophagy modulates keratocyte apoptosis and inflammation.

- Noninfectious (e.g., keratoconus): Dysregulated mitophagy contributes to oxidative damage and ECM thinning [18].
- Dystrophies: Aberrant protein aggregates engage autophagic clearance.

Corneal Stromal Dystrophies

1. Granular Corneal Dystrophy (GCD)
   - Pathogenesis: Characterized by hyaline deposits within the stromal layers, typically due to mutations in the *TGFBI*gene.
   - mTOR involvement:
     - mTORC1 may contribute to excessive protein synthesis and deposition of abnormal TGFBIp (transforming growth factor beta-induced protein).
     - Inhibition of autophagy reduces clearance of these deposits.
     - Promotes fibroblastic transformation of stromal keratocytes under stress.
2. Lattice Corneal Dystrophy (LCD)
   - Pathogenesis: Amyloid deposition in the stroma caused by mutated TGFBI or gelsolin.
   - mTOR involvement:
     - Supports amyloidogenic processing and inhibits autophagy-mediated clearance.
     - Chronic mTOR activation may exacerbate oxidative stress and keratocyte apoptosis.

3. Macular Corneal Dystrophy (MCD)

   - Pathogenesis: Caused by carbohydrate sulfotransferase 6 (*CHST6*) mutations, leading to accumulation of unsulfated keratan sulfate. Unsulfated keratan sulfate is a form of keratan sulfate that lacks normal sulfate groups, which are critical for its structural and functional integrity. In the cornea, sulfation is essential for maintaining proper hydration and transparency. Accumulation of unsulfated keratan sulfate, as seen in macular corneal dystrophy, leads to abnormal extracellular matrix composition, stromal clouding, and progressive visual impairment.
   - mTOR involvement:

     - Disrupted autophagy and lysosomal clearance mechanisms.
     - mTOR hyperactivity may impair keratocyte metabolic regulation and enhance stromal disorganization.

Therapeutic Implications
- mTOR inhibition (e.g., rapamycin):

  - May normalize ECM production and autophagic flux in epithelial and stromal dystrophies
  - Potentially reduces amyloid and hyaline accumulation
  - Inhibits inflammatory and fibrotic signaling cascades

- AMPK activation (e.g., metformin):

  - Counteracts mTORC1 activity
  - Enhances autophagy, reduces oxidative damage, and stabilizes keratocyte function

Alterations in mTOR activity have been shown to influence corneal stromal cell behavior, including proliferation rates, oxidative stress handling, and extracellular matrix (ECM) remodeling capacity. Indeed, KC-derived stromal cells exhibit altered ECM deposition and disrupted collagen organization—hallmarks that may be driven, at least in part, by aberrant mTOR signaling.

Corneal Endothelium [6]

The corneal endothelium is a single layer of hexagonally arranged, flattened cells lining the posterior surface of the cornea. Its primary function is to maintain corneal transparency by regulating stromal hydration through active ion transport and fluid movement. Endothelial cells have limited proliferative capacity; thus, cell loss due to aging, trauma, or disease can lead to corneal edema and vision impairment. Tight junctions and specialized ion pumps, particularly Na^+/K^+-ATPase, are essential for sustaining the cornea's transparency and optical clarity. Corneal endothelial cells play a critical role in maintaining corneal transparency and thickness through the active regulation of fluid and ion transport, thereby preventing stromal edema.

Modulation of mTOR signaling offers a promising therapeutic strategy to mitigate pathological matrix accumulation, cellular stress, degeneration, and fibrotic remodeling in corneal epithelial, stromal, and endothelial dystrophies.

Fuchs Endothelial Corneal Dystrophy (FECD)

mTOR influences endothelial cell survival and stress responses. Dysregulated signaling may contribute to endothelial apoptosis and ECM abnormalities in FECD [14].

Progressive loss of corneal endothelial cells occurs with the accumulation of guttae and Descemet membrane thickening. Impaired mitophagy leads to mitochondrial dysfunction, ROS accumulation, and cell death. Dysregulated mTOR signaling contributes to endothelial cell senescence and apoptosis [8].

- mTORC1 overactivation suppresses protective autophagy, leading to the accumulation of oxidative and metabolic stress.
- Impairs mitochondrial function and promotes fibrotic remodeling via TGF-β signaling pathways.

Congenital Hereditary Endothelial Dystrophy (CHED)

- Pathogenesis: Presents at birth or early childhood with diffuse corneal edema and thickened Descemet membrane
- mTOR involvement (theoretical):
  - Potential role in regulating endothelial cell metabolism and barrier function
  - May influence unfolded protein response and survival under cellular stress

Posterior Polymorphous Corneal Dystrophy (PPCD)

- Pathogenesis: Characterized by abnormal endothelial cells exhibiting epithelial-like features
- mTOR involvement:
  - Aberrant mTOR activity may facilitate metaplasia and proliferation of endothelial cells
  - May be linked to epithelial–mesenchymal transition and fibrotic gene expression

Therapeutic Implications

- mTOR inhibition (e.g., rapamycin):
  - May normalize ECM production and autophagic flux in epithelial, stromal, and endothelial dystrophies
  - Potentially reduces amyloid, hyaline, and fibrotic accumulation
  - Inhibits inflammatory and senescence-associated signaling cascades
- AMPK activation (e.g., metformin):
  - Counteracts mTORC1 activity
  - Enhances autophagy, reduces oxidative damage, stabilizes keratocyte and endothelial function

Bullous Keratopathy (BK)

Bullous keratopathy: Autophagic flux defects compromise cell survival.

- Pathogenesis: Characterized by chronic corneal endothelial dysfunction leading to stromal and epithelial edema with the formation of epithelial bullae
- mTOR involvement:
  - mTORC1 activation in response to cellular stress can contribute to endothelial decompensation and apoptotic loss.
  - Suppression of autophagy may impair clearance of damaged mitochondria and proteins in stressed endothelial cells.
  - Promotes inflammatory and fibrotic responses through the upregulation of TGF-β and proinflammatory cytokines.
  - May contribute to epithelial barrier compromise and abnormal epithelial–stromal interactions under chronic edema.

Therapeutic Implications

mTOR inhibition (e.g., rapamycin):

- May normalize ECM production and autophagic flux in epithelial, stromal, endothelial dystrophies, and bullous keratopathy
- Potentially reduces amyloid, hyaline, and fibrotic accumulation
- Inhibits inflammatory and senescence-associated signaling cascades

Summary of mTOR Effects on Cornea

Aspect	Normal function	Dysregulated function
Development	Supports epithelial stratification and stromal ECM synthesis	Structural defects, such as improper transparency
Homeostasis	Regulates turnover, repair, and metabolism	Chronic wounds and impaired epithelial integrity
Wound healing	Promotes repair and limits scarring	Delayed healing and excessive fibrosis
Neovascularization	Maintains avascularity	Promotes abnormal vascular growth

General Therapeutic Implications of Targeting mTOR in Corneal Disorders

1. mTOR Inhibitors for Fibrosis:
   - Rapamycin reduces stromal scarring by suppressing keratocyte proliferation and collagen deposition, preserving corneal transparency.
2. Anti-Angiogenic Therapy:
   - Targeting mTOR-driven VEGF expression can mitigate corneal neovascularization in conditions like infections or inflammation.
3. Enhancing Wound Healing:
   - Controlled activation of mTORC1 may accelerate epithelial repair in chronic corneal wounds, but overactivation must be avoided to prevent scarring.
4. Regenerative Medicine:
   - mTOR modulators can improve the efficacy of limbal stem cell therapies by supporting cell proliferation and differentiation without triggering fibrosis.

Bibliography

1. Anthony. The immunobiology of corneal HSV-1 infection and herpetic stromal keratitis. Clinic Microbiol Rev ASM J. 2024;37 https://doi.org/10.1128/cmr.00006-24.
2. BodaLi. Evodiamine promotes autophagy and alleviates oxidative stress in dry eye disease through the p53/mTOR pathway. IVOS. 2025;66 https://doi.org/10.1167/iovs.66.3.44.
3. Chang J. JAG1 mediates apoptosis in herpes simplex keratitis by suppressing autophagy via ROS/JAG1/NOTCH1/pULK1 signaling pathway. Cell Biol Toxicol. 2024; https://doi.org/10.1007/s10565-024-09968-0.
4. Durán-Cristiano. Omics in keratoconus: from molecular to clinical practice. J Clin Med. 2025; https://doi.org/10.3390/jcm14072459.

5. Gong J. Elucidating the mechanism of corneal epithelial cell repair: unraveling the impact of growth factors. Front Med. 2024; https://doi.org/10.3389/fmed.2024.1384500.
6. Hwang JS. Transcriptomic comparison of corneal endothelial cells in young versus old corneas. Nat Sci Rep. 2024; https://doi.org/10.1038/s41598-024-82423-6.
7. Jiande L. Rapamycin inhibits corneal inflammatory response and neovascularization in a mouse model of corneal alkali burn. Exp Eye Res. 2023;233 https://doi.org/10.1016/j.exer.2023.109539.
8. Jia-Xin. Therapeutic future of Fuchs endothelial corneal dystrophy: an ongoing way to explore. Taiwan J Ophthalmol. 2024; https://doi.org/10.4103/tjo.TJO-D-23-00115.
9. Jin M. Disrupted mitochondrial dynamics impair corneal epithelial healing in neurotrophic keratopathy. Int J Mol Sci. 2025; https://doi.org/10.3390/ijms26031290.
10. Jun I. Molecular pathogenesis of granular corneal dystrophy type 2 (GCD2) and TGFBI-related corneal dystrophies. TGFBI-related Corneal Dystrophies, Chapter; 2025. https://doi.org/10.1007/978-981-96-0131-8_8.
11. Chen K. The role of the PI3K/AKT signalling pathway in the corneal epithelium: recent updates. Cell Death Dis. 2022; https://doi.org/10.1038/s41419-022-04963-x.
12. Kempuraj. Autophagy in extracellular matrix and wound healing modulation in the cornea. Biomedicine. 2022; https://doi.org/10.3390/biomedicines10020339.
13. Krolo. The role of topical insulin in ocular surface restoration: a review. Surv Ophthalmol. 2024;69 https://doi.org/10.1016/j.survophthal.2024.04.003.
14. Chi M. MiR-23a-3p targets PTEN as a novel anti-ferroptosis regulator in Fuchs endothelial corneal dystrophy. Exp Eye Res. 2025;250 https://doi.org/10.1016/j.exer.2024.110180.
15. Martínez-Chacón. Autophagy modulation in animal models of corneal diseases: a systematic review. Mol Cell Biochem. 2020; https://doi.org/10.1007/s11010-020-03832-5.
16. Núñez. Sirtuins: emergent players in tissue and organ regeneration. Int J Transl Med; 2024. https://doi.org/10.3390/ijtm4040048.
17. Ramachandran. Inhibition of Unc-51-like-kinase is mitoprotective during Pseudomonas aeruginosa infection in corneal epithelial cells. ASM J. 2025; https://doi.org/10.1128/msphere.00537-24.
18. Ramachandran. The roles of autophagy and mitophagy in corneal pathology: current knowledge and future perspectives. Front Med. 2023;20 https://doi.org/10.3389/fmed.2023.1064938.
19. Robbins. Corneal treatment, repair, and regeneration: exosomes at rescue. Pharmaceutics. 2024;07 https://doi.org/10.3390/pharmaceutics16111424.
20. Saoncella. Nuclear Akt2 opposes limbal keratinocyte stem cell self-renewal by repressing a FOXO-mTORC1 signaling pathway. Stem Cells. 2014; https://doi.org/10.1002/stem.1565.
21. Shukal. Role of the AMPK signalling pathway in the aetiopathogenesis of ocular diseases. Hum Exp Toxicol. 2022; https://doi.org/10.1177/09603271211063165.
22. Stuard. The IGF/insulin-IGFBP axis in corneal development, wound healing, and disease. Front Endocrinol. 2020; https://doi.org/10.3389/fendo.2020.00024.
23. Vercammen. capacity of the innermost layer of the cornea. Transl Res. 2022;248 https://doi.org/10.1016/j.trsl.2022.05.003.
24. Volatier. UV protection in the cornea: failure and rescue. Biology. 2022; https://doi.org/10.3390/biology11020278.
25. Su W. Efficacious, safe, and stable inhibition of corneal neovascularization by AAV-vectored anti-VEGF therapeutics. Mol Ther Method Clinic Develop. 2021; https://doi.org/10.1016/j.omtm.2021.06.007.
26. Wang M. Expression distribution of keratins in normal and pathological corneas and the regulatory role of Krt17 on limbal stem cells. IVOS. 2025;66 https://doi.org/10.1167/iovs.66.4.55.
27. Li X. The mTOR signalling in corneal diseases: a recent update. Biochem Pharmacol. 2023;213 https://doi.org/10.1016/j.bcp.2023.115620.
28. Xia Y. Methylation in cornea and corneal diseases: a systematic review. Cell Death Dis. 2024; https://doi.org/10.1038/s41420-024-01935-2.

Chapter 6
mTOR Effect on the Anterior Segment of the Eye

Contents

Abstract The mechanistic target of rapamycin (mTOR) pathway plays a critical role in regulating cellular metabolism, growth, and survival within the anterior segment of the human eye, particularly in structures involved in aqueous humor dynamics. In the trabecular meshwork and Schlemm's canal, mTOR influences extracellular matrix remodeling, cytoskeletal organization, and cellular contractility—factors that are essential for maintaining aqueous outflow and intraocular pressure (IOP) homeostasis. Dysregulation of mTOR signaling in these angle structures has been implicated in increased outflow resistance and the pathogenesis of primary open-

K. T. Moazed, *mTOR Signaling in Ophthalmology*,
https://doi.org/10.1007/978-3-032-05044-1_6

angle glaucoma. Enhanced mTOR activity may contribute to trabecular meshwork fibrosis, oxidative stress, and reduced autophagy, all of which impair drainage function. Pharmacological inhibition of mTOR, particularly mTORC1, has demonstrated potential to restore trabecular outflow and reduce IOP by promoting autophagic clearance and cytoskeletal stability. While mTOR also plays roles in the cornea, lens, and conjunctiva, its dysregulation in the angle is of particular relevance to glaucomatous disease, making it a promising therapeutic target for early intervention and progression control.

Discussion

The mechanistic target of rapamycin (mTOR) plays a multifaceted role in the anterior segment of the eye, particularly within tissues critical for intraocular pressure (IOP) regulation and glaucoma pathogenesis. mTOR signaling influences cellular metabolism, autophagy, proliferation, and fibrotic remodeling across the corneal endothelium, trabecular meshwork (TM), Schlemm's canal, ciliary body, and iris.

In the trabecular meshwork, mTOR activation contributes to cytoskeletal changes, extracellular matrix (ECM) accumulation, and suppression of autophagy, leading to increased outflow resistance and elevated IOP—key features in primary open-angle glaucoma. In steroid-induced and uveitic glaucoma, mTOR promotes fibrotic and inflammatory responses that further impair aqueous humor drainage.

In the corneal endothelium and iris, mTOR modulates cell survival and wound healing, with dysregulation potentially affecting surgical outcomes and anterior segment integrity in glaucomatous eyes.

In the ciliary body, mTOR influences aqueous humor production by regulating epithelial cell function and mitochondrial activity. Aberrant signaling here may exacerbate IOP elevation in certain glaucomas (Fig. 6.1).

Glaucoma is a progressive optic neuropathy characterized by the apoptotic loss of retinal ganglion cells (RGCs), ultimately leading to irreversible vision impairment. A hallmark of this disease is optic nerve head cupping, axonal degeneration, and the death of RGCs. The etiology of glaucoma is multifactorial, involving elevated intraocular pressure (IOP); other influential factors are vascular dysregulation, oxidative stress, ischemic injury, glutamate-mediated excitotoxicity, and chronic inflammation.

Retinal ganglion cells (RGCs), the only projection neurons linking the eye to the brain, are essential for visual signal transmission. Their degeneration in diseases like glaucoma leads to irreversible vision loss. As postmitotic neurons, RGCs rely heavily on autophagy to clear damaged proteins and organelles, maintaining cellular homeostasis and survival.

A neuroretinal cell culture model offers a valuable platform for developing therapies targeting oxidative stress-induced damage in ocular diseases, particularly

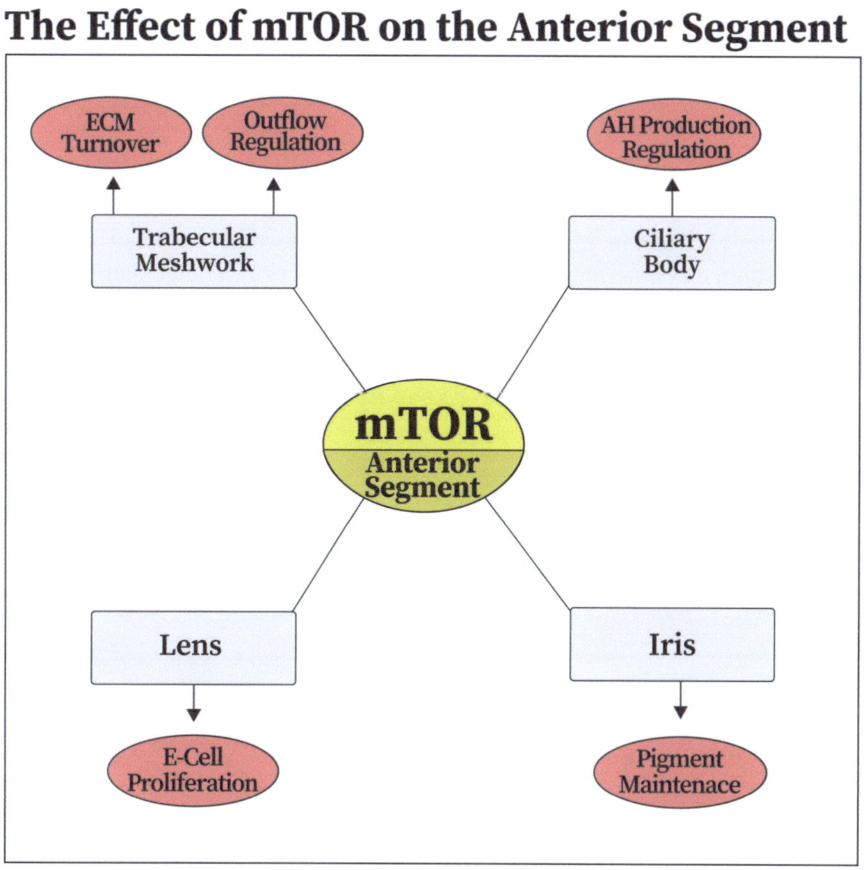

Fig. 6.1 The image above represents the effects of mTOR on different components on the anterior segment of the eye

glaucoma—a condition marked by progressive retinal ganglion cell degeneration and irreversible vision loss [7].

In this chapter, we will specifically address the angle structure and trabecular meshwork (TM), given their critical role in aqueous humor outflow and intraocular pressure (IOP) regulation and glaucoma. Other components of the anterior chamber will be discussed in subsequent chapters. Special attention is given to the mechanistic target of rapamycin (mTOR) pathway, whose dysregulation has emerged as a key contributor to glaucoma, one of the most prevalent and vision-threatening anterior segment disorders. Recent studies have demonstrated that mTOR signaling influences TM fibrosis, extracellular matrix remodeling, and cytoskeletal dynamics, all of which are central to the pathogenesis of elevated IOP and glaucomatous optic neuropathy. As such, targeting the mTOR pathway holds promise for novel therapeutic strategies in glaucoma management. The agents such as rapamycin hold therapeutic promise for restoring TM function, enhancing autophagic clearance, and reducing fibrosis, offering disease-modifying strategies beyond pressure-lowering agents.

mTOR Effect on Trabecular Meshwork

mTOR plays a role in maintaining trabecular meshwork (TM) cell function. Dysregulation may contribute to TM cell apoptosis and extracellular matrix remodeling, increasing outflow resistance and intraocular pressure (IOP) [21] (Fig. 6.2).

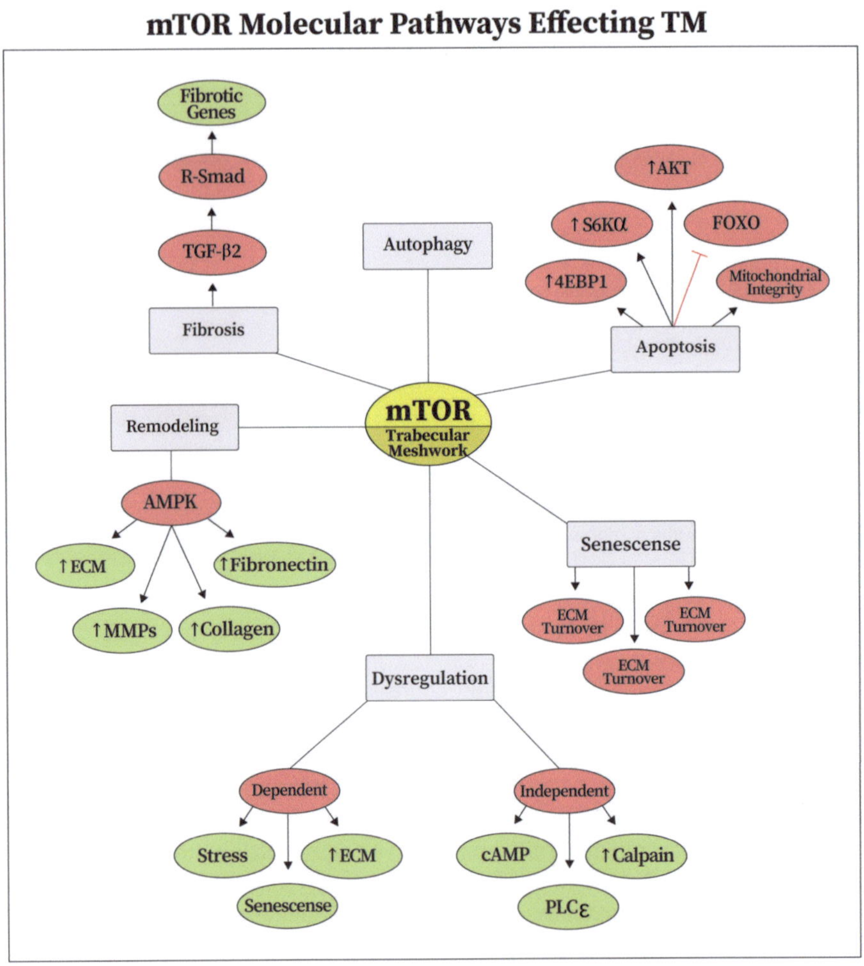

Fig. 6.2 The image illustrates how mTOR regulates various molecular pathways, influencing key cellular functions like autophagy, apoptosis, remodeling, and senescence. The dysregulation of mTORs effect is shown at the bottom

Autophagy and TM (mTOR signaling and autophagy regulation in the trabecular meshwork) [14]: mTOR signaling plays a pivotal role in modulating autophagy within the trabecular meshwork (TM), a key structure involved in aqueous humor outflow and intraocular pressure (IOP) regulation [8].

Autophagy is a tightly regulated, catabolic process that facilitates the degradation and recycling of damaged organelles and misfolded proteins, particularly under conditions of cellular stress such as oxidative injury or nutrient deprivation. This process is essential for maintaining intracellular homeostasis and has been implicated in a variety of physiological and pathological contexts, including inflammation, cancer, neurodegeneration, and fibrosis.

In the context of fibrotic diseases, the role of autophagy remains complex and somewhat paradoxical. While some studies suggest that autophagy may exert antifibrotic effects by degrading profibrotic mediators and limiting myofibroblast activation, other evidence indicates that it might contribute to fibrogenesis by promoting cell survival and persistent activation of fibrotic pathways.

In the trabecular meshwork (TM) of the eye—a critical structure for aqueous humor outflow and intraocular pressure regulation—fibrosis contributes to outflow resistance and the pathogenesis of glaucomatous damage. Transforming growth factor-beta 2 (TGF-β2), a cytokine enriched in the aqueous humor of glaucoma patients, is known to induce fibrotic responses in TM cells, including the increased production of extracellular matrix components such as fibronectin and collagen.

Whether autophagy plays a protective or detrimental role in this TGF-β2-driven fibrotic process remains unclear. Preliminary studies have raised the possibility that enhancing autophagic flux might counteract fibrotic remodeling by degrading excess extracellular matrix proteins or downregulating TGF-β2 signaling. Conversely, impaired or dysregulated autophagy may contribute to fibrotic progression and TM dysfunction.

Further investigation is needed to elucidate whether pharmacological or genetic activation of autophagy can mitigate TGF-β2-induced fibrotic changes in TM cells and whether targeting autophagic pathways might represent a novel therapeutic strategy for glaucoma management.

TGF-β2 and Fibrosis in the TM TGF-β2 is a key profibrotic cytokine that promotes a secretory and myofibroblast-like phenotype in cultured human trabecular meshwork (TM) cells. It is locally produced by ocular tissues such as the TM, iris, and ciliary body and exerts its effects through a dense network of receptors predominantly expressed in the TM. Upon receptor binding, TGF-β2 activates canonical Smad signaling pathways, particularly involving receptor-regulated Smads (R-Smads), including Smad1, 2, 3, 5, and 8. Among these, Smad3 plays a central role in mediating fibrotic responses, with its phosphorylation enhancing the transcription of downstream fibrotic genes [8].

AMPK Activation and Fibrotic Remodeling in Glaucoma Pathogenesis

At the molecular level, adenosine monophosphate-activated protein kinase (AMPK), a critical energy sensor, is increasingly recognized as a modulator of glaucomatous neurodegeneration. Phosphorylated AMPK levels are elevated in the optic nerves of glaucoma patients, indicating hyperactivation of this pathway. AMPK activation in this context has been associated with detrimental outcomes such as synaptic pruning and dendritic retraction in RGCs, contributing to their functional and structural decline [20].

In parallel, fibrotic remodeling of the trabecular meshwork (TM), a key site of aqueous humor outflow, is a major contributor to increased IOP in glaucoma. This remodeling is characterized by excessive deposition of extracellular matrix (ECM) components, including fibronectin, type I collagen, and matrix metalloproteinases (MMPs), as observed in both glaucomatous human aqueous humor and experimental animal models. These changes reduce aqueous outflow facility and elevate IOP, thereby exacerbating RGC stress [22].

Interestingly, AMPK signaling also appears to intersect with fibrotic pathways in the TM. Pharmacological activation of AMPK using 5-aminoimidazole-4-carboxamide ribonucleotide (AICAR) has been shown to attenuate the expression of cytoskeletal and ECM proteins in primary human TM cells. This effect is mediated, in part, by phosphorylation of RhoA at Ser188, a modification that suppresses RhoA activity and downstream fibrotic signaling. These findings suggest that AMPK activation may have dual and context-dependent roles—exacerbating neurodegeneration in RGCs while alleviating fibrotic obstruction in the TM.

Ocular hypertension induces hyperactivation of adenosine monophosphate-activated protein kinase (AMPK), resulting in dendrite retraction as well as synapse elimination via inhibition of mTORC1 in RGCs, linking mechanical stress to molecular dysregulation and RGC injury [3].

Additional signaling cascades, such as mitogen-activated protein kinases (MAPKs), exhibit spatiotemporal upregulation in both the retina and optic nerve under conditions of elevated IOP. These kinases contribute to stress-responsive gene expression and are implicated in the progressive nature of glaucomatous degeneration.

Together, these findings highlight the complex and bidirectional roles of metabolic and stress-response signaling pathways—particularly AMPK—in both the neurodegenerative and fibrotic aspects of glaucoma.

Trabecular Meshwork (TM) Senescence and Reactive Oxygen Species (ROS) [25]

In the trabecular meshwork (TM), increased levels of reactive oxygen species (ROS) contribute to cellular senescence and accelerate the aging process. One underlying cause of heightened ROS accumulation is the diminished activity of nuclear factor erythroid 2–related factor 2 (Nrf2), a master transcription factor that regulates the expression of antioxidant genes.

Elevated ROS levels activate several prosenescent signaling cascades, including:

- Mitogen-activated protein kinase (MAPK) pathway
- PI3K–AKT–mTOR signaling pathway
- Transforming growth factor-β (TGF-β) pathway

These pathways converge on the upregulation of cyclin-dependent kinase inhibitors such as p15^INK4b, p21^Cip1, and p27^Kip1, which mediate cell cycle arrest and promote a senescent phenotype in TM cells. The resulting senescence compromises TM function, impairs aqueous humor outflow, and contributes to intraocular pressure (IOP) dysregulation, a key pathogenic factor in glaucoma.

Dysregulation of mTOR in TM [15]

- mTOR-dependent dysregulation: There is a strong indication that the autophagic pathway in trabecular meshwork (TM) cells from glaucomatous eyes is dysregulated in a manner that is dependent on the mechanistic target of rapamycin (mTOR) signaling. Given mTOR's central role as a negative regulator of autophagy, its aberrant activation may suppress autophagic flux, thereby impairing the clearance of damaged organelles and protein aggregates. This dysfunction contributes to increased cellular stress, senescence, and extracellular matrix (ECM) accumulation, ultimately compromising aqueous humor outflow and elevating intraocular pressure (IOP). The evidence thus implicates mTOR-dependent autophagy impairment as a mechanistic link in TM pathology associated with glaucoma.
- mTOR-independent dysregulation: While mTORC1 activity classically suppresses autophagy under nutrient-rich conditions, emerging evidence suggests that autophagy in TM cells can also be activated via mTOR-independent mechanisms. Alternative signaling pathways—such as those mediated by cyclic AMP (cAMP), phospholipase C epsilon (PLCε), and calcium-dependent calpain activity—have been implicated in this noncanonical autophagic regulation. This dynamic interplay between mTOR and alternative autophagy-inducing pathways underscores a mechanotransductive response to stress within the TM, which may be critical for maintaining IOP homeostasis and preventing glaucomatous damage.

Role of mTOR in Apoptosis [2]

The mechanistic target of rapamycin (mTOR) plays a context-dependent dual role in apoptosis, influencing cell survival or death depending on the cellular environment and upstream signals. mTOR generally inhibits apoptosis under normal conditions, promoting survival. However, its dysregulation can lead to pro-apoptotic effects, particularly in neurodegenerative diseases like glaucoma.

Anti-apoptotic Role

mTORC1 and mTORC2 promote cell survival by:

- Activating protein synthesis (via S6K and 4EBP1)
- Enhancing Akt signaling (especially via mTORC2-mediated Akt phosphorylation at Ser473)
- Inhibiting pro-apoptotic factors like Bad, Bim, and FOXO transcription factors
- Supporting mitochondrial integrity and metabolic fitness

Pro-apoptotic Role (in Stress or Overactivation)

In some stress or disease contexts, dysregulated mTOR activity can contribute to:

- Mitochondrial dysfunction and increased reactive oxygen species (ROS)
- Inhibition of autophagy, leading to accumulation of damaged proteins and organelles
- Sensitization to apoptotic stimuli, especially in cancer or neurodegeneration

Apoptosis in Glaucoma

Hyperactivation of mTOR has been linked to retinal ganglion cell apoptosis via:

- Suppression of autophagy
- Increased oxidative stress
- Dysregulation of mitochondrial homeostasis

mTOR Suppression Effect on Trabecular Meshwork

mTOR suppression by rapamycin or metformin in the trabecular meshwork enhances autophagy, reduces fibrosis and ECM buildup, and improves aqueous outflow, aiding in intraocular pressure reduction.

Rapamycin [23]

- Intraocular Pressure Reduction: Rapamycin (Rapa) significantly lowers intraocular pressure (IOP) in mouse models of glucocorticoid-induced glaucoma (GIG).
- Antifibrotic Action: Rapa mitigates glucocorticoid-induced fibrosis in the trabecular meshwork (TM), a key contributor to outflow resistance and elevated IOP [10].
- Extracellular Matrix Regulation: Through inhibition of the mTORC1 pathway, Rapa reduces excessive deposition of extracellular matrix (ECM) proteins in the TM, thereby preserving the outflow facility [22].
- Cytoskeletal Remodeling: By suppressing mTORC2 signaling, Rapa modulates TM cytoskeletal architecture, potentially enhancing aqueous humor dynamics [17].

Metformin [16]

- Transforming growth factor-beta 2 (TGF-β2) is a well-established profibrotic cytokine that promotes the activation of myofibroblasts and the accumulation of extracellular matrix (ECM) proteins such as fibronectin and collagen, contributing to tissue fibrosis. In ocular tissues like the trabecular meshwork (TM), sustained TGF-β2 signaling is implicated in the pathogenesis of glaucoma due to ECM remodeling and increased outflow resistance.
- Metformin, a widely used antidiabetic drug, has been shown to counteract TGF-β2-induced fibrotic responses. One of its mechanisms involves the activation of the autophagy–lysosome pathway, an essential cellular process responsible for degrading long-lived proteins and damaged organelles. In fibrotic conditions, this pathway facilitates the clearance of aberrantly accumulated fibrotic proteins; specifically, metformin enhances autophagic flux, leading to increased formation of autophagosomes and their subsequent fusion with lysosomes.
- The autophagy–lysosome pathway activation results in the degradation of profibrotic proteins such as α-smooth muscle actin (α-SMA), fibronectin, and type I collagen. By restoring autophagic function, metformin reduces the cellular fibrotic burden and mitigates the structural and functional consequences of fibrosis. In experimental models of TGF-β2-induced fibrosis—including human trabecular meshwork cells—metformin treatment not only downregulates fibrotic gene expression but also upregulates key autophagy markers (e.g., LC3-II and

Beclin-1) while promoting the degradation of p62/sequestosome-1, a marker of active autophagy. These findings indicate that metformin's antifibrotic effects are, at least in part, mediated through its capacity to enhance autophagy and lysosomal degradation pathways.

Mechanism of Metformin Action via AMPK [9]

Metformin inhibits complex I of the mitochondrial respiratory chain, reducing ATP production. This increases the AMP/ATP ratio, thereby activating AMPK. Activated AMPK exerts multiple downstream effects:

- Inhibits mTORC1 signaling (key in cell growth and proliferation)
- Enhances insulin sensitivity by modulating GLUT4 translocation
- Promotes autophagy and mitochondrial biogenesis
- Suppresses lipogenesis and promotes fatty acid oxidation

Aqueous Humor Dynamics [18]

mTOR plays a pivotal role in maintaining aqueous humor outflow homeostasis by regulating cellular metabolism, cytoskeletal dynamics, and autophagic activity within the trabecular meshwork (TM). In the healthy eye, mTOR activity is tightly regulated to support TM cell viability, extracellular matrix (ECM) turnover, and cytoskeletal remodeling, all of which are critical for maintaining outflow resistance and intraocular pressure (IOP) within physiological ranges. mTOR signaling also affects aqueous humor production by influencing the metabolism and function of ciliary body epithelial cells. Overactive mTOR can lead to excessive aqueous humor production, contributing to elevated IOP.

Role of mTOR in Different Types of Glaucoma

mTOR activation contributes to glaucoma pathogenesis by upregulating HIF-1α and VEGF signaling in response to elevated intraocular pressure.

mTOR is increasingly recognized as a critical regulator of cellular homeostasis in the trabecular meshwork (TM), optic nerve head, and retinal ganglion cells (RGCs)—all of which are affected in various forms of glaucoma. Dysregulation of mTOR signaling contributes to disease progression through multiple mechanisms, including impaired autophagy, fibrotic remodeling, and neurodegeneration. The role of mTOR differs across glaucoma subtypes, reflecting the diverse pathophysiological features of each form.

Across multiple glaucoma subtypes, mTOR signaling emerges as a critical node linking metabolic stress, fibrotic remodeling, and neurodegeneration. Therapeutic targeting of mTOR particularly through isoform-specific inhibition or pathway modulation—holds promise for disease modification beyond IOP reduction (Fig. 6.3).

mTORC1 and mTORC2 play roles in retinal ganglion cell (RGC) survival. Dysregulated mTOR activity may lead to RGC apoptosis and optic nerve degeneration, contributing to glaucomatous vision loss.

1. Primary Open-Angle Glaucoma (POAG)

In POAG, increased mTOR activity in TM cells leads to reduced autophagic flux and excessive deposition of extracellular matrix (ECM), contributing to increased outflow resistance and elevated intraocular pressure (IOP). Additionally, chronic mTOR activation may promote TM cell senescence and oxidative stress, further compromising aqueous humor drainage. Targeted mTOR inhibition has shown potential in restoring TM function and lowering IOP in experimental models [5].

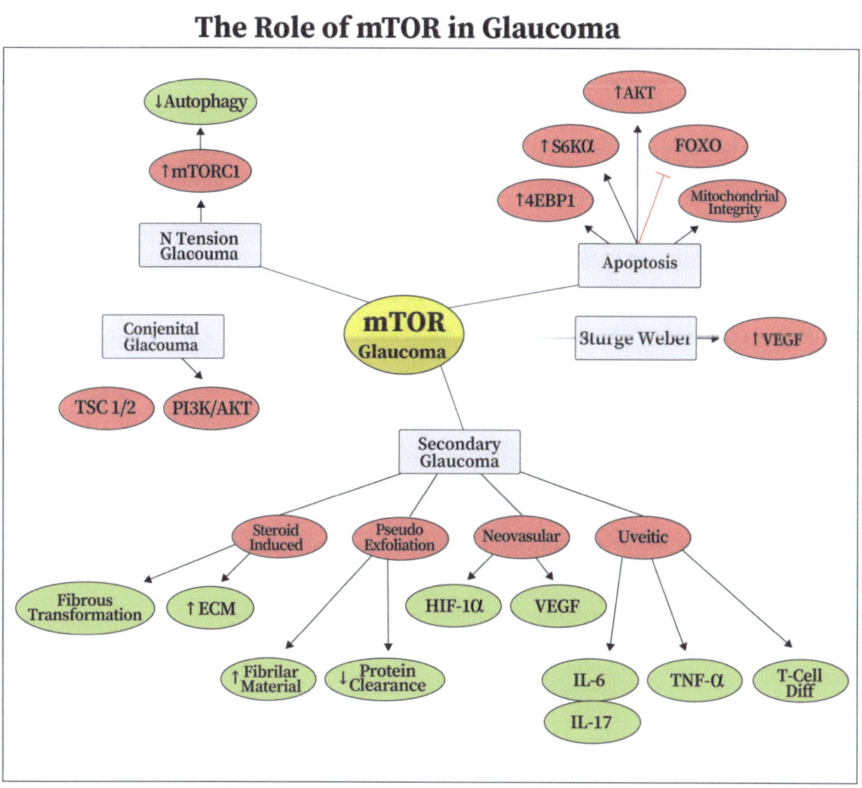

Fig. 6.3 The image illustrates how mTOR is involved in different types of glaucoma through distinct molecular pathways that influence disease progression and cellular responses

2. Normal-Tension Glaucoma (NTG)

Although IOP remains within normal limits, NTG involves progressive optic nerve damage and RGC death. In this context, mTOR dysregulation is primarily implicated in neuronal survival and axonal transport. Hyperactivation of mTORC1 may suppress protective autophagy in RGCs, rendering them more susceptible to mitochondrial dysfunction and apoptotic cell death. Restoring the mTOR–autophagy balance may help preserve RGC integrity in NTG.

3. Secondary Glaucoma

mTOR influences inflammatory and fibrotic processes involved in secondary glaucomas.

- *Steroid-Induced Glaucoma:* Glucocorticoids activate mTOR signaling, enhancing fibrotic transformation of TM cells and ECM accumulation. mTOR inhibitors such as rapamycin can mitigate steroid-induced TM fibrosis by promoting autophagy and reducing profibrotic signaling.
- *Pseudo-Exfoliation Glaucoma (PXG)*: Characterized by accumulation of fibrillar material in the anterior segment, PXG may involve impaired protein clearance mechanisms. Abnormal mTOR signaling may contribute to defective autophagy and ECM remodeling in the TM, although direct evidence remains limited.
- *Neovascular Glaucoma (NVG)*: In NVG, mTOR influences angiogenic signaling, particularly through the HIF-1α/VEGF pathway. mTOR inhibition may suppress pathologic neovascularization and inflammatory responses in the anterior chamber angle (hypoxia-inducible factor (HIF), a master regulator of angiogenesis) [11].

Uveitic Glaucoma mTOR contributes to inflammation-induced trabecular meshwork dysfunction and fibrosis. Its activation promotes immune cell proliferation, cytokine production, and fibrotic remodeling, all of which impair aqueous humor outflow and elevate IOP. mTORC1 and mTORC2 regulate immune cell activation, cytokine production (e.g., IL-6, IL-17, and TNF-α), and T-cell differentiation (Th1/Th17), contributing to persistent ocular inflammation. mTOR inhibitors may help modulate both inflammation and fibrosis in this context [24].

4. Congenital and Juvenile Glaucoma

The role of mTOR in developmental glaucomas is less well defined, but evidence suggests it may be involved in abnormal differentiation and maturation of TM and Schlemm's canal cells. Genetic alterations affecting upstream regulators of mTOR (e.g., TSC1/2 and PI3K/AKT pathway) may play a role in certain congenital forms [6].

mTOR and VEGF in Sturge–Weber Syndrome [1]

The mechanistic target of rapamycin (mTOR) pathway is a central regulator of cellular growth, metabolism, and angiogenesis. One of its downstream targets is vascular endothelial growth factor (VEGF), a key mediator of blood vessel formation. Under normal physiological conditions, mTOR signaling modulates VEGF expression in response to cellular energy status, oxygen availability, and growth signals.

In Sturge–Weber syndrome, a rare neurocutaneous disorder characterized by leptomeningeal angiomas and facial port-wine stains, hyperactivation of the mTOR pathway has been observed. This dysregulation is believed to contribute to excessive and abnormal angiogenesis, mediated in part by overexpression of VEGF.

Consequently, mTOR inhibitors such as rapamycin (sirolimus) and everolimus have been proposed as therapeutic agents. By inhibiting mTORC1 activity, these drugs may reduce VEGF expression and thereby suppress the pathological vascular proliferation associated with SWS. Preclinical models and early clinical data support the potential of mTOR inhibition to normalize vascular development and reduce disease burden in affected tissues.

Therapeutic Implications for mTOR in Anterior Segment and Glaucoma

1. *Trabecular Meshwork Protection:*
   - mTOR inhibitors may reduce ECM deposition and oxidative stress in TM cells, improving aqueous humor outflow and reducing IOP (Y.[23]).
2. *Aqueous Humor Suppression:*
   - Targeting mTOR in the ciliary body could modulate aqueous humor production, lowering IOP in glaucoma patients (Y. [23]).
3. *Neuroprotection:*
   - mTOR modulation may protect RGCs from apoptosis in glaucoma by enhancing autophagy and reducing oxidative stress [19].
4. *Antifibrotic Therapy:*
   - mTOR inhibitors can mitigate fibrosis in secondary glaucomas, particularly after surgical interventions.
   - Src modulator, a non-receptor tyrosine kinase, plays a pivotal role in regulating key cellular processes such as fibroblast activation, extracellular matrix (ECM) deposition, and cellular metabolism, positioning it as a potential therapeutic target in the treatment of glaucoma [4].

- c-Src is a key signaling molecule in several pathways activated by growth factors, integrins, cytokines, and hormones.
- It phosphorylates tyrosine residues on specific substrate proteins, regulating downstream signaling cascades.
- It interacts with proteins containing SH2 (Src homology 2) and SH3 domains, facilitating signal transduction.

Physiological Roles

- Cell growth and proliferation: Via MAPK and PI3K/Akt pathways.
- Cell adhesion and migration: Through interaction with focal adhesion kinase (FAK) and regulation of the cytoskeleton.
- Survival: Promotes anti-apoptotic signaling.
- Angiogenesis: Modulates VEGF signaling in endothelial cells.

Oncogenic Potential

- When mutated, overexpressed, or dysregulated, Src becomes constitutively active, leading to oncogenic transformation.
- Src activation is implicated in multiple cancers (e.g., breast, colon, lung, and prostate cancers) through enhanced cell proliferation, increased motility and invasiveness, and resistance to apoptosis.

Summary of mTOR Effects on the Anterior Segment and Glaucoma

Aspect	Normal function	Dysregulated function
Trabecular meshwork	Maintains ECM turnover and outflow resistance regulation	ECM accumulation, reduced outflow, and increased IOP
Ciliary body	Regulates aqueous humor production	Overproduction of aqueous humor
Retinal ganglion cells	Promotes survival under stress	Apoptosis and optic nerve degeneration
Lens	Supports epithelial cell function	Aberrant protein synthesis and cataract formation

Rho–ROCK Pathway Activation [12]

Several inhibitory molecules, including Nogo-A and myelin-associated glycoprotein (MAG), exert their effects on retinal ganglion cell (RGC) growth cones through the Rho/ROCK signaling cascade. Rho, a small GTPase of the Rho family, activates Rho-associated coiled-coil-containing protein kinase (ROCK), a key downstream effector extensively studied in the central nervous system. Activation of the Rho–ROCK pathway leads to the phosphorylation of multiple downstream targets, ultimately inhibiting neuronal survival and axonal regeneration. This inhibition is mediated, in part, through antagonistic interactions with the PI3K/Akt/mTOR signaling pathway.

mTOR Effect on Iris

mTORC1 supports the proliferation and maintenance of iris epithelial cells. Dysregulation may affect iris pigmentation and contribute to structural abnormalities [13].

mTOR Effect on Lens

mTOR regulates lens epithelial cell proliferation and differentiation into fiber cells. Dysregulated mTOR activity can lead to cataract formation due to aberrant protein synthesis and oxidative stress. This will be discussed in Chap. 7 of this book.

Bibliography

1. Shah A. Sturge–weber syndrome: a narrative review of clinical presentation and updates on management. J Clin Med. 2025;14 https://doi.org/10.3390/jcm14072182.
2. Xia, et al. Apoptosis in glaucoma: a new direction for the treatment of glaucoma (review). Mol Med Rep. 2024;29 https://doi.org/10.3892/mmr.2024.13207.
3. Belforte. AMPK hyperactivation promotes dendrite retraction, synaptic loss, and neuronal dysfunction in glaucoma. Mol Neurodegener. 2021;16 https://doi.org/10.1186/s13024-021-00466-z.
4. Bourke. Fibrosis and Src signalling in glaucoma: from molecular pathways to therapeutic prospects. Int J Mol Sci. 2025;26 https://doi.org/10.3390/ijms26031009.
5. Buonfiglio. Glaucoma and the ocular renin-angiotensin-aldosterone system: update on molecular signalling and treatment perspectives. Cell Signal. 2024;122 https://doi.org/10.1016/j.cellsig.2024.111343.
6. Faig. Functional genomics of primary congenital glaucoma by pathway analysis and functional characterization of CYP1B1 mutations. Vision Res. 2025;227 https://doi.org/10.1016/j.visres.2024.108534.

7. Fomo. Neuroretinal cell culture model as a tool for the development of new therapeutic approaches for oxidative stress-induced ocular diseases, with a focus on glaucoma. Cells. 2024; https://doi.org/10.3390/cells13090775.
8. Wang G. Autophagy activation ameliorates the fibrosis of trabecular meshwork cells induced by TGFβ2 through the promotion of fibrotic proteins degradation. Human Cell. 2024a; https://doi.org/10.1007/s13577-024-01141-3.
9. González-Casanova. New perspectives on the molecular action of metformin in the context of cellular transduction and adipogenesis. Int J Mol Sci. 2025;26 https://doi.org/10.3390/ijms26083690.
10. Igarashi. mTOR inhibitors potentially reduce TGF-β2-induced fibrogenic changes in trabecular meshwork cells. Scientific Reports. 2021; https://doi.org/10.1038/s41598-021-93580-3.
11. Zhou J. Role of mammalian target of rapamycin in regulating HIF-1α and vascular endothelial growth factor signals in glaucoma. Arch Physiol Biochem. 2018;127 https://doi.org/10.1080/13813455.2019.1609996.
12. Jing L. The role of the Rho/ROCK signaling pathway in inhibiting axonal regeneration in the central nervous system. Neural Regen Res. 2015; https://doi.org/10.4103/1673-5374.170325.
13. Moazed. Molecular biology of iris. Cham: Springer; 2020. https://doi.org/10.1007/978-3-030-45756-3_5.
14. Porter. mTOR-independent induction of autophagy in trabecular meshwork cells subjected to biaxial stretch. Biochim Biophys Acta. 2014; https://doi.org/10.1016/j.bbamcr.2014.02.010.
15. Porter. Autophagic dysregulation in glaucomatous trabecular meshwork cells. Molecular Basis of Disease. 2015;1852 https://doi.org/10.1016/j.bbadis.2014.11.021.
16. Ren J. Metformin alleviates fibrosis of trabecular meshwork cells induced by TGFβ2 through the activation of autophagy. Sage J. 2025; https://doi.org/10.1177/15593258251341598.
17. Sacchi. Fighting Bleb fibrosis after glaucoma surgery: updated focus on key players and novel targets for therapy. Int J Mol Sci. 2025; https://doi.org/10.3390/ijms26052327.
18. Shim. The physiological and pathophysiological roles of the autophagy lysosomal system in the conventional aqueous humor outflow pathway: more than cellular clean up. Prog Retin Eye Res. 2022;90 https://doi.org/10.1016/j.preteyeres.2022.101064.
19. Si Z. The role of RGC degeneration in the pathogenesis of glaucoma. Int J Biol Sci. 2025;21 https://doi.org/10.7150/ijbs.103222.
20. Rey V. From kinases to diseases: investigating the role of AMPK in human pathologies. Kinases Phosphatases. 2023;1 https://doi.org/10.3390/kinasesphosphatases1030012.
21. Watanabe. mTOR inhibitors modulate the biological nature of TGF-β2-treated or -untreated human trabecular meshwork cells in different manners. NIH, Biomedicines. 2024; https://doi.org/10.3390/biomedicines12112604.
22. Xiao Y-L. Autophagy mediates MMP-2 expression in glaucomatous trabecular meshwork cells. J Ophthalmol. 2022;2022 https://doi.org/10.1155/2022/6026464.
23. Song Y. Rapamycin protects glucocorticoid-induced glaucoma model mice against trabecular meshwork fibrosis by suppressing mTORC1/2 signaling. Eur J Pharmacol. 2025; https://doi.org/10.1016/j.ejphar.2025.177269.
24. Wang Y. Ocular immune-related diseases: molecular mechanisms and therapy. Med Comm. 2024b; https://doi.org/10.1002/mco2.70021.
25. Zhang Y. Aging, cellular senescence, and glaucoma. Aging Dis. 2024; https://doi.org/10.14336/AD.2023.0630-1.

Chapter 7
mTOR Role in the Lens

Contents

Abstract The mechanistic target of rapamycin (mTOR) plays an essential role in regulating cellular proliferation, differentiation, and metabolic homeostasis within the human lens. During lens development and maintenance, mTOR activity governs epithelial cell proliferation and fiber cell elongation, processes essential for preserving lens transparency and structural integrity. Dysregulation of mTOR signaling has been associated with age-related cataractogenesis, partly through impaired autophagy, oxidative stress accumulation, and altered protein homeostasis. Inhibition of mTOR, particularly mTORC1, has been shown to enhance autophagic flux, reduce reactive oxygen species, and stabilize crystallin proteins, thereby delaying cataract formation in experimental models. Thus, mTOR represents a key molecular integrator of growth and stress responses in the lens, with potential therapeutic implications for age-related and metabolic cataracts.

K. T. Moazed, *mTOR Signaling in Ophthalmology*,
https://doi.org/10.1007/978-3-032-05044-1_7

Discussion

The lens is a distinctive, encapsulated structure consisting of an anterior layer of cuboidal epithelial cells that overlies a core of elongated, transparent fiber cells. The differentiation of immature lens epithelial cells into these specialized, organelle-free, transparent fiber cells requires the precise coordination of multiple signaling, transcriptional, and translational pathways. Notably, this differentiation process continues throughout life. Disruptions in this lens differentiation program—whether during development or at later stages—can lead to the lens opacification and cataract formation.

The summary of the effect of mTOR in the lens can be explained by its involvement in:

1. *Lens development and growth*—regulating epithelial cell proliferation and fiber cell differentiation.
2. *Transparency and homeostasis*—maintaining metabolic balance and antioxidant defense.
3. *Autophagy and protein aggregation*—modulating protein turnover and preventing accumulation of damaged proteins.
4. *Injury and repair*—facilitating cellular regeneration after stress.
5. *Cataract formation*—where dysregulated mTOR activity contributes to oxidative stress, impaired autophagy, and lens opacification (Fig. 7.1).

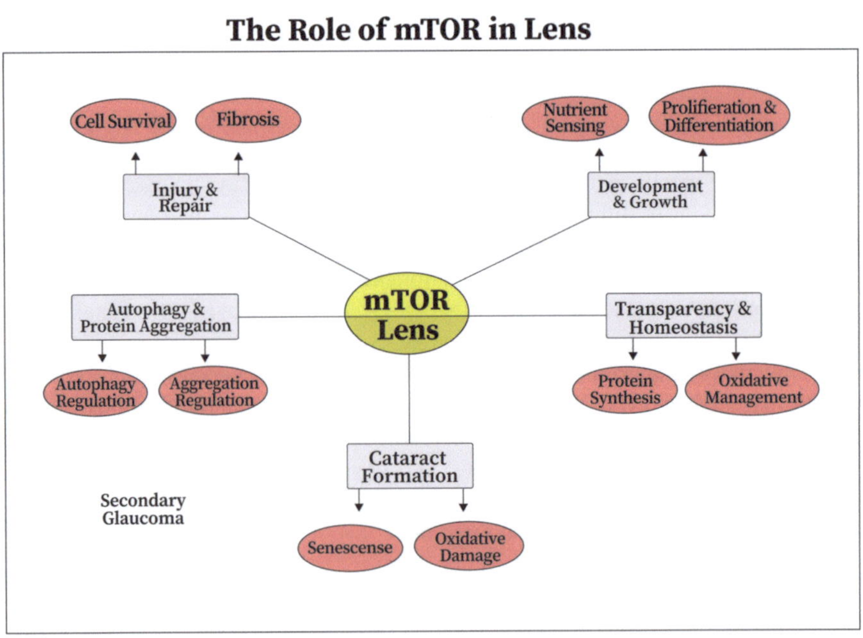

Fig. 7.1 The image illustrates the different roles of mTOR involved in lens development and maintenance

Role of mTOR in Lens Development and Maintenance

The mechanistic target of rapamycin (mTOR) is a central integrator of growth factor signals (especially FGF and IGF) and cellular nutrient status [2].

It plays essential roles in:

- *Lens Fiber Cell Differentiation:* mTORC1 activity promotes protein synthesis, including crystallins, and supports organelle degradation necessary for lens transparency.
- *Cell Growth and Elongation:* mTOR regulates cytoskeletal dynamics and biosynthetic processes critical for fiber cell elongation.
- *Metabolic Support:* Through mTORC2, it modulates AKT activation, contributing to cell survival and redox balance.
- *Lens Maintenance:* mTOR ensures homeostatic protein turnover, nutrient sensing, and stress response in lens epithelial cells.

Dysregulation of mTOR activity can contribute to aberrant fiber differentiation, accumulation of damaged proteins, and cataract formation, especially under conditions of oxidative or metabolic stress.

Lens Signaling Pathways

Here is a summary of the key signaling pathways involved in the development and maintenance of the human lens, with brief descriptions of their roles [11].

1. Fibroblast Growth Factor (FGF) Signaling
    - *Function:* Central to lens fiber cell differentiation. A gradient of FGF activity from anterior to posterior determines epithelial proliferation versus fiber differentiation.
    - *Pathways Involved:* Activates ERK/MAPK, PI3K/AKT, and PLCγ pathways to drive proliferation, survival, and expression of lens-specific proteins (e.g., crystallins).
2. Transforming Growth Factor Beta (TGFβ) Signaling
    - *Function:* Involved in lens development and wound response; promotes epithelial–mesenchymal transition (EMT) when dysregulated.
    - *Mechanism:* Activates Smad2/3–Smad4 complexes for transcriptional regulation; excessive activity is associated with anterior subcapsular cataract (ASC) and posterior capsule opacification (PCO).
3. Bone Morphogenetic Protein (BMP) Signaling
    - *Function:* Opposes TGFβ; maintains lens epithelial phenotype and inhibits EMT.

- *Mechanism:* Activates Smad1/5/8–Smad4 complexes. BMP7 is especially important for preventing fibrosis and promoting lens transparency.

4. Wnt/β-Catenin Signaling
   - *Function:* Regulates lens progenitor cell proliferation and anterior–posterior polarity during early development.
   - *Role in Maintenance:* Suppressed in lens fiber cells; misactivation can disrupt epithelial integrity or cause EMT.
5. Notch Signaling
   - *Function:* Maintains the balance between lens epithelial cell proliferation and differentiation.
   - *Mechanism:* Through Notch receptors and ligands (e.g., Jagged/Delta), it ensures proper spacing and timing of fiber cell differentiation.
6. Hedgehog (Hh) Signaling
   - *Function:* Regulates lens epithelial cell proliferation and lens vesicle formation during early development.
   - *Ligands:* Includes Sonic hedgehog (Shh); supports normal lens size and shape.
7. Retinoic Acid (RA) Signaling
   - *Function:* Modulates lens placode invagination and separation of the lens vesicle from the surface ectoderm.
   - *Role:* Works in concert with FGF and Wnt to control optic vesicle–lens interactions.
8. PI3K/AKT Signaling
   - *Function:* Promotes cell survival and metabolic activity, especially during lens fiber cell elongation and organelle degradation.
   - *Cross Talk:* Often activated downstream of FGF and IGF signaling.
9. ERK/MAPK Signaling
   - *Function:* Key effector of FGF-mediated lens fiber differentiation.
   - *Role:* Drives expression of crystallins and structural proteins and initiates cytoskeletal remodeling for fiber elongation.
10. Hippo-YAP/TAZ Signaling
    - *Emerging Role:* May regulate lens cell density, proliferation, and *mechanosensing* during development and wound healing.
    - *Status:* Still under active investigation in ocular biology.
11. JAK/STAT Signaling
    - *Function:* Involved in lens cell proliferation and response to inflammation or stress.

- *Evidence:* May contribute to fibrotic changes when chronically activated.

12. Insulin-like Growth Factor (IGF) Signaling

- *Function:* Promotes lens cell survival, growth, and metabolism.
- *Interaction:* Shares PI3K/AKT and MAPK pathways with FGF (Fig. 7.2).

Here, we focus exclusively on the most influential mTOR-regulated signaling pathways that are essential for the development and maintenance of the lens. Particular emphasis is placed on the molecular mechanisms underlying cataract formation, which serve as the hallmark of pathological changes leading to lens opacification.

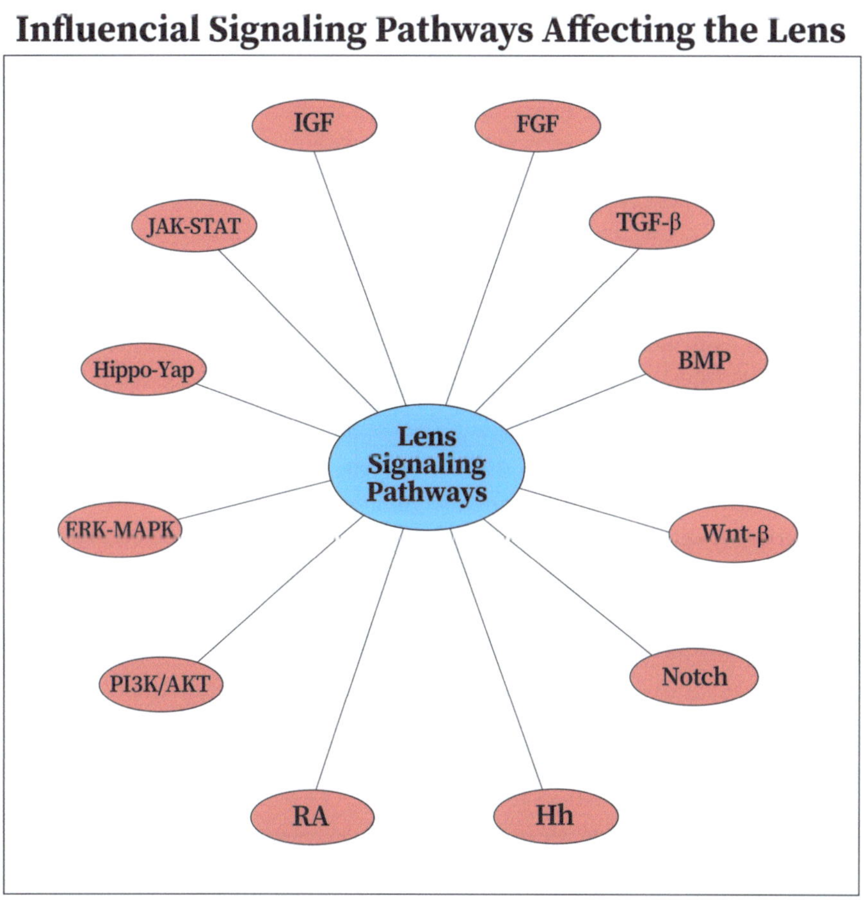

Fig. 7.2 The image illustrates the influential signaling pathways that are involved in the development and maintenance of the lens

FGF (Fibroblast Growth Factor) Signaling

Fibroblast growth factor (FGF) signaling acts as a graded morphogen-like cue in the lens, with its concentration varying across the tissue to provide critical spatial and temporal instructions for cell behavior [4].

This gradient regulates the transition from proliferation to differentiation within the lens epithelium. By activating downstream pathways such as ERK, PI3K/AKT, and PLCγ, FGF signaling coordinates a tightly controlled transcriptional program necessary for maintaining lens transparency and function. Perturbations in this signaling cascade—whether due to genetic mutations, metabolic stress, or aging—can contribute to the development of both congenital and age-related cataracts.

FGF Signaling in Lens Fiber Cell Differentiation

As the lens vesicle transitions into a mature, multilayered structure, FGF signaling becomes the central driver of cell fate determination within the lens. FGF not only regulates proliferation and survival of lens epithelial cells (LECs) but also plays a crucial role in initiating and sustaining differentiation into lens fiber cells, which are essential for lens transparency and refractive function.

- The lens epithelium exhibits a two-dimensional FGF gradient, both anteroposteriorly and from the anterior pole toward the equator.
- Anterior Epithelium: Cells here are exposed to low levels of FGF, maintaining a proliferative, undifferentiated epithelial phenotype.
- Equatorial Region: Cells experience intermediate-to-high FGF levels, initiating cell cycle exit and fiber cell differentiation.
- Posterior Lens Fiber Zone: Cells exposed to the highest FGF concentration undergo terminal differentiation, elongation, and crystallin gene expression.

This gradient is believed to arise from aqueous and vitreous humor-derived FGF, creating a signaling field across the lens epithelium.

Role of Adaptors

Fibroblast growth factor (FGF) signaling plays an essential role in lens development by orchestrating a complex network of molecular interactions that regulate cell proliferation, differentiation, and survival. One of the critical early events in FGF signaling is the phosphorylation of adaptor proteins that link activated FGF receptors to downstream effector pathways [14].

Shc1 (Src Homology 2 domain containing) is an adaptor protein that becomes phosphorylated on specific tyrosine residues upon FGF stimulation, creating binding sites for the Grb2 protein, which in turn recruits the guanine nucleotide exchange factor SOS, leading to activation of the Ras/MAPK pathway. This signaling axis is essential for lens vesicle morphogenesis and subsequent lens fiber cell differentiation.

In the context of this signaling network, Frs2 (FGF receptor substrate 2) and Shp2 (Src homology 2 domain-containing phosphatase 2) are also key adaptor proteins. Frs2 binds directly to activated FGF receptors and becomes phosphorylated, serving as a platform for assembling Grb2, Shp2, and other signaling molecules. Shp2 dephosphorylates specific sites and modulates the intensity and duration of FGF signaling, fine-tuning downstream outcomes.

The deletion of Shc1 exacerbates the lens vesicle defect observed when both Frs2 and Shp2 are absent, highlighting Shc1's critical collaborative role with Frs2 and Shp2 in recruiting Grb2. This suggests that Shc1 acts as a parallel adaptor that compensates for the loss of Frs2 or Shp2 by ensuring Grb2 recruitment and activation of downstream Ras/MAPK signaling. Without Shc1, the loss of Frs2 and Shp2 leads to a severe impairment of FGF signaling, thereby disrupting the coordinated cell behaviors necessary for normal lens morphogenesis.

Shc1 is a central component of the FGF signaling complex in the developing lens, acting in concert with Frs2 and Shp2 to integrate upstream FGF receptor signals and direct them toward the Grb2-Ras/MAPK axis, ultimately ensuring proper lens vesicle formation and development.

Signal Transduction Pathways Activated by FGF

FGF ligands (e.g., FGF1 and FGF2) bind to FGF receptors (FGFR1–4) on lens cells, leading to receptor dimerization and autophosphorylation, followed by activation of distinct intracellular cascades [3].

(a) ERK/MAPK Pathway:

- Prominent at intermediate to high FGF levels.
- Drives cell cycle exit and upregulation of lens-specific genes (e.g., crystallins and aquaporin 0).
- Promotes cytoskeletal reorganization, fiber cell elongation, and organelle degradation.

(b) PI3K/AKT Pathway [17]:

- Supports cell survival, metabolic activity, and contributes to lens fiber maturation.
- AKT activation is essential for resisting stress-induced apoptosis during the differentiation process.

(c) PLCγ Pathway [9]:

- Involved in calcium signaling and regulation of gene transcription.
- Though less characterized in the lens, it modulates differentiation and membrane remodeling.

FGF Role in Lens Morphogenesis and Cataractogenesis

Proper FGF signaling is indispensable for the highly ordered structure of the lens. Any dysregulation—due to genetic mutations in FGFRs, misexpression of ligands, or aberrant downstream activation—can impair:

- Lens polarity and elongation of fiber cells
- Crystallin expression, essential for transparency
- Cytoskeletal integrity, resulting in opacification (cataract)

Experimental models show that:

- Loss of FGF signaling leads to failure of fiber differentiation and disorganized lens architecture
- Constitutive activation of FGFRs can cause epithelial–mesenchymal transition-like changes, fibrosis, and anterior subcapsular cataract

PDGF (Platelet-Derived Growth Factor)

PDGF is a mitogenic signaling molecule that plays crucial roles in cell proliferation, survival, migration, and differentiation, particularly in development, wound healing, and angiogenesis. PDGF is a dimeric protein composed of two polypeptide chains (A, B, C, or D) that form homo- or heterodimers (e.g., PDGF-AA, -BB, -AB, -CC, or -DD). It signals through receptor tyrosine kinases (PDGFR-α and PDGFR-β) which dimerize upon ligand binding and undergo autophosphorylation, triggering downstream signaling cascades [21].

PDGF Key Functions in Development and Wound Healing

PDGF is critical for mesenchymal cell development, particularly in the formation of vascular smooth muscle, fibroblasts, and pericytes. In the lens, PDGF helps maintain the epithelial progenitor cell pool, counterbalancing prodifferentiation signals such as FGF.

PDGF promotes fibroblast proliferation, ECM production, and angiogenesis at injury sites. Overactivation of PDGF signaling is implicated in fibrosis, atherosclerosis, and some cancers, due to excessive proliferation and migration of mesenchymal cells.

Major Downstream Pathways Activated by PDGF

1. PI3K/AKT pathway—promotes cell survival and growth
2. MAPK/ERK pathway—supports cell proliferation and gene expression

3. PLCγ pathway—regulates calcium signaling and cell motility
4. STAT pathway—influences inflammatory gene expression

PDGF and Human Lens Development

Platelet-derived growth factor (PDGF) signals via the phosphoinositide 3-kinase (PI3K)/Akt pathway to enhance Notch signaling, thereby contributing to the maintenance of the progenitor state in lens epithelial cells [15]:

- Is active mainly in the anterior epithelial zone
- Signals via PI3K/AKT to enhance Notch signaling, helping maintain the progenitor state of lens epithelial cells
- Acts antagonistically to FGF, which drives differentiation via the ERK pathway

During lens development, precise spatial and temporal control of lens epithelial cell proliferation, differentiation, and maintenance of the progenitor pool is orchestrated by extracellular growth factors. Among these, fibroblast growth factor (FGF) and platelet-derived growth factor (PDGF) play opposing yet complementary roles through activation of distinct downstream signaling cascades [10].

1. FGF Signaling: Promotes Differentiation
   - FGF acts as a prodifferentiation signal, particularly at the equatorial region of the lens, where lens epithelial cells exit the cell cycle and begin to elongate into secondary lens fiber cells.
   - Downstream signaling bias:
     - FGF activates the Ras–MAPK (ERK) pathway, which is pivotal for:
       - Initiating lens fiber differentiation
       - Inducing the expression of fiber-specific proteins (e.g., crystallins and MIP/Aquaporin 0)
       - Promoting cytoskeletal remodeling and elongation
   - At higher concentrations, FGF also activates PI3K/AKT, supporting survival, but its main functional output is ERK-driven differentiation.
2. PDGF Signaling: Maintains Progenitor Identity
   - PDGF is more active in the anterior lens epithelium, where it helps preserve the lens epithelial progenitor pool
   - Downstream signaling bias:
     - PDGF preferentially activates the PI3K/AKT pathway, which:
       - Promotes cell survival and proliferation
       - Enhances Notch signaling, which is crucial for:
       - Inhibiting premature differentiation.

  - Maintaining the self-renewal capacity of lens progenitor cells.
- Notch activation, through PDGF-PI3K signaling, establishes a feedback loop to maintain epithelial phenotype and prevent differentiation signals from dominating prematurely.

3. Antagonistic Interplay

Fibroblast growth factor (fgf) and platelet-derived growth factor (PDGF) are key signaling molecules that regulate various cellular processes, including proliferation, differentiation, migration, and angiogenesis. Although both factors can promote cell growth and survival, they often exhibit antagonistic interplay in certain biological contexts, such as tissue repair, fibrosis, and tumorigenesis.

The interplay between FGF and PDGF is antagonistic but context-dependent, involving competitive receptor binding, downstream signaling biases, transcriptional regulation, and tissue-specific feedback mechanisms. Understanding this balance is crucial for developing targeted therapies in diseases characterized by dysregulated growth factor signaling, such as fibrosis, cancer, and proliferative retinopathies.

- FGF and PDGF antagonize each other through their divergent downstream biases:
  - FGF-ERK promotes differentiation, suppressing Notch expression.
  - PDGF-PI3K sustains Notch signaling, which inhibits ERK-mediated differentiation.
- This antagonism ensures that only lens epithelial cells at the appropriate position (equator) and developmental stage respond to differentiation cues, while anterior cells remain proliferative.

Receptor Cross Talk and Competition

- FGF binds primarily to FGFR1-4 receptors, activating pathways such as MAPK/ERK and PI3K/AKT, which drive proliferation and survival.
- PDGF binds to PDGFRα and PDGFRβ, similarly activating MAPK/ERK and PI3K/AKT pathways.
- These receptors can heterodimerize or compete for downstream signaling intermediates (e.g., GRB2, PLCγ, or PI3K), leading to signaling bias depending on the relative expression and activation status of FGF and PDGF receptors.

Downstream Signaling Bias

- FGF signaling often favors proliferation and migration in endothelial cells and fibroblasts, while PDGF signaling tends to stabilize the extracellular matrix and promote pericyte recruitment, favoring tissue remodeling.
- In some contexts, excessive FGF signaling can suppress PDGF-induced fibroblast differentiation or vice versa, depending on the tissue microenvironment.

Transcriptional Antagonism

- FGF signaling can induce transcriptional repressors (e.g., SPRY proteins) that negatively regulate PDGF receptor signaling and vice versa.
- This feedback ensures that one pathway does not excessively dominate, maintaining tissue homeostasis.

4. Developmental and Functional Significance

- FGF gradients across the lens help establish the transition zone between proliferating epithelial cells and differentiating fibers.
- PDGF and Notch provide a brake against overactivation of FGF-induced differentiation, preserving lens epithelial cell reservoirs.
- Disruption in this balance may result in:
  - Defective fiber cell elongation or maturation (if FGF is impaired)
  - Loss of epithelial integrity and progenitor depletion (if PDGF/Notch is suppressed)
  - Ultimately leading to lens malformations or cataract formation

FGF and PDGF Interaction

FGF and PDGF represent functionally opposing regulators in lens development. Through preferential activation of ERK/MAPK (FGF) versus PI3K/Notch (PDGF), they finely tune the spatiotemporal control of lens progenitor maintenance and differentiation. This mutual antagonism safeguards lens architecture and transparency by balancing epithelial proliferation with fiber cell formation [10] (Fig. 7.3).

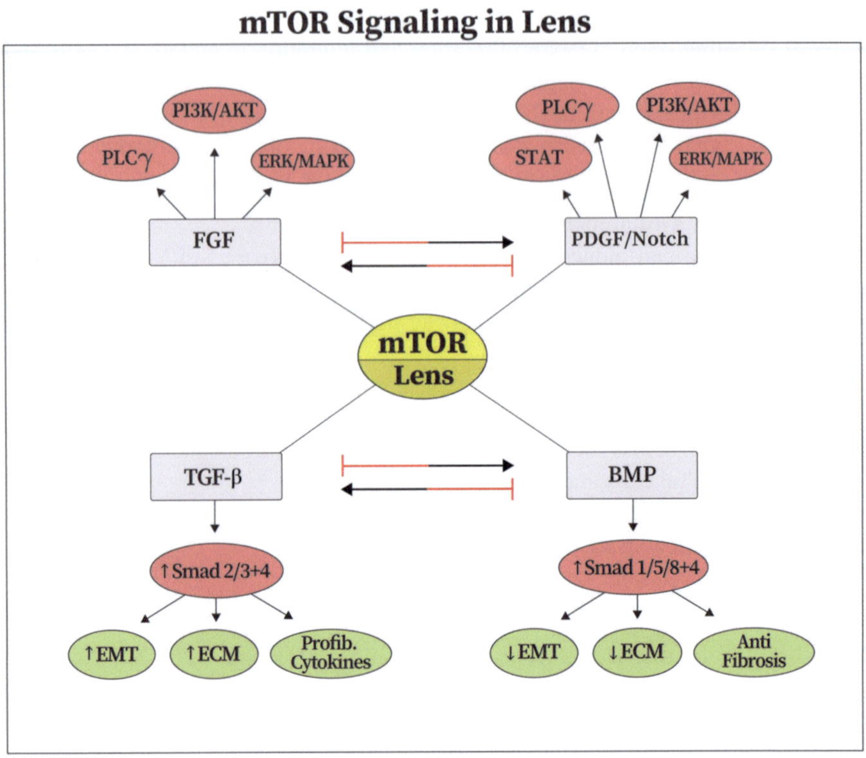

Fig. 7.3 The image depicts the complex and context-dependent antagonistic interplay of mTOR signaling pathways, highlighting how mTOR integrates signals from multiple pathways-including FGF, PDGF, Notch, TGFß, and BMP-to regulate cellular processes. These interactions illustrate both synergistic and opposing effects, emphasizing the dynamic nature of mTOR's role in cellular growth, differentiation, and homeostasis

TGFβ and BMP Signaling

The human lens is a transparent, avascular tissue that grows throughout life, maintaining its clarity through a tightly regulated balance of cell proliferation, differentiation, and extracellular matrix (ECM) remodeling. TGFβ and BMP signaling play opposing roles in these processes and are critically involved in lens development, maintenance, and pathologies, particularly posterior capsule opacification (PCO) and anterior subcapsular cataract (ASC) [7].

1. Receptor Signaling Mechanism in Lens Cells
   - *TGFβ and BMP ligands* are expressed in the ocular environment, including the aqueous humor and lens epithelial cells (LECs) [5].
   - These ligands bind to their respective type II receptors (TGFβRII or BMPRII), which recruit and phosphorylate type I receptors (ALKs).

2. Canonical Smad Signaling in the Lens [8]

   TGFβ Pathway (Profibrotic, Pro-EMT)

- In lens epithelial cells (LECs) [16].
  - TGFβ activates Smad2/3, which then form complexes with Smad4 and translocate to the nucleus.
  - This induces the expression of genes associated with:
    - Epithelial-to-mesenchymal transition (EMT) (e.g., α-SMA, fibronectin).
    - ECM production (e.g., collagen types I and IV).
    - Profibrotic cytokines and integrins.
- Pathologically, TGFβ signaling is a key driver of anterior subcapsular cataract and PCO, as it promotes aberrant differentiation of LECs into myofibroblasts, leading to fibrosis and lens opacity.

BMP (Bone Morphogenetic Protein) Signaling: The bone morphogenetic protein (BMP) pathway modulates cellular growth, differentiation, and apoptosis. It is known for its antifibrotic properties and contributes to tissue homeostasis by inhibiting excessive extracellular matrix production and promoting balanced cell turnover [7].

- BMPs (e.g., BMP4 and BMP7) activate Smad1/5/8, forming complexes with Smad4.
- In lens cells:
  - BMP signaling supports normal epithelial phenotype, prevents EMT, and maintains lens transparency.

BMP7, in particular, has been shown to antagonize TGFβ-induced EMT and fibrosis in LECs.

3. Inhibitory Regulation in the Lens
   - Smad7 is upregulated in response to TGFβ and inhibits further TGFβ signaling by:
     - Blocking R-Smad phosphorylation
     - Recruiting Smurf2 to ubiquitinate TGFβRI
   - Smad6 preferentially inhibits BMP signaling and is also expressed in lens tissue.
   - These inhibitory Smads are critical in attenuating excessive fibrotic responses and maintaining cellular homeostasis in the lens.
4. Extracellular Modulation in the Ocular Microenvironment
   - The aqueous humor contains BMP antagonists such as noggin, gremlin, and chordin, which modulate the bioavailability of BMPs to LECs.

- BAMBI**,** a pseudo-receptor expressed in lens epithelium, inhibits both BMP and TGFβ signaling by acting as a dominant-negative receptor, especially during lens injury or fibrosis [13].

5. Functional Significance in the Lens

   - During embryonic lens development**,** BMP signaling promotes lens placode invagination and differentiation of lens fiber cells.
   - In adulthood, BMPs help preserve the quiescent state of lens epithelial cells**,** while dysregulated TGFβ signaling contributes to fibrosis, EMT, and cataract formation**.**
   - Thus, a tightly regulated balance between TGFβ and BMP signaling is essential for maintaining lens transparency and preventing fibrotic cataracts.

Clinical Implications

- Pharmacological modulation of TGFβ/BMP signaling is under investigation for preventing secondary cataracts (PCO)**.**
- BMP7 has been explored as a therapeutic counteragent to block TGFβ-driven fibrotic responses after cataract surgery.

As we mentioned, the mammalian target of rapamycin (mTOR) pathway plays a critical role in regulating cellular growth, proliferation, and survival. Its influence on the lens of the eye is complex and involves modulation of several key processes relevant to lens physiology and pathology:

1. mTOR Role in Lens Development and Growth

The mTOR–Wnt–Rac1 signaling axis functions as a central regulatory pathway orchestrating the cytoskeletal dynamics required for proper lens vesicle closure during ocular development. Activation of mTOR signaling integrates upstream Wnt cues with downstream Rac1-mediated modulation of actin cytoskeletal architecture. Through this coordinated signaling cascade, the pathway regulates cellular shape changes, junctional remodeling, and mechanical tension at the apical surface of the lens placode. Disruption in any component of this axis—whether through impaired mTOR activity, aberrant Wnt signaling, or deficient Rac1 activation—can compromise cytoskeletal contractility and lead to defective invagination and incomplete closure of the lens vesicle, thereby predisposing to congenital lens anomalies and cataract formation (Q. Wang, mTOR regulates Wnt signaling to promote tension-mediated lens vesicle closure 2025 [14]).

- Cell Proliferation and Differentiation: mTOR signaling regulates the proliferation and differentiation of lens epithelial cells into fiber cells, essential for proper lens development.
- Nutrient Sensing: mTOR serves as a nutrient sensor, ensuring the lens cells receive adequate amino acids, glucose, and other nutrients needed for their growth.

2. Transparency and Homeostasis

   – Protein Synthesis and Turnover: The lens is highly protein-dense, with crystallins being its primary structural proteins. mTOR promotes the synthesis of these proteins and plays a role in maintaining their stability and function, essential for lens transparency.
   – Oxidative Stress Management: mTOR signaling affects the lens's ability to manage oxidative stress, a critical factor in preserving its transparency and preventing cataract formation.

3. Cataract Formation

   – Oxidative Damage and Aging: Dysregulation of mTOR signaling can exacerbate oxidative damage and aging-related changes in the lens, contributing to cataractogenesis.
   – Senescence: Overactivation of mTOR has been linked to increased cellular senescence, which could promote lens opacity.

4. Autophagy and Protein Aggregation

   – Autophagy Regulation: mTOR inhibits autophagy, a cellular process that degrades and recycles damaged proteins and organelles. Proper autophagy is crucial in the lens to prevent the accumulation of damaged or aggregated proteins that leads to cataracts.
   – Protein Aggregation: Impaired autophagy due to mTOR hyperactivation may result in the accumulation of misfolded proteins, a hallmark of cataracts.

5. Lens Injury and Repair

   – Response to Injury: The mTOR pathway is activated in response to lens injury, promoting cell survival and repair. However, excessive activation may lead to maladaptive responses, such as fibrosis.

6. Therapeutic Implications

   – Rapamycin and Cataracts: The mTOR inhibitor rapamycin has shown potential in preclinical studies to prevent or delay cataract formation by reducing oxidative stress and promoting autophagy.
   – Balancing mTOR Activity: Modulating mTOR activity could be a promising strategy for maintaining lens health and managing age-related or diabetes-induced cataracts.

Investigations are ongoing into the role of mTOR signaling in specific lens disorders, including congenital cataracts and secondary cataracts following surgery, as well as its interaction with other signaling pathways such as Akt/PI3K and TGF-β in the context of lens pathology.

Pseudoexfoliation Syndrome (PEX)

Pseudoexfoliation syndrome (PEX) is a systemic, age-related disorder characterized by the abnormal production and accumulation of fibrillar extracellular material in ocular tissues, particularly on the lens capsule, iris, zonules, and trabecular meshwork. It is a leading cause of secondary open-angle glaucoma, with significant implications for intraocular pressure (IOP) regulation and optic nerve health [1].

One of the emerging pathogenic mechanisms implicated in PEX is mitochondrial dysfunction, specifically involving defects in mitochondrial quality control pathways, such as PINK1-mediated mitophagy.

Alterations in PINK1-mediated mitophagy disrupt mitochondrial quality control in the aging eye, contributing to oxidative stress, ECM dysregulation, and tissue degeneration seen in PEX. These findings underscore the role of mitochondrial homeostasis as a key target in understanding and potentially treating this complex ocular disorder [18].

PINK1-Parkin Pathway and Mitophagy

Mitochondrial serine/threonine kinase plays a central role in mitophagy, the selective autophagic degradation of damaged mitochondria [12].

- Under normal conditions, PINK1 is continuously imported into healthy mitochondria and degraded.
- Upon mitochondrial depolarization or oxidative stress, PINK1 accumulates on the outer mitochondrial membrane, where it recruits and activates Parkin, an E3 ubiquitin ligase.
- Activated Parkin ubiquitinates several mitochondrial outer membrane proteins, marking the organelle for degradation via the autophagy–lysosome pathway.

Relevance to PEX Pathophysiology

- *Oxidative stress* is a hallmark of PEX, with increased production of reactive oxygen species (ROS) in ocular tissues, especially the anterior segment.
- The *accumulation of damaged mitochondria* in PEX-affected cells—such as lens epithelial cells, trabecular meshwork cells, and ciliary epithelium—suggests inefficient mitophagy.
- *Altered PINK1 expression or function* has been observed in experimental models and patient-derived tissues with PEX, implicating a compromised mitochondrial surveillance system.

Consequences of Impaired PINK1-Mediated Mitophagy in PEX

- Accumulation of dysfunctional mitochondria, leading to sustained ROS production.
- Increased oxidative damage to proteins, lipids, and DNA, contributing to extracellular matrix abnormalities and PEX fibril formation.
- Disruption of cellular energy homeostasis, particularly in metabolically active tissues like the trabecular meshwork, potentially impairing aqueous humor outflow and elevating IOP.
- Enhanced cellular senescence and apoptosis, which may contribute to zonular instability, lens dislocation, and optic nerve vulnerability.

Therapeutic Implications

- Enhancing PINK1-Parkin-mediated mitophagy may represent a novel therapeutic strategy to restore mitochondrial quality control in PEX.
- Agents that activate mitophagy (e.g., urolithin A, resveratrol, or AMPK activators) are being investigated in other degenerative diseases and could hold potential in ocular applications.
- Understanding the interplay between genetic risk factors for PEX (e.g., LOXL1 variants) and mitochondrial dynamics may further clarify the disease's systemic and ocular manifestations.

mTOR and UVB-Induced Cataract Formation

UVB-induced oxidative stress is a major contributor to cataract formation, primarily through ROS-mediated DNA damage and apoptotic death of lens epithelial cells. The downregulation of TRIM69 and upregulation of p53 represent a key molecular axis in this process, implicating TRIM69 as a potential cytoprotective factor in the lens. Further exploration of this pathway may open new avenues for preventive or protective strategies against UV-related cataracts [19].

There is a potential mechanistic association between mTOR signaling and the TRIM69–p53 axis in UVB-induced lens epithelial cell (LEC) damage and cataractogenesis, although this relationship is not yet fully elucidated in the lens specifically. Here is a summary of how mTOR may interface with UVB-induced stress, TRIM69, p53, and apoptosis in human lens epithelial cells.

While direct experimental evidence linking mTOR to TRIM69 in the lens is currently lacking, the known interactions between mTOR, oxidative stress, p53, and cell death support a plausible connection. Given mTOR's central role in lens homeostasis, further research into this triad (mTOR–TRIM69–p53) could reveal novel insights into UV-induced cataractogenesis and potential therapeutic targets.

mTOR and Oxidative Stress Response

The mechanistic target of rapamycin (mTOR) is a nutrient-sensing kinase that regulates cell growth, protein synthesis, autophagy, and survival. Under oxidative stress (e.g., from UVB exposure), mTOR activity is modulated [20].

- mTORC1 suppression can promote autophagy, which helps clear damaged organelles like mitochondria.
- Chronic activation, however, may impair autophagic flux and enhance susceptibility to apoptosis in stress-vulnerable cells such as LECs.

mTOR and p53 Cross Talk

p53 can inhibit mTOR signaling under stress conditions via activation of AMPK or induction of TSC2, leading to growth arrest or autophagy [6].

Conversely, mTOR can also modulate p53 activity:

- mTORC1 promotes translation of MDM2, a negative regulator of p53, thereby repressing p53 activation under homeostatic conditions.
- Under stress, suppression of mTOR may allow p53 accumulation and transcriptional activation of apoptotic genes.

Possible mTOR Link to TRIM69

Although direct studies on TRIM69 and mTOR in lens cells are limited, the following theoretical links can be proposed.

TRIM family proteins, including TRIM69, often function as E3 ubiquitin ligases that regulate stress response pathways, including:

- p53 stability and activity, either by direct ubiquitination or through regulation of MDM2,
- mTOR pathway components, as seen with other TRIMs (e.g., TRIM21 and TRIM8) that modulate AKT/mTOR or AMPK pathways,

Downregulation of TRIM69 under UVB stress might relieve inhibition on p53 and/or affect upstream regulators of mTOR, shifting the cell toward apoptosis instead of survival or autophagy.

mTOR's Role in Lens Epithelial Cell Survival and Cataract Prevention

- mTOR supports LEC survival, protein synthesis (e.g., crystallins), and organelle clearance during fiber cell differentiation.
- Dysregulated mTOR signaling has been implicated in age-related cataract, where chronic oxidative stress leads to impaired autophagy, accumulation of damaged proteins, and lens opacity.
- Hence, a delicate balance of mTOR activity is essential—too much or too little can contribute to lens pathology.

Summary Hypothetical Model

- UVB exposure → ↑ ROS → ↓ TRIM69 → ↑ p53 → ↑ apoptosis.
- Under this stress:
  - p53 may suppress mTOR, limiting cell survival and autophagy.
  - mTOR suppression may facilitate p53 activation.
- TRIM69 downregulation may disrupt this balance, indirectly affecting mTOR signaling and promoting cataract formation.

Bibliography

1. Aydemir. Evidence of mitophagy in lens capsule epithelial cells of patients with pseudoexfoliation syndrome. J Glaucoma. 2024;34 https://doi.org/10.1097/IJG.0000000000002484.
2. Brennan. Autophagy requirements for eye lens differentiation and transparency. Cells. 2023;12 https://doi.org/10.3390/cells12030475.
3. Clark. Diverse Fgfr1 signaling pathways and endocytic trafficking regulate early mesoderm development. NIH, bioRxiv. 2024; https://doi.org/10.1101/2024.02.16.580629.
4. Collins. Crk proteins transduce FGF signaling to promote lens fiber cell elongation. elife. 2018;7 https://doi.org/10.7554/eLife.32586.
5. Coomson. Receptor signaling mechanism in lens cells. Cell Biol Dev Biol. 2025; https://doi.org/10.7554/eLife.106519.
6. Cui D. The cross talk between p53 and mTOR pathways in response to physiological and genotoxic stresses. Front Cell Dev Biol. 2021;9 https://doi.org/10.3389/fcell.2021.775507.
7. Shu D. Insights into bone morphogenetic protein—(BMP-) signaling in ocular lens biology and pathology. Cells. 2021;10 https://doi.org/10.3390/cells10102604.
8. Flokis. FGF-2 differentially regulates lens epithelial cell behaviour during TGF-β-induced EMT. Cells. 2023; https://doi.org/10.3390/cells12060827.
9. Goetz. Exploring mechanisms of FGF signalling through the lens of structural biology. Nat Rev Mol Cell Biol. 2013;14 https://doi.org/10.1038/nrm3528.
10. Li H. Lens differentiation is controlled by the balance between PDGF and FGF signaling. PLOS, Biology. 2019;17 https://doi.org/10.1371/journal.pbio.3000133.

11. Henry. Cell signaling pathways in vertebrate lens regeneration. Published in "New Perspectives in Regeneration". Curr Top Microbiol Immunol. 2015; https://doi.org/10.1007/82_2012_289.
12. Wu J. PINK1-Parkin pathway and mitophagy. Bioengineering. 2025;12 https://doi.org/10.3390/bioengineering12060563.
13. Liton. Autophagy in the eye: from physiology to pathophysiology. Autophagy Reports. 2023;2 https://doi.org/10.1080/27694127.2023.2178996.
14. Wang Q. Shc1 cooperates with Frs2 and Shp2 to recruit Grb2 in FGF-induced lens development. Cell Biol Develop Biol. 2025; https://doi.org/10.7554/eLife.103615.2.
15. Reardon. Hyperactive Pdgfrβ signaling induces cataractogenesis via Tgfβ and Stat5-Igf1. SSRN. 2025; https://papers.ssrn.com/sol3/papers.cfm?abstract_id=5193745
16. Sisto. Epigenetic regulation of EMP/EMT-dependent fibrosis. Int J Mol Sci. 2024;25 https://doi.org/10.3390/ijms25052775.
17. Teven. Fibroblast growth factor (FGF) signaling in development and skeletal diseases. Genes Dis. 2014;1 https://doi.org/10.1016/j.gendis.2014.09.005.
18. Liu X. PINK1-Parkin pathway and mitophagy. Exp Eye Res. 2025;258 https://doi.org/10.1016/j.exer.2025.110437.
19. Rong X. TRIM69 inhibits cataractogenesis by negatively regulating p53. Redox Biol. 2019;22 https://doi.org/10.1016/j.redox.2019.101157.
20. Qin Y. Cellular senescence in health, disease, and lens aging. Pharmaceuticals. 2025;18 https://doi.org/10.3390/ph18020244.
21. Liu Z. The lens epithelium as a major determinant in the development, maintenance, and regeneration of the crystalline lens, vol. 92. Progress in Retinal and Eye Research; 2023. https://doi.org/10.1016/j.preteyeres.2022.101112.

Chapter 8
mTOR Role in the Retina

Contents

Abstract The mechanistic target of rapamycin (mTOR) is a central regulator of cellular metabolism, growth, and survival and plays an essential role in maintaining retinal structure and function. Within the retina, a highly metabolically active and layered neural tissue, mTOR signaling governs diverse physiological processes, including neurogenesis, synaptic connectivity, photoreceptor maintenance, and metabolic adaptation. Dysregulation of mTOR signaling has been implicated in a wide array of retinal pathologies such as age-related macular degeneration, diabetic retinopathy, retinitis pigmentosa, and glaucoma. This chapter reviews the spatial and functional dynamics of mTOR complexes (mTORC1 and mTORC2) across retinal cell types, explores their cross talk with key metabolic and stress–response pathways, and discusses emerging therapeutic strategies targeting mTOR to preserve retinal integrity and function in both degenerative and proliferative retinal diseases.

K. T. Moazed, *mTOR Signaling in Ophthalmology*,
https://doi.org/10.1007/978-3-032-05044-1_8

Discussion

Retinal development begins with the morphogenetic transformation of the eye primordia through a coordinated process of invagination, leading to the formation of bilateral optic vesicles. These vesicles extend from the forebrain and undergo further invagination upon interaction with the overlying surface ectoderm, resulting in the formation of the bilayered optic cup. The inner layer of this structure differentiates into the neural retina, responsible for phototransduction and signal processing, while the outer layer gives rise to the non-neural retinal pigmented epithelium (RPE), which plays a vital role in photoreceptor maintenance and visual cycle homeostasis. Studies using a range of vertebrate model organisms—including mouse, zebrafish, and Xenopus—have identified a complex network of signaling pathways that regulate distinct stages of retinal induction, proliferation, and differentiation.

Among these, the Wnt signaling pathway has emerged as a critical regulator, with spatially and temporally restricted activity required for proper retinal specification, morphogenesis, and maturation. Wnt/β-catenin signaling pathway is critical for the proliferation of reprogrammed progenitor cells [9].

Dysregulation of Wnt signaling has been associated with developmental anomalies such as coloboma, retinal dysplasia, and impaired optic cup formation, underscoring its essential role in orchestrating retinal architecture and cellular identity [5].

The mechanistic target of rapamycin (mTOR) is a central regulator of cellular metabolism, growth, survival, and autophagy. mTOR functions mainly through two distinct complexes—mTORC1 and mTORC2—which differ in their composition, upstream regulators, and downstream targets. mTORC1 integrates signals from nutrients, growth factors, and cellular energy status to control protein synthesis, autophagy inhibition, and lipid metabolism. In contrast, mTORC2 primarily responds to growth factors and regulates cytoskeletal organization, cell survival, and AKT phosphorylation [13].

Within the retina—a highly specialized and metabolically demanding neural tissue—mTOR signaling is critical for maintaining cellular homeostasis, energy balance, and stress response. Dysregulation of mTOR activity has been implicated in several retinal diseases, including age-related macular degeneration (AMD), diabetic retinopathy, and glaucoma.

The components of the mTOR pathway are differentially distributed across various retinal layers and cell types. For instance:

- *Retinal pigment epithelium (RPE)* cells utilize mTORC1 to regulate phagocytosis of photoreceptor outer segments and manage oxidative stress (discussed in the next chapter).
- *Photoreceptors* depend on mTOR signaling for outer segment renewal, energy metabolism, and protection from light-induced damage.
- *Müller glia*, the principal glial cells of the retina, use mTOR to coordinate neuroprotection, gliosis, and metabolic support to neurons.

- *Retinal ganglion cells (RGCs)* exhibit mTOR activity relevant to axonal growth, survival, and response to injury.

Together, these spatially and functionally distinct roles underscore the essential and context-specific functions of mTOR signaling in the retina. mTOR plays a dual role in the retina, supporting normal function and homeostasis while contributing to the pathogenesis of various retinal diseases when dysregulated. Strategic modulation of mTOR signaling is a promising avenue for therapeutic development. Understanding these roles provides insights into both physiological retinal maintenance and pathophysiological mechanisms underlying degenerative retinal disorders.

mTOR in Retinal Development and Physiology

During retinal development, mTOR signaling governs the proliferation and differentiation of retinal progenitor cells (RPCs). mTORC1 activity promotes cell cycle progression and biosynthetic growth of RPCs, while temporal modulation of its activity is essential for the transition from proliferation to differentiation into various retinal cell types, including photoreceptors, interneurons, and ganglion cells. mTORC1 serves as a master regulator of growth, differentiation, and laminar organization in hiPSC-derived retinal organoids. Its precise spatiotemporal activation is indispensable for recapitulating human retinal development in vitro. Modulating mTORC1 activity may offer strategies to improve organoid fidelity or model retinal developmental disorders.

Role of mTORC1 Activity in Early Retinal Development (Fig. 8.1)

mTORC1 serves as a master regulator of growth, differentiation, and laminar organization in hiPSC-derived retinal organoids. Its precise spatiotemporal activation is indispensable for recapitulating human retinal development in vitro. Modulating mTORC1 activity may offer strategies to improve organoid fidelity or model retinal developmental disorders [15].

1. Regulation of Progenitor Cell Proliferation

During the early stages of retinal development, mTORC1 is essential for maintaining the proliferative capacity of retinal progenitor cells (RPCs). It integrates signals from growth factors (e.g., insulin and IGF-1) and nutrients (notably amino acids) to drive protein synthesis, ribosomal biogenesis, and cell cycle progression. In hiPSC-derived organoids, mTORC1 activity ensures an adequate pool of RPCs necessary for proper retinal tissue expansion and laminar patterning.

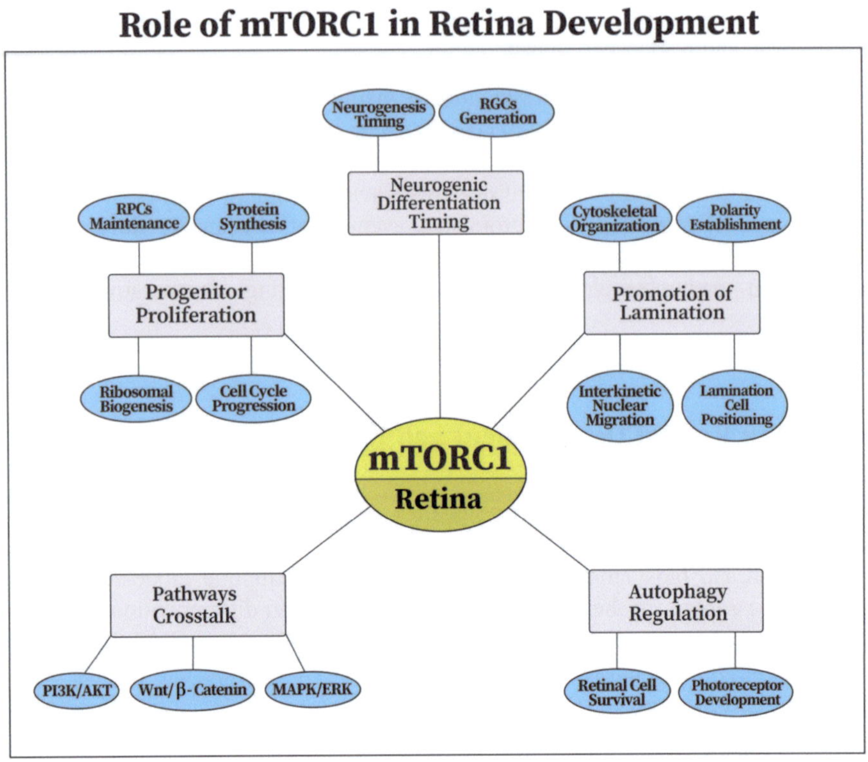

Fig. 8.1 The image illustrates the role of mTORC1 in regulating cellular growth of the retina, promoting differentiation, and maintaining proper laminar organization within retinal organoids, highlighting its importance in retinal development and tissue architecture

2. Control of Neurogenic Differentiation Timing

mTORC1 influences the timing of neurogenesis by modulating the expression of proneural genes such as ATOH7, which are critical for the generation of retinal ganglion cells (RGCs). Hyperactivation or inhibition of mTORC1 can disturb the temporal sequence of retinal cell birth, thereby impairing stratification and the proper formation of retinal layers.

3. Promotion of Retinal Lamination

mTORC1 activity supports cytoskeletal organization and polarity establishment, which are required for interkinetic nuclear migration and cell positioning during lamination. Disruption of mTORC1 signaling (e.g., via rapamycin treatment) in retinal organoids results in disorganized retinal layers and defective outer segment morphogenesis in photoreceptors.

4. Interaction with Other Pathways

mTORC1 cross talks with PI3K/AKT, Wnt/β-catenin, and MAPK/ERK pathways to coordinate proliferation, differentiation, and metabolic programming. In retinal organoids, this integration is crucial for the stepwise maturation of layered retinal architecture.

5. Autophagy Regulation

By suppressing autophagy under nutrient-rich conditions, mTORC1 ensures high biosynthetic activity. However, tightly controlled autophagy is needed for retinal cell survival and photoreceptor development. In mTORC1-dysregulated organoids, aberrant autophagic flux may contribute to defective lamination or early degeneration.

Role of mTORC2 Activity in Early Retinal Development (Fig. 8.2)

Role of mTORC2 Activity During Early Retinal Development and Lamination in Human-Induced Pluripotent Stem Cell (hiPSC)-Derived Retinal Organoids

mTORC2, though less studied than mTORC1, plays a crucial and complementary role in orchestrating early retinal development and lamination in hiPSC-derived retinal organoids. Its activity modulates key processes involving cytoskeletal organization, cell polarity, metabolic regulation, and neuronal differentiation.

mTORC2 plays a fundamental but distinct role from mTORC1 in early retinal development within hiPSC-derived organoids. It regulates cytoskeletal remodeling, polarity, and survival, all of which are indispensable for retinal lamination and neuronal positioning. Therapeutic modulation of mTORC2 could enhance organoid maturation or model retinal developmental disorders involving polarity defects and neurogenesis failure.

1. Cytoskeletal Architecture and Retinal Lamination

mTORC2 regulates the organization of the actin cytoskeleton by activating downstream effectors such as Rho GTPases (e.g., Rac1 and Cdc42) and protein kinase C-α (PKCα). In retinal organoids, proper cytoskeletal dynamics are essential for:

- Apical–basal polarity of neuroepithelial cells
- Interkinetic nuclear migration of retinal progenitors
- Accurate stratification of neuronal layers

Disruption of mTORC2 (e.g., via Rictor knockdown) leads to impaired laminar organization, with mispositioned retinal ganglion cells (RGCs) and a breakdown of apical Adherens junctions.

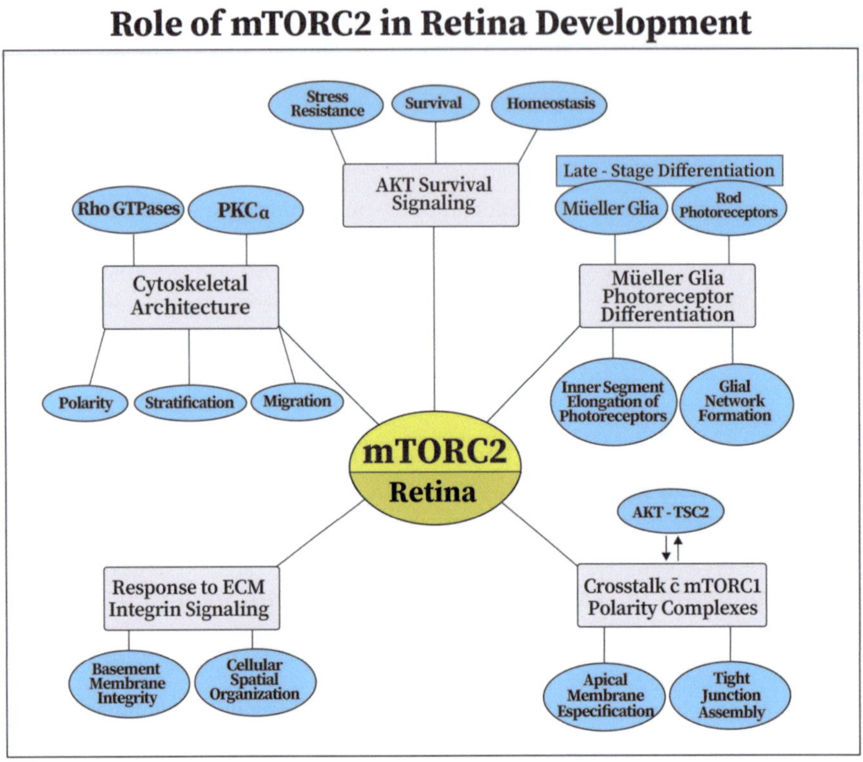

Fig. 8.2 The image depicts how mTORC2 activity influences early stages of retinal development and contributes to the proper lamination and structural organization in retinal organoids derived from human-induced pluripotent stem cells (hiPSCs)

2. AKT Phosphorylation and Survival Signaling

mTORC2 is the major kinase responsible for phosphorylating AKT at Ser473, a modification required for full AKT activation. This enhances:

- Cell survival during early retinal neurogenesis
- Metabolic homeostasis in differentiating progenitors
- Resistance to stress, particularly during the formation of complex 3D structures in organoids

Reduced mTORC2 activity increases apoptosis and results in hypoplastic retinal organoids.

3. Promotion of Müller Glia and Photoreceptor Differentiation

Emerging data suggest mTORC2 supports late-stage progenitor cell differentiation, especially toward Müller glia and rod photoreceptors. In retinal organoids, delayed or deficient mTORC2 signaling may hinder proper elongation of photoreceptor inner segments or the formation of supportive glial networks, both essential for long-term structural stability.

4. Cross Talk with mTORC1 and Polarity Complexes

mTORC2 activity interacts with polarity protein complexes such as Par3/Par6/aPKC, influencing apical membrane specification and tight junction assembly. This is critical in establishing the retinal neuroepithelium's layered organization in vitro. mTORC2 may also modulate mTORC1 indirectly via feedback loops involving AKT-TSC2 signaling.

5. Response to Extracellular Matrix (ECM) and Integrin Signaling

mTORC2 responds to mechanical and ECM signals through integrins, which are pivotal during retinal invagination and optic vesicle formation in organoids. This mechanotransduction function may guide the spatial organization of differentiating cells and support basement membrane integrity.

mTOR Role in Photoreceptor Maturation

In photoreceptor maturation, mTOR activity is essential for the biosynthesis of phototransduction components and the energy-demanding renewal of outer segments. Sustained mTOR signaling supports photoreceptor survival, especially under conditions of metabolic or oxidative stress, by regulating autophagy, mitochondrial dynamics, and protein turnover [6].

mTOR also contributes to synaptogenesis and the formation of retinal neural circuits by modulating protein synthesis and cytoskeletal dynamics. These processes are critical for the establishment of precise connectivity between retinal neurons during development and synaptic maintenance throughout life [12].

Within Müller glia, mTOR orchestrates metabolic support for neurons, including glucose metabolism, amino acid supply, and antioxidant defense. This glial–neuronal coupling is essential for maintaining retinal homeostasis, particularly in the face of environmental and metabolic stressors. mTOR signaling is required for the formation of proliferating Müller glia-derived progenitor cells in the chick retina [25].

Although not discussed in depth here, mTOR also regulates phagocytosis in the retinal pigment epithelium (RPE), particularly in the daily clearance of photoreceptor outer segments—a topic that will be addressed in the following chapter.

mTOR and Metabolism in the Retina

The retina is among the most metabolically active tissues in the body, requiring tightly coordinated energy production and nutrient utilization to support visual function, phototransduction, and cellular maintenance. The mechanistic target of rapamycin (mTOR) plays a central role in regulating these metabolic processes by integrating signals from nutrients, energy status, and growth factors [14].

These mechanisms highlight the dual role of mTOR as both a sensor and effector in retinal stress adaptation. Fine-tuned regulation of mTOR activity is therefore essential not only for normal retinal physiology but also for protection against degenerative diseases such as age-related macular degeneration, glaucoma, and inherited retinal dystrophies.

mTORC1, in particular, is a key regulator of glycolysis, promoting glucose uptake and glycolytic enzyme expression in retinal cells, especially in photoreceptors and Müller glia. This is critical given the retina's reliance on aerobic glycolysis (Warburg-like metabolism) to meet its high biosynthetic and energetic demands. mTORC1 accelerates retinal development via the immunoproteasome [8].

In addition to glucose metabolism, mTOR governs lipid metabolism, facilitating lipid synthesis and storage necessary for membrane biogenesis, outer segment renewal in photoreceptors, and protection against lipotoxicity. mTORC1 activation enhances the expression of sterol regulatory element-binding proteins (SREBPs), key transcription factors that control lipid biosynthetic genes [22, 23].

mTOR also supports mitochondrial biogenesis and function, ensuring efficient ATP production and redox homeostasis. Through transcriptional coactivators such as PGC-1α, mTOR influences mitochondrial replication, respiration, and turnover—processes essential for photoreceptor and RPE cell survival [19].

Furthermore, mTOR operates within a broader network of nutrient-sensing pathways, including reciprocal interactions with AMP-activated protein kinase (AMPK), sirtuin 1 (SIRT1), and the insulin/IGF-1 axis. These pathways coordinate cellular responses to nutrient availability, stress, and aging. For example, AMPK negatively regulates mTORC1 during energy stress, promoting catabolic pathways such as autophagy, while insulin and IGF-1 signaling promote mTORC1 activation to support anabolic growth [17].

Through these interconnected mechanisms, mTOR ensures metabolic adaptability and energy sufficiency in the retina, aligning nutrient availability with the functional demand. Dysregulation of mTOR-mediated metabolism has been implicated in the pathogenesis of retinal diseases such as diabetic retinopathy, age-related macular degeneration, and retinitis pigmentosa.

mTOR in Retinal Stress Responses and Autophagy

Maintaining cellular homeostasis in the retina requires a delicate balance between biosynthesis and degradation, especially in the face of constant light exposure, oxidative stress, and high metabolic demand. A key player in this balance is the mechanistic target of rapamycin (mTOR), which regulates autophagy, oxidative stress responses, and mitochondrial quality control across multiple retinal cell types [10].

Autophagy, a conserved lysosome-dependent degradation pathway, is essential for retinal health. In photoreceptors and the retinal pigment epithelium (RPE), basal autophagy supports turnover of damaged organelles and protein aggregates under physiological conditions. Stress-induced autophagy, triggered by nutrient deprivation, oxidative damage, or inflammation, becomes critical for cell survival and recovery. mTORC1 is a principal inhibitor of autophagy initiation; its inactivation during stress enables the activation of ULK1 and the autophagic cascade, facilitating cytoprotective clearance mechanisms [4].

Oxidative stress, which results from excess reactive oxygen species (ROS), is a major contributor to retinal degeneration. mTOR signaling modulates antioxidant responses by integrating inputs from redox-sensitive pathways. Under mild oxidative conditions, mTOR activity supports survival by promoting protein synthesis and antioxidant defenses. However, in the context of severe or chronic stress, sustained mTORC1 activation may impair autophagy and exacerbate cellular injury. Conversely, mTOR inhibition can promote protective autophagy and improve cellular resilience [18].

Mitophagy: A critical aspect of the retinal stress response is *mitochondrial quality control*, particularly through mitophagy, the selective autophagic removal of damaged mitochondria. The PINK1/Parkin pathway plays a central role in tagging dysfunctional mitochondria for degradation. mTOR signaling influences this pathway indirectly by modulating general autophagy levels and mitochondrial biogenesis. By maintaining a balance between mitochondrial renewal and degradation, mTOR helps preserve mitochondrial integrity and prevent retinal cell death [3].

mTOR in Retinal Degenerative Diseases (Fig. 8.3)

The mechanistic target of rapamycin (mTOR) plays a complex and disease-specific role in the pathogenesis of several major retinal degenerative disorders. As a master regulator of metabolism, protein synthesis, autophagy, and cell survival, mTOR's dysregulation can contribute to either protective or pathological outcomes, depending on the cellular context and disease stage.

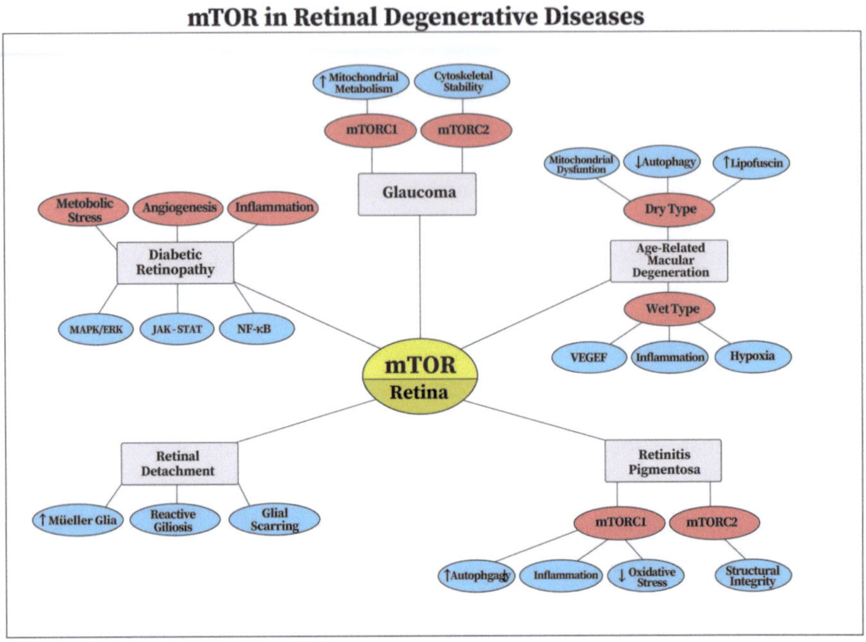

Fig. 8.3 The image illustrates the complex and highly specific role of mTOR in the pathogenesis of several major retinal degenerative disorders, highlighting how its signaling pathways contribute to disease onset, progression, and cellular dysfunction within different retinal layers. It emphasizes the involvement of mTOR in regulating key processes such as cell survival, autophagy, metabolism, and inflammation, all of which play crucial roles in the development and severity of conditions like age-related macular degeneration, diabetic retinopathy, retinal detachment, glaucoma, and retinitis pigmentosa

Age-Related Macular Degeneration (AMD)

In AMD, mTOR exerts dual and context-dependent effects within the retinal pigment epithelium (RPE) and the choroidal vasculature. In the dry (atrophic) form, impaired autophagy due to chronic mTORC1 activation leads to RPE degeneration, mitochondrial dysfunction, and accumulation of toxic debris such as lipofuscin. In contrast, in the wet (neovascular) form, mTOR signaling promotes choroidal neovascularization by stimulating angiogenic factors such as VEGF, especially under hypoxic or inflammatory conditions. Targeting mTOR must therefore balance RPE preservation with the suppression of abnormal vessel growth [11].

Diabetic Retinopathy

Hyperglycemia chronically activates mTOR signaling in retinal endothelial cells and glia, contributing to metabolic stress, inflammation, and pathological angiogenesis.

The PI3K/Akt/mechanistic target of rapamycin (mTOR) pathway is a critical signaling pathway for cell survival and proliferation, particularly in pathological angiogenesis, a hallmark of PDR. In PDR, the typical hypoxic conditions seen trigger the activation of this pathway through growth factors like IGF-1, leading to increased VEGF expression and promoting abnormal neovascularization [1].

Role of NF-κB Signaling in Diabetic Eye Disease

The NF-κB (nuclear factor kappa-light-chain-enhancer of activated B cells) signaling pathway plays a central role in mediating inflammation and immune responses in the diabetic eye. Upon activation by hyperglycemia-induced stressors—such as oxidative stress, advanced glycation end-products (AGEs), and inflammatory cytokines—NF-κB promotes the transcription of proinflammatory mediators including inducible nitric oxide synthase (iNOS) and intercellular adhesion molecules (ICAMs). These factors are pivotal in the pathogenesis of diabetic retinopathy (DR) and diabetic macular edema (DME).

NF-κB-driven inflammation facilitates leukostasis, apoptosis of retinal cells, and disruption of the blood–retina barrier (BRB), contributing to vascular leakage and neurodegeneration—hallmark features of DR and DME.

Moreover, mTOR signaling is vital for the hypoxia-induced proliferation of vascular cells, including smooth muscle and endothelial cells, by increasing their sensitivity to growth factors. In diabetic keratopathy, hyperglycemia inhibits the PI3K/Akt pathway, which is crucial for cellular survival and regeneration. Elevated mTORC1 activity promotes the expression of proinflammatory cytokines, impairs autophagy, and enhances VEGF-driven vascular proliferation, which disrupt the blood–retina barrier and accelerate retinal damage. Inhibition of mTOR in experimental models has shown promise in reducing vascular leakage and inflammatory responses [2].

JAK-STAT and MAPK/ERK Signaling Pathways in Diabetic Retinopathy

The JAK-STAT (Janus kinase-signal transducer and activator of transcription) signaling pathway plays a critical role in regulating key cellular functions such as proliferation, differentiation, apoptosis, and inflammatory responses. In the diabetic retina, the activation and upregulation of STAT family proteins—notably STAT1, STAT3, and STAT5—are associated with pathological changes that impair the blood–retina barrier (BRB). These STAT proteins influence tight junction integrity, promote endothelial cell injury, and disrupt retinal pigment epithelium (RPE) function. Moreover, STAT signaling contributes to the activation of proinflammatory microglia and circulating immune cells, leading to capillary occlusion, further compromising vascular homeostasis and exacerbating BRB breakdown.

Parallel to JAK-STAT, the mitogen-activated protein kinase (MAPK) signaling cascade is pivotal in coordinating cellular processes such as gene transcription, cell proliferation, survival, and apoptosis. Of particular relevance is the MAPK/ERK (extracellular signal-regulated kinase) branch, which is critically involved in the pathophysiology of diabetic retinopathy (DR). ERK activity in neuroretinal tissues provides neuroprotection, supporting essential interactions between the neuroretina and RPE, thereby preserving the structural and functional integrity of the inner BRB. However, suppression of ERK signaling disrupts this interaction, promotes subretinal fluid accumulation, and accelerates DR progression.

Conversely, chronic diabetic stressors such as advanced glycation end-products (AGEs) activate the MAPK/ERK pathway through engagement with RAGE (receptor for AGE). This results in increased oxidative stress and upregulation of proinflammatory cytokines, adhesion molecules, and angiogenic regulators, thereby promoting vascular endothelial damage, retinal lesions, and inflammation-driven neurovascular degeneration.

The mitogen-activated protein kinase (MAPK) pathway is integral to a wide range of physiological processes, including gene expression, cell proliferation, differentiation, survival, and apoptosis. Within this cascade, the MAPK/ERK (extracellular signal-regulated kinase) signaling axis plays a pivotal role in mediating both normal retinal function and disease-related mechanisms.

In the context of diabetic retinopathy (DR), the MAPK/ERK pathway regulates cell cycle progression and contributes to chronic inflammation, a hallmark of the diabetic retinal environment. ERK activation is particularly significant in neuroretinal tissues, where it serves a neuroprotective role by facilitating the structural and functional interaction between the neuroretina and the retinal pigment epithelium (RPE). This interaction is vital for preserving the integrity of the inner blood–retina barrier (BRB).

When ERK signaling is suppressed or dysregulated, this neuroretina–RPE cross talk is disrupted, leading to subretinal fluid accumulation, compromised BRB function, and **accelerated disease progression** in diabetic retinopathy.

Retinitis Pigmentosa (RP)

RP involves progressive photoreceptor degeneration, often due to inherited mutations. mTOR signaling becomes dysregulated as photoreceptors attempt to adapt to declining metabolic capacity. Aberrant mTOR activation or suppression can both be harmful, indicating a need for metabolic reprogramming strategies to maintain energy homeostasis, and delay cell death. Interventions targeting mTOR may preserve photoreceptors by enhancing autophagy and mitochondrial turnover [21].

mTOR signaling plays a role in retinitis pigmentosa (RP), particularly important in photoreceptor survival, metabolism, and degeneration. As mTOR is a key regulator of cellular metabolism, protein synthesis, and autophagy, photoreceptors—particularlyrods—exhibit exceptionally high metabolic demands.

Dysfunction in nutrient sensing (via mTORC1) may contribute to progressive degeneration.

In RP, mutations in photoreceptor genes lead to metabolic stress, and mTOR activity is often dysregulated, exacerbating cell death.

mTORC1 activation can lead to photoreceptor apoptosis due to metabolic imbalance.

Rapamycin (mTORC1 inhibitor) has been studied in models of RP:

- It reduces oxidative stress and inflammation.
- It promotes autophagy, clearing damaged cellular components.
- Some studies show protection against rod degeneration, while others caution that excessive inhibition may disrupt retinal homeostasis.

mTORC2 is involved in cytoskeletal organization and cell survival.

- Loss of mTORC2 signaling may affect retinal structural integrity, making photoreceptors more vulnerable to degeneration.

mTOR is a double-edged sword in RP, and dysregulated activation contributes to photoreceptor stress and degeneration. Careful modulation of mTOR (via autophagy enhancement or metabolic support) may offer neuroprotective benefits in RP.

Retinal Detachment

Following retinal detachment, mTOR is rapidly activated in Müller glial cells, initiating a response that supports cell survival and reactive gliosis. While mTOR-dependent proliferation of Müller cells may aid short-term repair and neuroprotection, excessive or prolonged activation can contribute to glial scarring and structural disorganization. mTORC1 induced retinal progenitor cell over proliferation leads to accelerated mitotic aging and degeneration of descendent Müller glia [16].

Thus, modulating mTOR activity may help limit maladaptive gliosis while preserving beneficial glial functions [25].

Glaucoma

Glaucoma is characterized by the progressive loss of retinal ganglion cells (RGCs) and optic nerve axons. RGCs are highly dependent on mTOR signaling for survival, protein synthesis, and axonal regeneration. mTORC1 activity supports neurotrophic responses and mitochondrial metabolism, while mTORC2 regulates cytoskeletal stability. Targeted modulation of mTOR, particularly in conjunction with autophagy or neuroprotective agents, may enhance RGC resilience and promote axon repair following injury [24].

mTOR and Retinal Angiogenesis

Angiogenesis in the retina is a tightly regulated process essential for vascular development and oxygen delivery but becomes pathologic when dysregulated. The mechanistic target of rapamycin (mTOR), particularly through its interaction with hypoxia-responsive and growth factor pathways, plays a pivotal role in driving retinal neovascularization in disease states.

A key mediator of mTOR-driven angiogenesis is the mTOR–vascular endothelial growth factor (VEGF) axis. mTORC1 promotes the transcription and translation of VEGF—a principal angiogenic cytokine—by enhancing protein synthesis machinery and facilitating the stabilization and activity of hypoxia-inducible factors (HIFs). In conditions of hypoxia or oxidative stress, mTORC1 supports HIF-1α accumulation, which transcriptionally activates VEGF and other pro-angiogenic genes, leading to pathological vessel growth.

This mechanism is particularly relevant in proliferative diabetic retinopathy (PDR), where chronic hyperglycemia and inflammation stimulate mTOR activity, resulting in persistent VEGF overexpression and pathological retinal neovascularization. The neovessels are often fragile and leaky, contributing to retinal edema and hemorrhage.

Similarly, in retinopathy of prematurity (ROP), immature retinal vasculature is highly sensitive to oxygen fluctuations. Hyperoxia, followed by hypoxia triggers mTOR-mediated HIF-1α stabilization and VEGF expression, leading to aberrant neovascular tufts that threaten retinal structure and function [20].

Beyond VEGF, mTOR integrates signals from nutrient availability, growth factors, and cytokines, coordinating a broader angiogenic program involving endothelial cell proliferation, migration, and survival. Both mTORC1 and mTORC2 are involved—mTORC1 primarily promotes protein synthesis and VEGF production, while mTORC2 regulates cytoskeletal dynamics and endothelial cell motility via AKT and PKC pathways.

Guanylate-binding protein 2 (GBP2), a member of the dynamin superfamily of large GTPases, has emerged as a negative regulator of pathological angiogenesis. Recent evidence indicates that GBP2 downregulates the expression of vascular endothelial growth factor A (VEGFA), a critical mediator of neovascularization, by inhibiting the AKT/mTOR signaling pathway—a key axis that promotes endothelial cell proliferation, survival, and vascular permeability. In experimental models of retinal neovascular disease, overexpression of GBP2 led to significant suppression of aberrant angiogenic activity, including reduced endothelial cell sprouting and neovessel formation. Mechanistically, GBP2 interferes with phosphorylation events within the AKT/mTOR cascade, thereby attenuating the downstream translation of pro-angiogenic factors such as VEGFA. These findings collectively suggest that GBP2 modulates pathological retinal angiogenesis via the AKT/mTOR/VEGFA axis. Given its ability to disrupt a central pro-angiogenic signaling pathway, GBP2 may represent a promising molecular target for the development of novel therapeutic strategies aimed at controlling neovascular complications in retinal diseases such as proliferative diabetic retinopathy, age-related macular degeneration, and retinopathy of prematurity [22, 23].

Given its central role, mTOR is a potential therapeutic target for modulating angiogenesis in ischemic and proliferative retinal diseases. Pharmacological inhibition of mTOR has shown efficacy in reducing neovascularization in experimental models, offering adjunctive or alternative strategies to anti-VEGF therapies.

Signaling Pathways and Cross Talk (Fig. 8.4)

The mTOR signaling pathway functions as a central node in a highly interconnected network of intracellular signals that coordinate growth, metabolism, and stress responses. Its activity is finely regulated by cross talk with several key pathways, ensuring that cellular outcomes are appropriately tailored to environmental conditions such as nutrient availability, energy status, and oxidative stress.

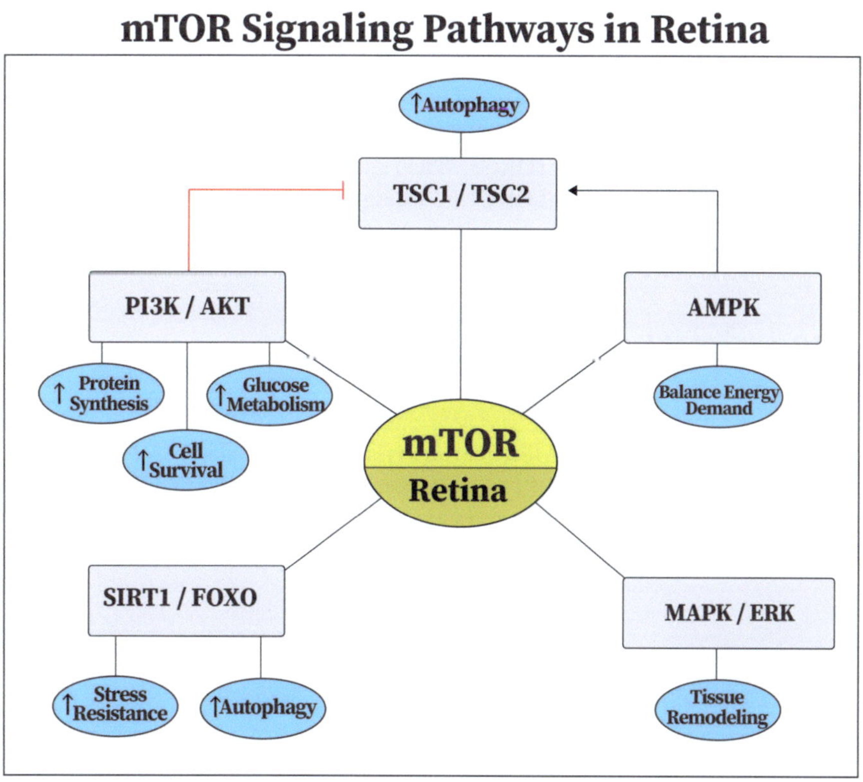

Fig. 8.4 The image represents the mTOR signaling pathway, which functions as a central node in a highly interconnected network of intracellular signals. It coordinates growth, metabolism, autophagy, and stress responses, playing a critical role in maintaining cellular homeostasis and adaptation to environmental changes

Collectively, these signaling interactions ensure that mTOR activity is not static but dynamically modulated in response to both internal and external signals. This integrative signaling network enables the retina to maintain homeostasis under physiological conditions and adapt to metabolic and environmental stress.

PI3K/AKT/mTOR Axis

The PI3K/AKT pathway is a principal upstream activator of mTORC1. Growth factors such as insulin and IGF-1 activate PI3K, leading to AKT phosphorylation. Activated AKT inhibits the TSC1/TSC2 complex, a negative regulator of mTORC1, thereby relieving its suppression and enabling mTORC1 activation. This axis is fundamental in promoting protein synthesis, glucose metabolism, and cell survival across retinal cells, particularly in development and response to injury.

TSC1/TSC2 Complex

The TSC1/TSC2 heterodimer acts as a critical integration point for multiple upstream signals. It functions as a GTPase-activating protein (GAP) for Rheb, a small GTPase that activates mTORC1. When energy is low or stress is high, TSC1/TSC2 is activated to inhibit mTORC1, reducing anabolic processes and promoting autophagy.

AMP-Activated Protein Kinase (AMPK)

AMPK is an energy-sensing kinase that antagonizes mTORC1 during energetic stress or caloric restriction. AMPK phosphorylates and activates TSC2 and directly phosphorylates raptor, an mTORC1 component, thereby inhibiting mTORC1 activity. In the retina, this regulation helps balance energy demand and availability, especially under hypoxic or glucose-deprived conditions.

MAPK/ERK Pathway

The MAPK/ERK pathway, commonly activated by mitogens and FGF signaling, also intersects with mTOR regulation. ERK can phosphorylate and inhibit TSC2, similar to AKT, leading to mTORC1 activation. This cross talk coordinates cell cycle progression and differentiation, particularly in retinal progenitor cells and during tissue remodeling.

Role of FGF Signaling in Retinal Development and Regeneration

Within the layered architecture of the developing retina, fibroblast growth factor (FGF) signaling exhibits remarkable versatility, orchestrating processes such as neurogenesis, tissue patterning, and cell survival. During early retinal development, FGF signaling is essential for promoting the proliferation of retinal progenitor cells, thereby ensuring the proper formation of distinct retinal layers.

As development progresses, FGF signaling assumes a neuroprotective role, particularly in safeguarding photoreceptors from degeneration. In regenerative species such as zebrafish, it is also critically involved in Müller glia-mediated retinal regeneration, facilitating the reprogramming of glial cells into multipotent progenitors.

In contrast, the mammalian retina, which has limited regenerative capacity, shows promising responses to exogenous FGF stimulation, which can evoke a regeneration-like program, thereby highlighting a potential therapeutic strategy for degenerative retinal diseases such as retinitis pigmentosa.

In three-dimensional models such as retinal organoids, FGF signaling reveals a tightly regulated interplay between spatial patterning, cell fate specification, and neuroprotection—underscoring its multifaceted role and therapeutic relevance in retinal biology.

SIRT1, FOXO, and Caloric Restriction

SIRT1, a NAD^+-dependent deacetylase, is activated during caloric restriction and low-energy states. It modulates transcription factors such as FOXO, which promote stress resistance, autophagy, and metabolic adaptation. SIRT1 and FOXO indirectly inhibit mTORC1, contributing to enhanced autophagy and cell survival under stress. This regulatory axis plays a key role in retinal aging and protection against degenerative diseases. Longevity factor FOXO3a is a potential therapeutic target for age-related ocular diseases such as retinopathy [7].

mTOR as a Therapeutic Target in Retinal Diseases

Given its central role in regulating cell growth, metabolism, autophagy, inflammation, and angiogenesis, the mechanistic target of rapamycin (mTOR) has emerged as a promising therapeutic target in a wide range of retinal disorders. These include age-related macular degeneration (AMD), diabetic retinopathy, retinitis pigmentosa, retinal detachment, and glaucoma. Modulating mTOR signaling offers opportunities to restore homeostasis, reduce pathological neovascularization, and promote neuroprotection.

Rapamycin and mTOR Inhibitors

Rapamycin (sirolimus) is a macrolide compound that selectively inhibits mTORC1 through binding to FKBP12, thereby blocking downstream anabolic processes and promoting autophagy. Its analogs, known as rapalogs (e.g., everolimus and temsirolimus), have been developed to improve pharmacokinetic profiles and therapeutic applications. In preclinical retinal models, these agents have shown efficacy in reducing neovascularization, mitigating photoreceptor degeneration, **and** enhancing autophagic clearance in stressed or damaged cells.

Clinical Trials and Experimental Models

Several experimental models and early-phase clinical trials have investigated mTOR inhibition in retinal diseases. Intravitreal or subconjunctival delivery of rapamycin has demonstrated suppression of choroidal neovascularization in AMD models and attenuation of vascular leakage in diabetic retinopathy. In models of retinal detachment and optic nerve injury, mTOR inhibition has been shown to modulate Müller glial activation, reduce gliosis, and promote retinal ganglion cell survival.

Systemic Versus Local mTOR Inhibition

A major challenge in targeting mTOR for retinal therapy lies in balancing efficacy with safety. Systemic administration of mTOR inhibitors may lead to off-target effects, including immunosuppression, delayed wound healing, and metabolic disturbances. In contrast, local delivery (e.g., intravitreal injection) offers targeted modulation of mTOR signaling within the eye while minimizing systemic toxicity. However, local administration requires optimization of formulation, dosing frequency, and drug stability to ensure sustained therapeutic action.

Combination Therapies

mTOR inhibitors are also being explored in combination therapies to enhance efficacy. Co-administration with anti-VEGF agents may provide synergistic effects in neovascular AMD and proliferative diabetic retinopathy by concurrently targeting angiogenic and metabolic pathways. Similarly, combining mTOR inhibitors with antioxidants or neuroprotective agents may augment photoreceptor and RGC survival in degenerative conditions by addressing oxidative stress and mitochondrial dysfunction.

Overall, the therapeutic targeting of mTOR represents a multifaceted approach to treating retinal diseases. While promising, its clinical translation requires precise control of dosing, delivery method, and combination strategy to maximize benefit and minimize risk. Ongoing studies will help define the optimal therapeutic windows and patient populations most likely to benefit from mTOR-based interventions.

Therapeutic Implications in Summary

mTOR Inhibitors

Rapamycin: As an mTOR inhibitor, rapamycin has shown potential in treating retinal diseases by reducing:

- Pathological angiogenesis (e.g., in DR and AMD).
- Inflammation and oxidative stress.
- However, prolonged inhibition of mTOR may impair normal retinal cell function, highlighting the need for targeted or intermittent therapies.

Nutritional and Metabolic Interventions

- Caloric restriction and exercise, both of which modulate mTOR activity, have demonstrated protective effects on retinal health.

Gene and Drug Therapies

- mTOR modulation via genetic tools or small molecules is being investigated to enhance cell survival in retinal degeneration (e.g., RP and glaucoma).

Research Frontiers

- Understanding mTOR's cross talk with other pathways, such as PI3K/Akt, AMPK, and HIF-1α, is critical to developing targeted therapies for retinal diseases.
- Exploring how mTOR activity affects retinal progenitor cell therapies and retinal organoids could advance regenerative medicine approaches for vision restoration.

Bibliography

1. Barone. The role of immune cells and signaling pathways in diabetic eye disease: a comprehensive review. Biomedicine. 2024;12 https://doi.org/10.3390/biomedicines12102346.
2. Casciano. The role of the mTOR pathway in diabetic retinopathy. Front Med. 2022;9 https://doi.org/10.3389/fmed.2022.973856.
3. Datta. Mitophagy initiates retrograde mitochondrial-nuclear signaling to guide retinal pigment cell heterogeneity. Autophagy. 2022;19 https://doi.org/10.1080/15548627.2022.2109286.
4. Fan J-L. Ghrelin inhibits autophagy mediated by AKT/mTOR pathway to ameliorate retinal angiogenesis induced by high glucose stress. Int J Ophthalmol. 2024; https://doi.org/10.18240/ijo.2024.05.01.
5. Nguyen H. Selective activation of the Wnt-signaling pathway as a novel therapy for the treatment of diabetic retinopathy and other retinal vascular diseases. Pharmaceutics. 2022;14 https://doi.org/10.3390/pharmaceutics14112476.
6. Hanna. Beyond genetics: the role of metabolism in photoreceptor survival, development and repair, vol. 10. Front Cell Dev Biol; 2022. https://doi.org/10.3389/fcell.2022.887764.
7. Hao X-D. Longevity factor FOXO3a: a potential therapeutic target for age-related ocular diseases. Life Sci. 2024; https://doi.org/10.1016/j.lfs.2024.122769.
8. Choi J. mTORC1 accelerates retinal development via the immunoproteasome. Nat Commun. 2018;9 https://doi.org/10.1038/s41467-018-04774-9.
9. Wan J. HB-EGF is necessary and sufficient for Müller glia dedifferentiation and retina regeneration. Dev Cell. 2012;22 https://doi.org/10.1016/j.devcel.2011.11.020.
10. Chang K. The interplay of autophagy and oxidative stress in the pathogenesis and therapy of retinal degenerative diseases. Cell Biosci. 2022; https://doi.org/10.1186/s13578-021-00736-9.
11. Kaarniranta. Autophagy in age-related macular degeneration. Autophagy. 2022; https://doi.org/10.1080/15548627.2022.2069437.
12. LiCausi. Role of mTOR complexes in neurogenesis. Int J Mol Sci. 2018;19 https://doi.org/10.3390/ijms19051544.
13. Losiewicz. mTORC1 and mTORC2 expression in inner retinal neurons and glial cells. Exp Eye Res. 2021;197 https://doi.org/10.1016/j.exer.2020.108131.
14. Pan. Photoreceptor metabolic reprogramming: current understanding and therapeutic implications. Commun Biol. 2021;4 https://doi.org/10.1038/s42003-021-01765-3.
15. Lee SH. Role of mTORC1 activity during early retinal development and lamination in human-induced pluripotent stem cell-derived retinal organoids. Cell Death Discovery. 2022;8 https://doi.org/10.1038/s41420-022-00837-5.
16. Lim S. mTORC1-induced retinal progenitor cell overproliferation leads to accelerated mitotic aging and degeneration of descendent Müller glia. Developmental Biology. 2022;10 https://doi.org/10.7554/eLife.70079.
17. Sadria. Interactions among mTORC, AMPK and SIRT: a computational model for cell energy balance and metabolism. Cell Commun Signal. 2021;19 https://doi.org/10.1186/s12964-021-00706-1.
18. Shu Y. Role of oxidative stress in ocular diseases: a balancing act. Meta. 2023;13 https://doi.org/10.3390/metabo13020187.
19. Steketee. Mitochondrial dynamics regulate growth cone motility, guidance, and neurite growth rate in perinatal retinal ganglion cells in vitro. IVOS. 2012;53 https://doi.org/10.1167/iovs.12-10298.
20. Tomita. Metabolism in retinopathy of prematurity. Life. 2021;11 https://doi.org/10.3390/life11111119.
21. Liu W. Retinitis pigmentosa: progress in molecular pathology and biotherapeutical strategies. Int J Mol Sci. 2022;23 https://doi.org/10.3390/ijms23094883.
22. Xu X. GBP2 inhibits pathological angiogenesis in the retina via the AKT/mTOR/VEGFA axis. Microvascular Res. 2024a;154 https://doi.org/10.1016/j.mvr.2024.104689.

23. Xu J. The formation and renewal of photoreceptor outer segments. Cells. 2024b;13 https://doi.org/10.3390/cells13161357.
24. Wen Y. mTORC2 activation protects retinal ganglion cells via Akt signaling after autophagy induction in traumatic optic nerve injury. Experiment Molecul Med. 2019;51 https://doi.org/10.1038/s12276-019-0298-z.
25. Zelinka. mTor signaling is required for the formation of proliferating Müller glia-derived progenitor cells in the chick retina. PMC/Development. 2016; https://doi.org/10.1242/dev.133215.

Chapter 9
mTOR Effect in Retinal Pigment Epithelium (RPE)

Contents

Abstract The mechanistic target of rapamycin (mTOR) signaling pathway plays a fundamental role in the regulation of cellular metabolism, autophagy, and survival within the human retinal pigment epithelium (RPE), a monolayer critical for photoreceptor support and visual function. mTOR integrates environmental signals such as nutrient availability, oxidative stress, and growth factors to modulate protein synthesis, mitochondrial function, and lysosomal activity in RPE cells. Dysregulation of mTOR particularly chronic hyperactivation of mTORC1—has been implicated in the pathogenesis of age-related macular degeneration (AMD), leading to impaired autophagic flux, accumulation of damaged organelles, increased inflammatory signaling, and deposition of lipofuscin and drusen formation. Conversely, selective mTOR inhibition has been shown to enhance autophagy, improve cellular clearance mechanisms, and protect against RPE degeneration in experimental models. Given the RPE's central role in retinal homeostasis, precise regulation of mTOR signaling is essential for maintaining retinal integrity and represents a promising therapeutic target in degenerative retinal diseases such as diabetic retinopathy and retinitis pigmentosa. Although the retinal pigment epithelium (RPE) is anatomically considered a part of the retina, its distinct and essential physiological roles warrant a dedicated chapter for detailed discussion.

K. T. Moazed, *mTOR Signaling in Ophthalmology*,
https://doi.org/10.1007/978-3-032-05044-1_9

Discussion

The retinal pigment epithelium (RPE), located between retinal photoreceptors and choroidal capillaries, is a single layer of pigmented cells that are of critical importance for the eye. The RPE plays key roles in maintaining the structure and function of the retina; phagocytosis; barrier formation; transportation of nutrients, ions, and water; absorption of light; protection of retinal cells against photo-oxidation; visual cycle maintenance; and production of various factors. Impaired RPE structure or function plays important roles in many ocular pathologies, such as age-related macular degeneration (AMD), retinitis pigmentosa (RP), diabetic retinopathy (DR), and proliferative vitreoretinopathy (PVR).

The retinal pigment epithelium (RPE) plays a central role in managing a substantial daily influx of nutrients and metabolic byproducts. This includes the phagocytosis of lipid- and protein-rich photoreceptor outer segments, the clearance of metabolic "waste" such as lactate released by the neural retina, and the uptake of nutrients delivered via the choroidal circulation. Beyond acting as a conduit for nutrient transfer to the neural retina, the RPE also contributes actively to retinal metabolism by recycling and generating metabolites through lysosomal degradation and mitochondrial oxidative processes. Together, these activities establish a finely tuned metabolic ecosystem between the outer retina and the RPE. The metabolic flexibility of RPE cells—i.e., their ability to utilize a broad spectrum of substrates such as glucose, galactose, lactate, fatty acids, succinate, proline, glutamine, and other amino acids—is essential for maintaining retinal homeostasis. Disruption of this balance, particularly due to mitochondrial or lysosomal dysfunction within the RPE, can precipitate retinal degeneration [17].

Mitochondria–Melanosome Interactions and Their Role in RPE Health

Melanosomes are lysosome-related organelles derived from endosomal precursors, which undergo a well-defined maturation process progressing through stages I to IV, characterized by increasing levels of melanin synthesis and deposition [28]. As melanosomes mature and are transported toward the cell periphery, they require substantial energetic support, primarily in the form of ATP. To meet this demand, the mitochondrial network dynamically repositions itself in close proximity to maturing melanosomes, facilitating efficient ATP delivery. These mitochondria–melanosome interactions are particularly critical during periods of active melanosome biogenesis and are notably disrupted in conditions of melanosomal dysfunction.

In the retinal pigment epithelium (RPE), proper melanosome function is essential for maintaining cellular health and visual function. Melanosomes serve as a protective reservoir against oxidative stress, mitigating the damaging effects of reactive oxygen species (ROS) generated by high metabolic activity, daily phagocytosis of photoreceptor outer segments, and photo-oxidative stress. Thus, disruptions in melanosome maturation or mitochondrial association may compromise RPE homeostasis and contribute to retinal degenerative diseases, including age-related macular degeneration (AMD) [10].

mTOR Dysregulation in the RPE

The key mTOR dysregulations involves RPE metabolism, autophagy, inflammation, oxidative stress, angiogenesis, and barrier function. Each disorder involves distinct but overlapping molecular pathways, emphasizing the importance of targeted therapeutic interventions that stabilize RPE function, cellular metabolism, and overall retinal homeostasis.

Highlights: mTOR Dysregulation in the Retinal Pigment Epithelium (RPE)

Central Metabolic Regulator

mTOR (mechanistic target of rapamycin) integrates signals from nutrients, growth factors, and cellular energy status to regulate RPE homeostasis, including protein synthesis, autophagy, and mitochondrial function.

Disruption of Autophagy

- Hyperactivation of *mTORC1* suppresses autophagy, a critical process for RPE cells to degrade phagocytosed photoreceptor outer segments and damaged organelles.
- Impaired autophagic flux leads to accumulation of lipofuscin and cellular debris, contributing to RPE dysfunction and AMD pathogenesis.

Oxidative Stress Vulnerability

- mTOR hyperactivation increases mitochondrial oxidative stress and reduces antioxidant capacity.
- Suppressed autophagy and mitochondrial quality control render RPE cells more susceptible to ROS-mediated damage.

Dysregulated Lipid and Nutrient Metabolism

- mTOR influences lipid biosynthesis and nutrient transport in RPE.
- Dysregulation contributes to lipid accumulation, metabolic inflexibility, and subretinal drusenoid deposits.

VEGF Overexpression and Neovascularization

- Aberrant mTOR signaling upregulates HIF-1α and VEGF-A, promoting angiogenesis.
- This is particularly relevant in neovascular AMD, where pathological CNV originates from RPE-driven VEGF release.

Inflammation and Senescence

- Chronic mTOR activation fosters a proinflammatory, senescent RPE phenotype via NF-κB and SASP (senescence-associated secretory phenotype) signaling.
- Contributes to chronic inflammation seen in AMD and other retinal degenerative conditions.

Cross Talk with Other Signaling Pathways

- mTOR activity in RPE is modulated by PI3K/AKT, AMPK, TSC1/2, and MAPK pathways.
- Diabetic retinopathy and aging can shift this balance, exacerbating RPE dysfunction.

Role of mTORC1 and mTORC2 in the Retinal Pigment Epithelium (RPE)

The mechanistic target of rapamycin (mTOR) exists in two distinct multiprotein complexes, mTORC1 and mTORC2, each with unique components, activation mechanisms, and downstream targets. In the retinal pigment epithelium (RPE)—a metabolically active and highly specialized monolayer essential for photoreceptor support, immune privilege, and metabolic exchange—both complexes play critical, yet distinct, roles in maintaining cellular homeostasis, function, and survival.

Elevated activity of mTORC1 and mTORC2 signaling pathways in the retinal pigment epithelium (RPE) has been shown to also disrupt glucose metabolism, resulting in phenotypic and molecular changes that resemble age-related macular degeneration (AMD). Recent studies have implicated impaired glycolysis as a contributing factor in AMD pathogenesis [4].

Together, mTORC1 and mTORC2 coordinate a finely tuned balance of growth, survival, and metabolic adaptation in the RPE. While necessary for normal cellular function, dysregulated mTOR signaling—whether excessive or deficient—can precipitate oxidative stress, impaired autophagy, barrier dysfunction, and neovascularization, all of which are implicated in the pathophysiology of age-related macular degeneration and other retinal diseases. Therapeutic strategies targeting mTOR pathways must therefore consider the distinct roles of mTORC1 and mTORC2 to avoid exacerbating disease processes while preserving essential RPE functions.

Elevated mTORC1 and mTORC2 signaling in the retinal pigmented epithelium alters glucose metabolism, leading to a pathology resembling age-related macular degeneration [10] (Fig. 9.1).

mTORC1 Role in RPE

mTORC1 is composed of mTOR, raptor, mLST8, PRAS40, and DEPTOR and is primarily activated by growth factors, amino acids, and energy status via the PI3K/AKT and TSC1/2 pathways. It regulates protein synthesis, lipid metabolism, autophagy, and mitochondrial function.

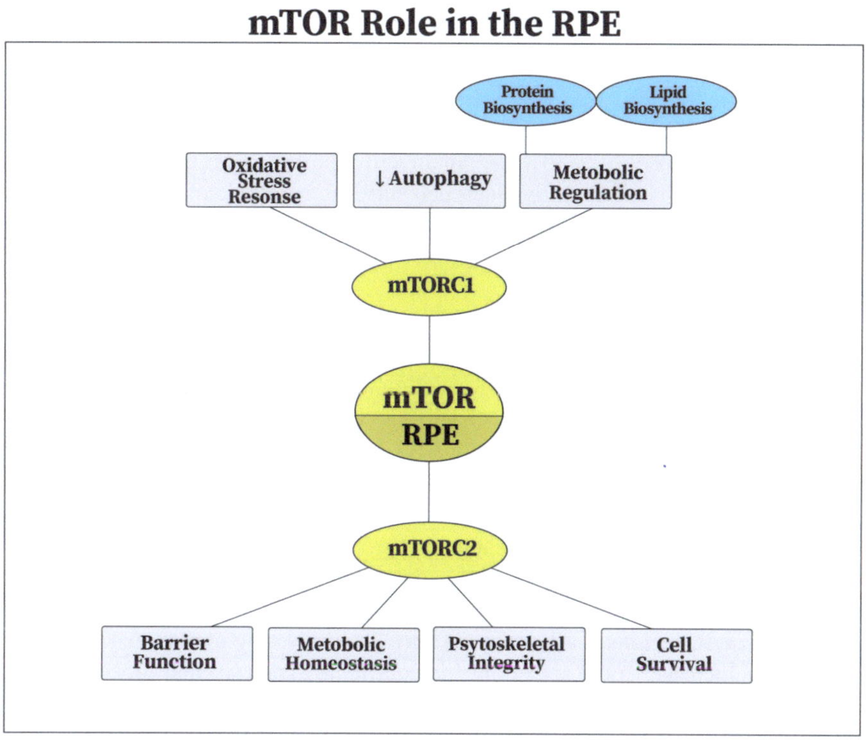

Fig. 9.1 The image illustrates the role of mTOR in the retinal pigment epithelium (RPE), where it exists in two distinct multiprotein complexes: mTORC1 and mTORC2. Both complexes play critical, yet distinct, roles in maintaining cellular homeostasis, function, and survival

mTORC1 Key Functions in RPE:

- *Metabolic Regulation:* mTORC1 supports anabolic metabolism, including lipid and protein biosynthesis, necessary for the daily phagocytosis of photoreceptor outer segments. Proper mTORC1 activity ensures the recycling of photoreceptor outer segments (POS), which is critical for retinal homeostasis [25].
- *Autophagy Inhibition*: Under nutrient-rich conditions, mTORC1 inhibits autophagy by phosphorylating ULK1. Dysregulation of autophagy in the RPE impairs degradation of photoreceptor debris, contributing to drusen formation and AMD pathogenesis.
- Defective autophagy due to dysregulated mTORC1 activity contributes to the accumulation of toxic waste products such as lipofuscin [18].
- *Oxidative Stress Response*: mTORC1 influences mitochondrial biogenesis and antioxidant defenses. Hyperactivation can increase ROS production and reduce stress resilience. mTORC1 influences the antioxidant defense systems in the RPE, helping to mitigate oxidative damage [30].

- *Neovascularization*: mTORC1 signaling pathway regulates macrophages in choroidal neovascularization [38].

mTORC2 Role in RPE

mTORC2 comprises mTOR, Rictor, mLST8, SIN1, and Protor-1/2. Unlike mTORC1, it is insensitive to acute rapamycin exposure and is activated predominantly by growth factors. It regulates cell survival, cytoskeletal organization, and metabolism through downstream targets such as AKT (Ser473), SGK1, and PKC isoforms.

mTORC2 Key Functions in RPE

- *Cell Survival and Cytoskeletal Integrity:* mTORC2 promotes RPE cell survival by activating AKT and modulating actin cytoskeleton dynamics, which are essential for maintaining barrier function and polarity.
- *Metabolic Homeostasis*: Through AKT and SGK1, it contributes to glucose uptake, ion transport, and lipid metabolism, processes vital for maintaining RPE functionality under stress.
- *Barrier Function*: mTORC2 helps preserve tight junction integrity and apical–basal polarity, crucial for the outer blood–retinal barrier and nutrient transport between the choroid and retina.
- *Disease Association:* Aberrant mTORC2 activity may alter cytoskeletal stability, increase VEGF secretion, and contribute to neovascular processes, particularly in the context of wet AMD.

Summary of Diseases Associated with mTOR Dysregulation in the Retinal Pigment Epithelium (RPE)

The most common retinal pathologies such as age-related macular degeneration (AMD), retinitis pigmentosa (rp), diabetic retinopathy (DR), and proliferative vitreoretinopathy (PVR) illustrate diverse yet interconnected dysregulations of RPE [31].

A brief preview is presented below, followed by a detailed description of each subject (Fig. 9.2).

Age-Related Macular Degeneration (AMD)

AMD involves progressive dysfunction and loss of central vision, significantly related to abnormalities in the RPE layer. Despite significant advances, the precise molecular mechanisms underlying these pathological processes in AMD remain incompletely understood.

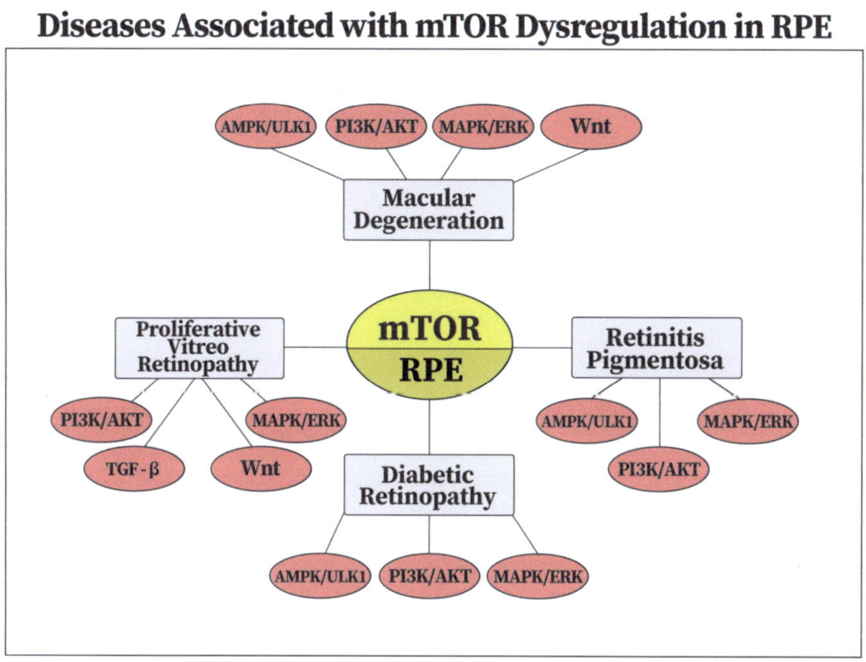

Fig. 9.2 The image highlights the major diseases associated with mTOR dysregulation in the retinal pigment epithelium (RPE), illustrating the distinct signaling pathways implicated in the development and progression of each condition

Key RPE Dysfunctions

- *Oxidative Stress:* Chronic accumulation of reactive oxygen species (ROS).
- *Autophagic Impairment:* Reduced clearance of damaged organelles, proteins, and lipids.
- *Inflammation and Complement Activation:* Chronic inflammatory state damages RPE cells.
- *Metabolic Dysfunction:* Inefficient clearance of photoreceptor outer segments and drusen formation.
- *Angiogenic Imbalance:* Excess VEGF causes neovascularization in wet AMD.

Main Molecular Pathways

- *mTOR, AMPK/ULK1* (autophagy and metabolic control)
- *PI3K/AKT* (angiogenesis and oxidative stress)
- *MAPK/ERK and Wnt* (inflammation and fibrosis)

Retinitis Pigmentosa (RP)

RP describes genetic retinal dystrophies primarily affecting photoreceptors, secondarily damaging RPE.

Key RPE Dysfunctions

- *Phagocytic Dysfunction:* Reduced clearance of photoreceptor outer segments
- *Oxidative Damage:* Progressive oxidative injury to RPE cells
- *Barrier Dysfunction:* Loss of RPE integrity, secondary to oxidative stress and metabolic dysregulation
- *Apoptosis*: Secondary RPE cell death due to chronic metabolic burden

Main Molecular Pathways

- *AMPK/ULK1* (autophagy impairment)
- *PI3K/AKT, MAPK/ERK* (oxidative stress response, apoptosis)

Diabetic Retinopathy (DR)

DR arises from sustained hyperglycemia-induced damage to retinal vessels and neurons, significantly impacting RPE function.

Key RPE Dysfunctions

- *Metabolic Stress:* Chronic glucose toxicity, oxidative stress, and AGE accumulation
- *Barrier Breakdown:* Disruption of tight junction integrity, leading to retinal edema
- *Inflammatory Response:* Increased cytokine and chemokine secretion
- *Angiogenesis*: Elevated VEGF levels promoting pathological neovascularization

Main Molecular Pathways

- *PI3K/AKT* (vascular permeability and VEGF-driven angiogenesis)
- *MAPK/ERK* (inflammation and cell survival/apoptosis)
- *mTOR/AMPK/ULK1* (autophagy and metabolic regulation)

Proliferative Vitreoretinopathy (PVR)

PVR is a complication following retinal detachment or trauma, characterized by the pathological proliferation, migration, and epithelial–mesenchymal transition (EMT) of RPE cells.

Key RPE Dysfunctions

- *Epithelial–Mesenchymal Transition (EMT)*: Transformation of differentiated RPE cells into migratory, fibroblast-like cells forming fibrotic membranes
- *Aberrant Proliferation and Migration:* Excessive cellular proliferation and migration into vitreous, leading to scar tissue formation

- *Fibrotic Response:* Increased extracellular matrix production causing retinal traction and re-detachment
- *Chronic Inflammation*: Elevated cytokine and growth factor secretion perpetuating fibrosis and cellular migration

Main Molecular Pathways
- *Wnt/β-catenin signaling* (EMT and cellular migration)
- *MAPK/ERK signaling* (cellular proliferation and fibrosis)
- *PI3K/AKT signaling* (cell survival, migration, and EMT)
- *TGF-β signaling* (fibrosis and EMT induction)

Therapeutic Approaches Across Disorders
- *Antioxidants and Anti-inflammatory Agents* (AMD, RP, DR, and PVR)
- *Autophagy Activators* (AMPK activators for AMD, RP, and DR)
- *Anti-VEGF Therapies* (AMD, DR, and selectively in PVR)
- *Gene Therapy* (primarily RP)
- *EMT Inhibitors and Antifibrotic Agents* (primarily PVR)

Physiological Role of mTOR in RPE

The mammalian target of rapamycin (mTOR) plays an essential role in maintaining the physiological integrity and function of the retinal pigment epithelium (RPE), a monolayer of post-mitotic, metabolically active cells critical to retinal homeostasis. Through its two functionally distinct complexes, mTORC1 and mTORC2, mTOR orchestrates a broad range of cellular processes within the RPE. These include the fine-tuned modulation of autophagy, which is essential for the clearance of damaged organelles and aggregated proteins; the regulation of oxidative stress responses, protecting RPE cells from reactive oxygen species generated by light exposure and high metabolic demand; and the promotion of anabolic processes such as protein and lipid synthesis necessary for cellular maintenance and renewal. Moreover, mTOR signaling contributes to the regulation of energy homeostasis and broader metabolic functions, aligning nutrient availability with cellular activity. Importantly, mTOR activity also supports the daily phagocytosis of shed photoreceptor outer segments, a vital function for sustaining photoreceptor health and visual cycle continuity. Dysregulation of mTOR in the RPE has been increasingly implicated in the pathogenesis of various retinal degenerative diseases, underscoring its central role in retinal physiology (Fig. 9.3).

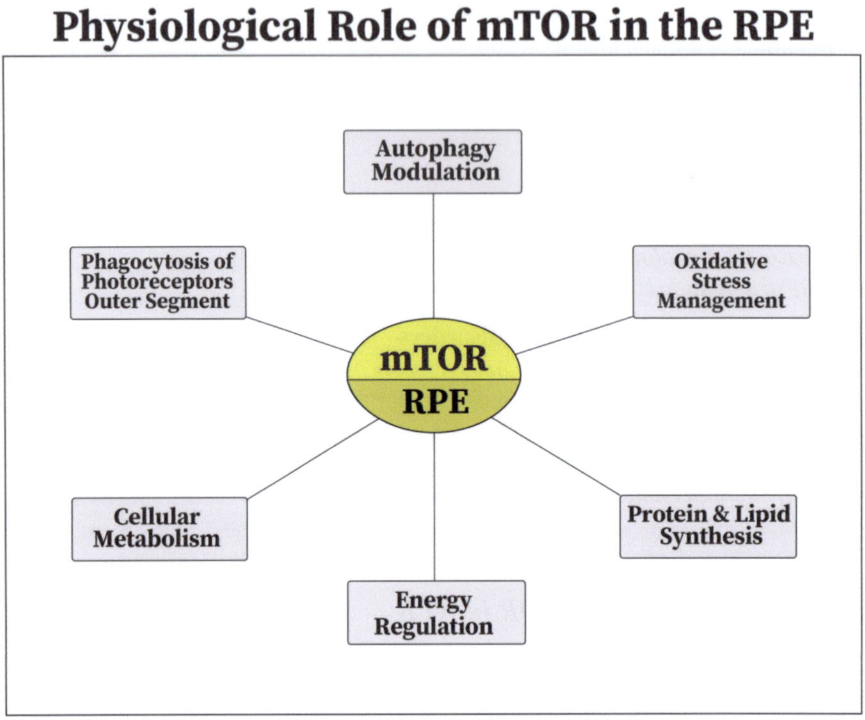

Fig. 9.3 The image illustrates the physiological role of mTOR in the retinal pigment epithelium (RPE). Five key interactions are depicted, each contributing to distinct aspects of RPE function and homeostasis

Detailed Description of Diseases Associated with mTOR Dysregulation in the Retinal Pigment Epithelium (RPE)

mTOR Role in Macular Degeneration

AMD primarily affects people over the age of 50 and is divided into two major forms: Dry (atrophic AMD), which accounts for 85–90% of the cases and involves the gradual thinning and breakdown of the macular tissues, with drusen (small yellow deposits) accumulating beneath the retina. Although dry AMD may progress slowly, it can lead to geographic atrophy and severe central vision loss. Wet (neovascular) AMD accounts for 10–15% of cases but is more severe and more likely to lead to severe vision loss. It characterized by abnormal growth of blood vessels under the retina, leading to leakage of blood and fluid, which progresses rapidly without prompt treatment [20].

mTOR plays a significant role in the physiology of the retinal pigment epithelium (RPE), which is essential for maintaining retinal health. Dysfunction in mTOR signaling has been implicated in the development of age-related macular degeneration (AMD) and other retinal diseases.

Age-related macular degeneration (AMD) is a significant public health concern, particularly in aging populations. It has affected approximately 20 million people in the US and 196 million people worldwide. It is characterized by the degeneration of the macula, the central portion of the retina, leading to a gradual loss of central vision. AMD is a leading cause of severe vision impairment in older people and is expected to affect approximately 288 million people worldwide by 2040 [14].

mTOR Dysregulation in Macular Degeneration

mTOR plays a crucial role in the retinal pigment epithelium (RPE) by regulating autophagy, metabolism, and oxidative stress. Dysregulated mTORC1 activity can impair RPE function, leading to the formation of drusen (early AMD) due to autophagy inhibition, RPE cell death and geographic atrophy (advanced dry AMD), and, finally, neovascularization (wet AMD) through increased VEGF expression. In this chapter, we review the function of RPE and the effect of molecular pathways involved in these processes, with much emphasis on macular degeneration, which is due to overactive mTORC1 and drusen formation (early AMD), RPE cell death and geographic atrophy (advanced AMD), and neovascular AMD (wet AMD).

Targeting mTOR with inhibitors like rapamycin may offer therapeutic potential by restoring autophagy and reducing abnormal angiogenesis.

- *RPE Metabolism and Function*: The RPE requires active mTOR signaling to manage lipid metabolism, autophagy, and mitochondrial function. Proper mTORC1 activity ensures the recycling of photoreceptor outer segments (POS), which is critical for retinal homeostasis. RPE cell death and geographic atrophy (advanced AMD) due to persistent mTORC1 hyperactivity promotes RPE degeneration by impairing mitochondrial function and autophagy. This can lead to geographic atrophy (GA), a severe form of dry AMD characterized by the progressive loss of RPE cells and photoreceptors [16].
- *Inflammation and Immune Dysregulation*: Inflammation and immune dysregulation are central to the early pathogenesis of age-related macular degeneration (AMD). Drusen—the hallmark extracellular deposits of dry AMD—are enriched with proinflammatory constituents, including apolipoprotein E, coagulation factors, acute-phase proteins, immunoglobulin G (IgG), and complement activators. The presence of these molecules reflects localized immune activation and positions chronic, low-grade inflammation as a critical driver of disease initiation. Accumulating evidence implicates dysregulated inflammatory cascades and immune imbalance in both drusen formation and AMD progression. These pathological processes are characterized by the deposition of extracellular material, activation of the innate immune system, and recruitment of microglia and macrophages to subretinal and choroidal compartments. The ensuing inflammatory milieu exacerbates cellular stress and tissue damage, further advancing retinal degeneration [36].
- *Oxidative Stress Response*: mTORC1 influences the antioxidant defense systems in the RPE, helping to mitigate oxidative damage, which is a contributing factor

to AMD. LAMTOR1-Mediated Regulation of mTORC1 and Autophagy in Oxidative Stress Response in AMD. Neovascular AMD (wet AMD): In some cases, mTORC1 dysregulation enhances the expression of vascular endothelial growth factor (VEGF), driving the formation of abnormal blood vessels beneath the retina. This process is associated with neovascular (wet) AMD, which leads to rapid and severe vision loss if untreated [33]. Oxidative stress is a well-established pathogenic driver of age-related macular degeneration (AMD), contributing to RPE cell damage and degeneration. To counteract oxidative stress and maintain cellular homeostasis, autophagy plays a critical cytoprotective role by facilitating the degradation of damaged organelles and oxidized macromolecules [6].

- Oxidative stress serves as a central pathogenic mechanism in age-related macular degeneration (AMD), driving cellular damage and protein modification in the retina. One key oxidative product is 2-(ω-carboxyethyl) pyrrole (CEP), which forms covalent adducts with proteins, altering their structure and function. With aging, cumulative low-level oxidative injuries lead to the modification and cross-linking of endogenous proteins, resulting in misfolded aggregates and the accumulation of CEP-adducted proteins. These aberrant proteins contribute to the formation of drusen—extracellular, lipoproteinaceous deposits that are toxic to retinal cells. In parallel, lipofuscin, another hallmark of aging, accumulates within the retinal pigment epithelium (RPE). Composed of lipid–protein complexes formed through photo-oxidative reactions, lipofuscin exerts phototoxic effects and further amplifies oxidative damage, contributing to RPE dysfunction and AMD progression.
- *Autophagy Regulation*: mTORC1 suppresses autophagy under nutrient-rich conditions to maintain energy balance. In the RPE, defective autophagy due to dysregulated mTORC1 activity contributes to the accumulation of toxic waste products such as lipofuscin. Overactive mTORC1 and Drusen Formation (Early AMD): Excessive mTORC1 activity inhibits autophagy, leading to the accumulation of drusen—lipid and protein deposits that accumulate beneath the RPE. Drusen formation is a hallmark of early AMD and contributes to chronic inflammation and RPE dysfunction. A key regulator of autophagy is the late endosomal/lysosomal adaptor, MAPK and mTOR activator 1 (LAMTOR1). LAMTOR1 acts as a scaffold protein on the lysosomal membrane and governs the mechanistic target of rapamycin complex 1 (mTORC1) signaling in response to amino acid availability. Under conditions of amino acid sufficiency, LAMTOR1 recruits mTORC1 to the lysosome, leading to its activation and suppression of autophagy. Conversely, during amino acid deprivation, LAMTOR1 facilitates the disassembly or inactivation of mTORC1, thereby promoting autophagy initiation. This nutrient-sensing axis is especially relevant in the context of AMD, where impaired autophagy and increased oxidative damage synergize to exacerbate RPE dysfunction and retinal degeneration. Modulating LAMTOR1-mediated mTORC1 activity represents a potential strategy to restore autophagic flux and mitigate oxidative stress in the aging retina.

- *Angiogenesis and Choroidal Neovascularization (CNV)*: The novel identification of ALKBH5 upregulation as a critical molecular alteration in AMD highlights its role in RPE dysfunction and subsequent choroidal neovascularization (CNV). Targeting ALKBH5 could represent an innovative and potent therapeutic strategy to halt or reverse AMD progression, preserving vision and improving patient outcomes [35].

ALKBH5 (AlkB homolog 5) is an RNA demethylase that catalyzes the removal of N6-methyladenosine (m6A) modifications from messenger RNA (mRNA). As a member of the AlkB family of dioxygenases, ALKBH5 plays a key role in epitranscriptomic regulation, influencing RNA stability, splicing, export, and translation.

In the context of retinal pigment epithelium (RPE) and retinal disease:

- Upregulation of ALKBH5 has been observed in conditions such as age-related macular degeneration (AMD).
- Elevated ALKBH5 activity is associated with oxidative stress, impaired autophagy, lipid metabolism dysregulation, and VEGF-A overproduction.
- These alterations contribute to RPE dysfunction, angiogenesis, and disease progression.

Elevated ALKBH5 levels induce several critical pathological alterations in RPE cells:

- ALKBH5 overexpression results in compromised mitochondrial membrane potential (depolarization).
- This dysfunction increases susceptibility to oxidative injury and reduces cellular energy efficiency, further exacerbating AMD pathology.
- Increased ALKBH5 expression correlates with higher reactive oxygen species (ROS) generation.
- Elevated oxidative stress damages proteins, lipids, and DNA in RPE cells, significantly disrupting their cellular integrity and function.
- Autophagy, a critical cellular degradation mechanism for removing damaged cellular components, becomes severely disrupted with ALKBH5 elevation.
- Impaired autophagy results in the accumulation of damaged organelles, increased cellular debris, and cellular senescence.
- ALKBH5 dysregulation disturbs lipid metabolism, leading to lipid accumulation and formation of intracellular lipid droplets.
- Dysregulated lipid metabolism further exacerbates oxidative stress and cellular dysfunction, contributing to drusen formation—an AMD hallmark.
- ALKBH5 overexpression significantly elevates VEGF-A secretion from RPE cells.
- Increased VEGF-A is a principal driver of CNV, promoting the proliferation, migration, and abnormal vascular tube formation in endothelial cells.
- Elevated VEGF-A secretion from dysfunctional RPE cells due to ALKBH5 overexpression strongly influences choroidal endothelial cells.
- Endothelial cell proliferation initiates abnormal vessel growth.

- Enhanced migration facilitates invasive neovascularization.
- Tube formation and angiogenesis cause the formation of pathological CNV lesions beneath the retina.

Therapeutic Potential: Targeting mTOR in AMD

Rapamycin, via its inhibition of mTOR signaling, partially alleviates deficits in energy metabolism caused by genetic variation in retinal pigment epithelial (RPE) cells. mTOR activity is intimately linked to cellular aging and age-related pathologies, including age-related macular degeneration (AMD). Chronic elevation of mTOR activity, coupled with increased levels of proinflammatory cytokines and cellular stress markers, may exacerbate aging processes and promote AMD pathogenesis. Furthermore, oxidative stress alone is sufficient to trigger dedifferentiation of RPE cells through the activation of the Akt/mTOR signaling cascade. Importantly, these deleterious effects are attenuated by pharmacological inhibition of mTOR with rapamycin, underscoring its potential as a therapeutic strategy to counteract oxidative damage and preserve RPE function in AMD [39].

1. *Rapamycin (mTOR Inhibitor):*
   - *Rapamycin* or other mTOR inhibitors have been explored to reduce mTORC1 overactivity, promoting *autophagy* and reducing *RPE stress*. However, careful control is necessary, as excessive inhibition can impair normal cellular functions.
   - *Light irradiation* can induce autophagy in ARPE-19 cells, and rapamycin can upregulate the activity of autophagy [32].
2. *Combination Therapies*:
   - Therapies targeting both *mTOR* and *VEGF* pathways hold promise for treating *wet AMD* by mitigating both *angiogenesis* and RPE dysfunction.
   - Metformin use was associated with decreased odds of developing AMD in a dose-dependent manner, with the greatest benefit at low-to-moderate dosages [5]. Interestingly, population-based studies have revealed that patients receiving metformin are less likely to develop age-related macular degeneration (AMD) [37].
   - Rapamycin, via inhibition of mTOR, partially reverts the deficit in energy metabolism caused by FH loss in RPE cells [27]. Furthermore, mTOR activity is closely linked to aging and age-related diseases.

mTOR Role in Retinitis Pigmentosa (RP)

Retinitis pigmentosa (RP) is a group of inherited retinal dystrophies affecting approximately 2.5 million individuals globally, with the prevalence ranging from 1 in 3500 to 1 in 5000 across various populations. The disease is marked by the progressive degeneration of photoreceptors—initially rods, followed by cones—resulting in severe visual impairment and eventual bilateral blindness. RP is genetically heterogeneous, with mutations in at least 83 genes identified to date, 58 of which are associated with autosomal recessive inheritance. In most cases, a mutation in a single gene is sufficient to cause disease, representing a major cause of inherited blindness. The majority of these mutations are localized to photoreceptor cells (rods and cones), although a smaller proportion also affects the retinal pigment epithelium (RPE), contributing to the complex pathophysiology of RP.

Dysregulated mTOR signaling contributes critically to RPE dysfunction by suppressing autophagy, increasing oxidative stress, disrupting cellular metabolism, and compromising barrier integrity. Therapeutically targeting the mTOR pathway offers a promising avenue to delay retinal degeneration and preserve vision in RP [34].

mTOR signaling dysregulation significantly contributes to the pathogenesis of retinitis pigmentosa (RP), a heterogeneous group of inherited retinal dystrophies characterized by progressive photoreceptor degeneration and eventual blindness. Although the primary genetic defects in RP directly affect photoreceptors, secondary impairment of retinal pigment epithelium (RPE) function, involving mTOR dysregulation, plays a crucial role in exacerbating disease progression.

- Impaired Autophagy: Autophagy maintains RPE cellular health by degrading damaged mitochondria, proteins, and photoreceptor outer segments.

  Hyperactivation of mTORC1 suppresses autophagy, causing accumulation of damaged cellular components, which leads to RPE stress, dysfunction, and apoptosis.

  Increased oxidative damage and metabolic stress exacerbate photoreceptor degeneration and RPE cell death [3].
- Metabolic Dysregulation: Efficient metabolic regulation through balanced mTOR activity supports photoreceptor nutritional demands. mTOR hyperactivation causes aberrant metabolism and impaired mitochondrial bioenergetics, resulting in elevated oxidative stress in the RPE. Chronic metabolic stress in RPE cells accelerates secondary photoreceptor loss [9].
- Cellular Stress and Oxidative Damage: RPE cells maintain retinal homeostasis by continuously phagocytosing photoreceptor outer segments, preventing debris accumulation [15]. Aberrant mTOR activity hampers clearance mechanisms due to autophagy suppression, leading to accumulated oxidative debris, lipofuscin, and drusen-like deposits [29].
- Chronic inflammation further degrades RPE integrity, exacerbating photoreceptor degeneration. Altered RPE Barrier Integrity: mTOR signaling maintains cellular junction integrity, crucial for RPE barrier function. Excessive or sustained mTOR signaling disrupts tight junctions, compromising the RPE barrier. Leakage, inflammation, and impaired nutrient/waste exchange occur, damaging photoreceptors and the retinal architecture [22].

Molecular and Cellular Mechanisms of mTOR Dysregulation in RP

Genetic Mutation In retinitis pigmentosa (RP), genetic mutations—such as those in *RHO*, *PDE6B*, and *RPE65*—primarily affect photoreceptors but secondarily impose metabolic stress on retinal pigment epithelial (RPE) cells, disrupting autophagy regulation [21].

mTORC1 Hyperactivation In retinal pigment epithelial (RPE) cells, hyperactivation of mTORC1 promotes the accumulation of metabolic byproducts, leading to impaired cellular homeostasis. Elevated oxidative stress and persistent cellular damage serve as additional stimuli that perpetuate aberrant mTORC1 signaling, thereby exacerbating RPE dysfunction [2].

mTOR Downstream Pathophysiological Effects

- Reduced AMPK Activation: Disrupts cellular energy sensing, compromising ATP homeostasis and stress adaptation
- Suppressed ULK1-mediated autophagy initiation: Inhibits autophagic flux, leading to accumulation of damaged organelles and protein aggregates
- Enhanced proinflammatory signaling: Promotes chronic inflammation, exacerbating retinal degeneration and accelerating disease progression

Therapeutic Implications: mTOR Modulation

- *mTOR Inhibitors (e.g., Rapamycin and Everolimus)* [40]:
- Potential therapeutic strategy by restoring autophagy and mitigating oxidative stress.
- *AMPK Activators (e.g., Metformin)* [1]:
- Indirectly attenuate excessive mTORC1 signaling, restoring metabolic and autophagic balance.
- *Combined Therapy Approaches:*
- Using mTOR inhibitors with antioxidants, autophagy stimulators, or gene therapy can synergistically improve outcomes in RP models [11].

mTOR Role in Diabetic Retinopathy (DR)

mTOR Signaling in Diabetic Retinopathy: A Central Integrator of Neurodegeneration and Metabolic Stress

Diabetic retinopathy (DR) is a prevalent microvascular and neurodegenerative complication of diabetes mellitus, affecting approximately 30–40% of diabetic individuals. By 2030, it is projected that the global population impacted by DR will reach 191 million. DR is widely acknowledged as the leading cause of diabetes-related visual impairment among the working-age population worldwide. Without timely prevention and effective management, DR poses a substantial socioeconomic burden. In recent years, intravitreal administration of antivascular endothelial growth factor (VEGF) agents has emerged as a major therapeutic advance, significantly reducing retinal neovascularization and alleviating diabetic macular edema.

However, the efficacy of anti-VEGF therapy is limited to a subset of patients, necessitates frequent intravitreal injections, and may diminish over time, highlighting the need for alternative or adjunctive treatment strategies.

In diabetic retinopathy (DR), chronic hyperglycemia induces a cascade of metabolic and cellular disturbances that culminate in retinal neurodegeneration. The mammalian target of rapamycin (mTOR) signaling pathway plays a central role in orchestrating these pathogenic events by integrating multiple anabolic and catabolic processes.

Specifically, mTOR regulates autophagy, modulates the oxidative stress response, governs pathways of programmed cell death, and influences the release of proinflammatory cytokines. These processes are tightly interconnected and contribute collectively to the progressive dysfunction and loss of retinal neurons and glia.

Through its dual complexes, mTORC1 and mTORC2, the pathway serves as a nutrient and energy sensor, responding to hyperglycemic stress by altering cellular homeostasis. In the diabetic retina, dysregulated mTOR activity may lead to insufficient autophagy, excessive ROS accumulation, heightened inflammatory signaling, and ultimately, neuronal apoptosis—key features of early DR pathogenesis.

In DR, chronic hyperglycemia leads to persistent mTOR pathway dysregulation, impairing autophagy, exacerbating inflammation, increasing VEGF production, and causing barrier dysfunction in the RPE [8].

Microglia, the resident immune cells of the retina, play a pivotal role in the pathogenesis of diabetic retinopathy (DR). Their activation is governed by complex immunometabolism mechanisms. In the early stages of DR, microglia often adopt a proinflammatory M1 phenotype, characterized by a metabolic shift from oxidative phosphorylation to aerobic glycolysis to meet increased energy demands. This metabolic reprogramming supports the production of proinflammatory cytokines and reactive oxygen species (ROS), amplifying local inflammation and oxidative stress. Emerging evidence indicates that, in addition to altering core metabolic pathways, activated microglia undergo significant reorganization of their redox systems, further contributing to the inflammatory milieu and neurovascular injury characteristic of DR.

Reactive oxygen species (ROS) play a dual role in diabetic retinopathy (DR), acting both as signaling molecules and mediators of oxidative damage. In retinal microglia, ROS generation is closely linked to metabolic reprogramming and inflammatory activation. One of the primary sources of ROS is the NADPH oxidase 2 (NOX2) system, which not only contributes to oxidative stress but also promotes glycolytic metabolism. This is achieved through activation of the AKT/mTOR signaling pathway, which facilitates the translocation of glucose transporter 4 (GLUT4) to the cell membrane, enhancing glucose uptake and driving aerobic glycolysis.

Conversely, cellular antioxidant systems such as the thioredoxin (Trx) pathway and the nuclear E2-related factor 2 (NRF2) signaling axis play protective roles by counteracting oxidative stress and maintaining microglia in an anti-inflammatory, homeostatic state. NRF2 activation leads to the transcription of antioxidant response element (ARE)-driven genes, supporting redox balance and suppressing proinflammatory gene expression. Together, the dynamic interplay between ROS generation and antioxidant defenses dictates microglial phenotype and function in DR, influencing both neuroinflammation and retinal vascular integrity [7].

Therapeutically targeting mTOR signaling represents a promising strategy to limit the progression of DR by restoring retinal cellular homeostasis, reducing pathological angiogenesis, and preserving visual function. mTOR signaling dysregulation is significantly implicated in the pathogenesis and progression of diabetic retinopathy (DR), a severe complication of diabetes characterized by progressive retinal microvascular damage, neuronal degeneration, and retinal pigment epithelium (RPE) dysfunction.

While endothelial cell dysfunction and microvascular leakage are central features, retinal pigment epithelium (RPE) cells also contribute significantly to disease progression, particularly through epithelial–mesenchymal transition (EMT) and fibrosis. Among intracellular mediators, the AKT (protein kinase B) isoforms play distinct roles in DR pathophysiology:

- *AKT1*: Downregulation is linked to vascular endothelial damage and impaired cell survival.
- *AKT2*: Predominantly expressed in insulin-responsive tissues and involved in glucose metabolism, but its role in RPE-related retinal fibrosis has remained poorly understood.

AKT2 is a key driver of EMT and fibrosis in diabetic RPE, distinct from the protective vascular role of AKT1. The PI3K/AKT2/ERK axis emerges as a central profibrotic pathway in DR and a promising therapeutic target to limit vision-threatening fibrotic complications in advanced diabetic retinopathy [12].

Mechanisms of mTOR Dysregulation in DR

In the context of diabetes, chronic hyperglycemia leads to sustained activation of the mechanistic target of rapamycin complex 1 (mTORC1), contributing to retinal pathology through several interconnected mechanisms:

- Nutrient and Metabolic Stress:

  Elevated glucose levels serve as energy-rich signals that activate mTORC1, disrupting cellular homeostasis. This activation impairs autophagic flux and contributes to metabolic inflexibility and cellular dysfunction in retinal cells.
- Oxidative Stress and Mitochondrial Dysfunction:

  Hyperglycemia increases the production of reactive oxygen species (ROS), which in turn activate mTOR signaling pathways. This creates a feedback loop that exacerbates mitochondrial dysfunction and heightens cellular stress responses.

- Chronic Inflammation:
  High glucose conditions induce the release of proinflammatory cytokines such as interleukin-1β (IL-1β) and tumor necrosis factor-alpha (TNF-α), which further stimulate mTOR activity. This contributes to a proinflammatory microenvironment and enhances the progression of diabetic retinopathy (DR).
- Dysregulation of Insulin and IGF-1 Signaling:
  Persistent insulin resistance and alterations in insulin-like growth factor-1 (IGF-1) signaling potentiate aberrant mTOR activation. This dysregulation impairs cellular repair processes and accelerates tissue damage within the retina.

Consequences of mTOR Dysregulation in the Retinal Pigment Epithelium (RPE) in Diabetic Retinopathy (DR)

A. Impaired Autophagy

- Hyperactivation of mTORC1 inhibits autophagy, preventing the clearance of dysfunctional mitochondria, damaged proteins, and lipid aggregates within RPE cells.
- The accumulation of these toxic byproducts leads to elevated cellular stress, oxidative damage, and chronic inflammation, thereby accelerating RPE degeneration and compromising retinal homeostasis.

B. Increased Angiogenesis and Vascular Permeability

- Persistent mTORC1 activity upregulates the expression and secretion of vascular endothelial growth factor (VEGF).
- Elevated VEGF levels drive pathological neovascularization, disrupt vascular integrity, and increase retinal vascular permeability, contributing to macular edema and the progression toward proliferative diabetic retinopathy (PDR).

C. Enhanced Inflammation and Cellular Senescence

- mTOR signaling amplifies the production of proinflammatory cytokines, including IL-6 and TNF-α, intensifying local retinal inflammation.
- Chronic mTOR activation promotes cellular senescence in RPE cells, marked by permanent cell cycle arrest and a senescence-associated secretory phenotype (SASP), which further propagates tissue dysfunction and degeneration.

D. Barrier Dysfunction and Breakdown

- Sustained mTOR activity compromises tight junction integrity in the RPE, weakening the outer blood–retinal barrier (BRB).
- This loss of barrier function increases paracellular permeability, facilitating fluid accumulation, neuronal damage, and vascular injury within the retina.

Cross Talk Between mTOR and Other Signaling Pathways in Diabetic Retinopathy (DR)

- AMPK/ULK1 Signaling:
  AMP-activated protein kinase (AMPK) serves as a critical energy sensor that negatively regulates mTORC1 and activates ULK1 to initiate autophagy. In diabetic conditions, AMPK activity is diminished due to nutrient surplus and metabolic inflexibility. This suppression disrupts ULK1-mediated autophagy initiation, exacerbating cellular stress and mitochondrial dysfunction in retinal cells.
- PI3K/AKT Pathway:
  Chronic hyperglycemia activates the PI3K/AKT pathway, which in turn reinforces mTORC1 signaling. This persistent activation aggravates metabolic dysregulation, enhances proinflammatory cytokine production, and promotes pathological angiogenesis—all key contributors to DR progression.
- MAPK/ERK Pathway:
  The MAPK/ERK cascade interacts synergistically with mTORC1, particularly under hyperglycemic and inflammatory conditions. This cross talk amplifies the expression of angiogenic factors such as VEGF and proinflammatory mediators, furthering vascular leakage, neuroinflammation, and structural retinal damage.

Therapeutic Potential and Intervention

Targeting mTOR pathway dysregulation is increasingly considered beneficial in managing DR:

- mTOR Inhibitors (e.g., Rapamycin and Everolimus):
  Suppress VEGF-driven angiogenesis, restore autophagy, reduce inflammation, and improve RPE cellular health in experimental DR models.
- Combination Therapies:
  Utilizing mTOR inhibitors alongside anti-VEGF therapies, antioxidants, and metabolic regulators (e.g., AMPK activators), these offer synergistic therapeutic benefits.
- Dietary and Pharmacologic AMPK activation:
  AMPK activation indirectly inhibits mTOR, enhancing autophagy, reducing inflammation, and mitigating metabolic and oxidative stress.

mTOR Role in Proliferative Vitreoretinopathy (PVR)

Proliferative vitreoretinopathy (PVR) is a fibrotic complication of retinal detachment and ocular trauma characterized by the proliferation, migration, and contraction of retinal pigment epithelial (RPE) cells, glial cells, and myofibroblasts. Recent studies implicate aberrant mTOR signaling—particularly mTORC1—as a critical contributor to the pathological cellular behaviors underpinning PVR development.

The Hippo signaling pathway interacts with multiple other signaling networks to influence the development of proliferative vitreoretinopathy (PVR). In particular, dysregulated activity of the Hippo pathway effectors, Yes-associated protein (YAP) and the transcriptional co-activator with PDZ-binding motif (TAZ), contributes to pathological RPE proliferation, epithelial–mesenchymal transition (EMT), and fibrotic membrane formation [13].

In addition to promoting neovascularization, the Hippo signaling pathway plays a crucial role in regulating subretinal fibrosis and fibrovascular scar formation in age-related macular degeneration (AMD). Central to this process are the downstream effectors YAP (Yes-associated protein) and TAZ (transcriptional co-activator with PDZ-binding motif), which drive both epithelial–mesenchymal transition (EMT) and endothelial–mesenchymal transition (EndMT)—key events in the pathogenesis of fibrotic AMD.

Several studies have highlighted the influence of YAP/TAZ on cytoskeletal remodeling and mesenchymal transdifferentiation. For instance, reduced nuclear retention of TAZ and its transcriptional partner ZEB1 has been shown to inhibit stress fiber formation in porcine RPE cells, suggesting a regulatory role in actin dynamics and cellular contractility. Moreover, under hypoxic condition—a common feature of the diseased retina—YAP expression and nuclear activity are markedly increased in human umbilical vein endothelial cells (HUVECs), further implicating the Hippo pathway in hypoxia-induced vascular remodeling and EndMT.

A. Enhanced Cell Proliferation and Survival

- mTORC1 hyperactivation in RPE and Müller glial cells promotes unchecked cell cycle progression and resistance to apoptosis through downstream effectors such as S6K1 and 4E-BP1.
- This pro-proliferative environment facilitates the expansion of fibrocellular membranes on both retinal surfaces, contributing to retinal traction and detachment recurrence.

B. Epithelial-to-Mesenchymal Transition (EMT)

- mTOR signaling is involved in driving EMT in RPE cells, a key step in PVR pathogenesis.
- Upregulation of transcription factors such as Snail, Twist, and ZEB1—partially mediated by mTOR/PI3K/AKT and mTOR/MAPK cross talk—promotes the loss of epithelial markers (e.g., E-cadherin) and acquisition of mesenchymal traits (e.g., α-SMA), enhancing cell motility and contractility.

C. Autophagy Suppression and Fibrosis

- mTORC1 negatively regulates autophagy, leading to the accumulation of damaged organelles and stress signaling that further potentiates fibrotic responses.
- Inhibition of autophagy in RPE cells has been linked to increased extracellular matrix (ECM) deposition and fibrotic membrane formation.

D. Inflammatory Signaling and mTOR Cross Talk

- Proinflammatory cytokines (e.g., TNF-α and IL-6) in the vitreous stimulate mTOR pathways, reinforcing a cycle of inflammation, proliferation, and ECM remodeling.
- mTOR also modulates the activity of NF-κB and STAT3, promoting a persistent inflammatory and fibrogenic state.

E. Therapeutic Implications

- Targeting mTOR signaling—especially mTORC1—with inhibitors such as rapamycin or dual mTOR/PI3K inhibitors has shown promise in preclinical models by suppressing RPE proliferation, EMT, and membrane contraction.
- However, optimal delivery routes (e.g., sustained-release intraocular systems) and combination strategies (e.g., with anti-inflammatory or antifibrotic agents) are critical for translating these findings into effective clinical therapies.

Mechanisms of mTOR Dysregulation in PVR

Proliferative vitreoretinopathy (PVR) develops as a pathological wound healing response, driven by excessive retinal pigment epithelial (RPE) cell activation, migration, proliferation, and epithelial-to-mesenchymal transition (EMT) in response to injury and inflammation. Aberrant activation of the mechanistic target of rapamycin (mTOR) pathway—particularly mTORC1 and mTORC2—is central to these maladaptive cellular processes.

Several upstream mechanisms contribute to mTOR dysregulation in the context of PVR:

- Trauma and Inflammatory Stimuli:

  Retinal injury and surgical manipulation induce the release of proinflammatory cytokines such as transforming growth factor-beta (TGF-β), platelet-derived growth factor (PDGF), vascular endothelial growth factor (VEGF), and interleukins. These cytokines activate mTOR signaling predominantly via the PI3K/AKT axis, triggering RPE cell proliferation, survival, and matrix remodeling.
- Enhanced Growth Factor Signaling:

In the vitreous of eyes with PVR, elevated levels of growth factors (e.g., PDGF, epidermal growth factor [EGF], VEGF, and TGF-β) robustly stimulate both mTORC1 and mTORC2. This activation supports abnormal RPE proliferation, cytoskeletal remodeling, and EMT—hallmark features of fibrocellular membrane formation and contraction.

- Hypoxia and Metabolic Stress:
  Post-injury ischemia and localized hypoxia activate mTOR signaling as a compensatory response aimed at restoring energy balance and supporting cell survival. However, in the context of PVR, this activation becomes maladaptive, enhancing pathological cellular behavior and promoting fibrotic remodeling.

Consequences of mTOR Dysregulation in RPE during PVR

A. Epithelial–Mesenchymal Transition (EMT)

- mTOR signaling (particularly via mTORC2 and its downstream effector AKT) drives RPE cell transformation into mesenchymal, migratory fibroblast-like cells.
- EMT is characterized by the downregulation of epithelial markers (e.g., E-cadherin) and upregulation of mesenchymal markers (e.g., α-SMA, fibronectin, and vimentin), processes strongly promoted by mTOR signaling.

B. Aberrant Cell Proliferation and Migration

- Hyperactivated mTORC1 enhances protein synthesis and cellular proliferation, leading to the uncontrolled growth of RPE cells within the vitreous cavity.
- mTOR signaling enhances migratory capacity through the reorganization of cytoskeletal elements (regulated by mTORC2) and increased extracellular matrix interactions.

C. Fibrotic Response and Extracellular Matrix (ECM) Production

- mTOR activation promotes excessive ECM deposition (collagen and fibronectin), forming rigid fibrocellular membranes that contract and induce tractional retinal detachment.
- The sustained mTOR activation potentiates profibrotic signaling cascades (notably TGF-β/Smad signaling), further aggravating fibrosis.

D. Inflammation and Chronic Cellular Stress

- mTOR dysregulation enhances the secretion of proinflammatory cytokines, perpetuating inflammatory and fibrotic responses.
- Chronic inflammation promotes persistent RPE activation, proliferation, and EMT, exacerbating membrane formation.

Interaction with Other Pathways in PVR

- TGF-β/Smad Signaling:
- mTOR acts synergistically with TGF-β signaling, potentiating EMT and fibrosis.
- PI3K/AKT Pathway:
- Functions upstream of mTOR, activating mTORC1/mTORC2 pathways and amplifying proliferative and migratory responses.
- MAPK/ERK Pathway:
- Interacts with mTOR to further stimulate cellular proliferation, migration, and fibrotic ECM production.
- Wnt/β-catenin Pathway:
- Cooperatively involved in promoting EMT and fibrotic responses of RPE cells in PVR.

Therapeutic Implications and Potential Interventions

Given mTOR's pivotal role, therapeutic strategies targeting mTOR signaling offer significant potential for treating PVR:

- mTOR Inhibitors (Rapamycin/Everolimus):
- Effective in experimental models by suppressing EMT, RPE proliferation, fibrotic membrane formation, and inflammation.
- Antifibrotic Therapies:
- Combination of mTOR inhibitors with TGF-β inhibitors may synergistically limit fibrosis and EMT.
- EMT-Targeted Therapies:
- Drugs specifically targeting mTORC2 or downstream AKT pathways could mitigate pathological cellular migration and proliferation.

Signaling Pathways in RPE

The key signaling pathways in the retinal pigment epithelium (RPE) and their physiological and pathological relevance (Fig. 9.4).

AMPK/ULK1 Signaling Pathways

AMPK plays a pivotal role in maintaining retinal pigment epithelium (RPE) health, primarily through its regulatory influence on autophagy, cellular metabolism, and stress response mechanisms. The AMPK/ULK1 signaling axis is vital for

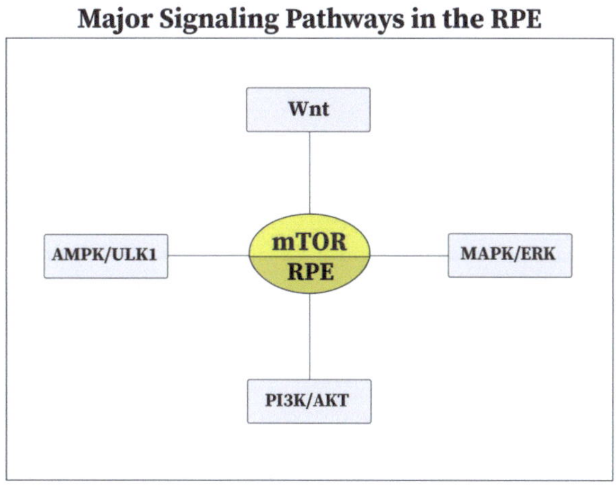

Fig. 9.4 The image illustrates the essential signaling pathways affecting retinal pigment epithelium (RPE) homeostasis

maintaining RPE cell health by modulating autophagy, metabolism, and stress responses. Dysfunction of this pathway contributes significantly to retinal diseases such as AMD and diabetic retinopathy. Therapeutic strategies aimed at enhancing AMPK/ULK1 signaling present promising opportunities for protecting and improving retinal health [41].

Overview of AMPK/ULK1 Signaling Pathway

- *AMP-Activated Protein Kinase (AMPK)*:
  - Acts as an energy sensor, activated under conditions of low cellular energy (high AMP/ATP ratio), stress, caloric restriction, hypoxia, or oxidative stress.
  - Upon activation, it regulates various metabolic pathways to restore cellular energy balance.
- *Unc-51-Like Autophagy Activating Kinase 1 (ULK1)*:
  - A serine/threonine kinase homologous to yeast Atg1, serving as a critical initiator of autophagy.
  - AMPK activates ULK1 by phosphorylation under nutrient stress conditions, promoting autophagy initiation.

Mechanism of AMPK/ULK1 Activation

- Under conditions of metabolic or oxidative stress:
  - Increased AMP binds to AMPK, facilitating its phosphorylation and activation by upstream kinases (e.g., liver kinase B1 [LKB1]).
  - Activated AMPK phosphorylates ULK1 at specific residues, promoting ULK1-mediated initiation of autophagy.

- AMPK simultaneously inhibits mTORC1 activity, further enhancing ULK1 activation and autophagic induction.

Role of AMPK/ULK1 Signaling in the RPE

Autophagy Regulation

- Autophagy is critical for RPE cells to remove damaged mitochondria, misfolded proteins, and oxidative stress-induced cellular debris.
- AMPK-activated ULK1 signaling initiates the autophagic process, maintaining cellular homeostasis, reducing oxidative stress, and protecting against degeneration.

Metabolic Homeostasis

- AMPK signaling promotes energy conservation, enhances mitochondrial function, and optimizes glucose and lipid metabolism.
- Essential in the RPE to maintain metabolic efficiency, crucial given its high-energy demand and role in supporting retinal photoreceptors.

Cell Survival and Stress Response

- Activation of AMPK/ULK1 signaling enhances the resilience of RPE cells under stress conditions (oxidative stress, nutrient deprivation, and aging).
- Provides cytoprotective effects by promoting autophagy-mediated clearance of toxic components, thus preventing apoptosis and degeneration.

Pathological Implications in Retinal Disorders

Age-Related Macular Degeneration (AMD)

- Dysfunctional AMPK/ULK1 signaling results in impaired autophagy, accumulation of damaged organelles (especially mitochondria), increased oxidative stress, and RPE cell degeneration.
- Restoring or enhancing AMPK/ULK1 signaling is a potential therapeutic strategy to mitigate AMD progression by boosting cellular clearance mechanisms.

Diabetic Retinopathy (DR)

- Altered AMPK signaling contributes to metabolic dysregulation, increased inflammation, and oxidative stress, accelerating retinal damage.
- Activation of AMPK can restore metabolic balance, improve autophagy, and decrease pathological inflammation and angiogenesis.

Proliferative Vitreoretinopathy (PVR)

- Regulation of autophagy and EMT processes via AMPK/ULK1 can influence the RPE cell behavior, potentially modulating pathological proliferation and migration characteristic of PVR.

Cross Talk with Other Pathways

- *mTOR Signaling*:
  - AMPK antagonizes mTORC1 signaling, promoting autophagy and inhibiting cellular growth and proliferation under stress.
- *PI3K/AKT Pathway*:
  - Counterbalances AKT-mediated anabolic effects, enhancing metabolic flexibility.
- *MAPK/ERK Pathway*:
  - Integrates with AMPK signaling during stress response and metabolic regulation.

Therapeutic Potential

- *Pharmacological Activators of AMPK (e.g., Metformin and AICAR)*:
  - Evaluated to promote autophagy, reduce oxidative stress, and protect RPE cells in retinal diseases. [37]
- *Dietary Interventions (e.g., Caloric Restriction and Intermittent Fasting)*:
  - Can naturally enhance AMPK activation, potentially preserving RPE function and retinal health

AMP-activated protein kinase (AMPK) plays a vital role in maintaining retinal pigment epithelium (RPE) homeostasis. During aging or in the progression of retinal diseases, a series of morphological and functional alterations emerge in the RPE, including cellular hypertrophy, disruption of tight junctions, and impairment of the outer blood–retinal barrier. This barrier is essential for regulating the bidirectional transport of nutrients and metabolic waste between the choroid and the neural retina. Such structural deterioration compromises retinal homeostasis and contributes to the onset of RPE-related ocular pathologies. Notably, these pathological changes are associated with a marked reduction in AMPK activity [24].

As a central cellular energy sensor, AMPK is activated in response to metabolic stress and external stimuli. Once activated, AMPK modulates a wide range of signaling and metabolic pathways that collectively function to preserve energy balance and cellular integrity. It plays a protective role in the RPE by mitigating oxidative stress, suppressing inflammatory responses, and delaying degenerative changes. Furthermore, AMPK activation is implicated in key physiological processes within the RPE, including the regulation of apoptosis and autophagy. AMPK promotes autophagic flux through several downstream effectors and thereby contributes to cellular quality control. By attenuating apoptosis and cellular injury, AMPK activation supports RPE viability and function. These findings underscore the complex, multifaceted role of AMPK in safeguarding RPE cells against metabolic and oxidative damage.

ATM–AMPK–ULK1 Relationship in RPE Cells

Stress Activation

- Ataxia–telangiectasia mutated (ATM) is classically known for its role in DNA damage response, but it is also activated in response to oxidative stress independently of DNA damage.
- In RPE cells exposed to reactive oxygen species (ROS), ATM is activated and acts as a redox sensor.

ATM Activates AMPK

- Upon oxidative stress, ATM activates LKB1, a key upstream kinase of AMPK.
- This leads to phosphorylation and activation of AMPK, which are essential for restoring energy balance and promoting autophagy.

Regulation of Autophagy and Mitochondrial Function

- ATM–AMPK signaling promotes autophagy initiation (via ULK1), essential for the clearance of damaged mitochondria (mitophagy).
- This helps maintain mitochondrial homeostasis, which is critical for RPE health given their high metabolic demand.

Ataxia-telangiectasia mutated (ATM), a serine/threonine kinase primarily known for its role in the DNA damage response, has emerged as a critical regulator of cellular homeostasis in the retinal pigment epithelium (RPE) and is increasingly implicated in the pathogenesis of age-related macular degeneration (AMD). Beyond its canonical function in genomic stability, ATM exerts protective effects in the context of AMD by modulating several key cellular processes.

ATM activation promotes autophagy, thereby facilitating the clearance of damaged organelles and protein aggregates—an essential function in the metabolically active and post-mitotic RPE. Moreover, ATM helps preserve the integrity of the lysosomal–mitochondrial axis, which is crucial for maintaining energy production and preventing oxidative stress accumulation. Through these actions, ATM contributes to cellular senescence in a controlled, non-apoptotic manner, which may serve as a mechanism for limiting cell death under chronic stress conditions. In parallel, ATM signaling suppresses apoptosis, thereby preserving RPE cell viability and delaying retinal degeneration. Collectively, these findings highlight ATM as a multifaceted regulator of RPE survival and suggest its therapeutic relevance in mitigating AMD progression [23].

While no direct interaction between ALKBH5 and AMPK has been definitively proven in RPE cells, both are involved in overlapping cellular processes, especially autophagy and oxidative stress responses. ALKBH5 dysregulation may indirectly modulate AMPK signaling through its effects on stress and m6A-regulated gene networks. Further investigation is warranted to define this potential cross talk.

ALKBH5 (AlkB Homolog 5) is a member of the AlkB family of Fe(II)/α--ketoglutarate-dependent dioxygenases and functions as an RNA demethylase that specifically removes N6-methyladenosine (m^6A) modifications from RNA. m^6A is the most prevalent internal modification in eukaryotic mRNA and plays a crucial role in the regulation of RNA metabolism, including mRNA stability, splicing, export, translation, and degradation [35].

Key Functions of ALKBH5

m^6A Demethylation

- ALKBH5 catalyzes the oxidative demethylation of m^6A in mRNA, thereby influencing gene expression at the post-transcriptional level.
- By regulating m^6A levels, ALKBH5 modulates the fate of target RNAs, affecting cellular processes such as proliferation, differentiation, and stress responses.

Role in Autophagy and Metabolism

- In various cell types, including RPE cells, aberrant ALKBH5 expression has been linked to disrupted autophagy, lipid dysregulation, and oxidative stress.
- It is increasingly recognized that m^6A demethylases like ALKBH5 participate in metabolic reprogramming under stress or disease conditions.

Pathogenic Role in the Retina

- In RPE cells, overexpression of ALKBH5 is associated with:
  - Mitochondrial depolarization
  - Elevated oxidative stress
  - Impaired autophagy
  - Abnormal lipid metabolism
  - Upregulation of VEGF-A secretion
- These alterations collectively promote angiogenesis by stimulating endothelial cell proliferation, migration, and tube formation—hallmarks of wet AMD pathophysiology.

Implications in Disease

- Dysregulated ALKBH5 activity has been implicated in various diseases, including cancer, neurodegeneration, and ocular pathologies like age-related macular degeneration (AMD).
- Given its central role in post-transcriptional regulation, ALKBH5 is considered a potential therapeutic target, particularly in conditions where m^6A imbalance contributes to pathogenesis.

The retinal pigment epithelium (RPE) is crucial for retinal health and vision maintenance, functioning via multiple interconnected signaling pathways.

AKT/mTOR Signaling Pathways

The AKT/mTOR pathway is essential for RPE cell metabolism, survival, and angiogenic regulation. Its dysregulation contributes to the pathogenesis of major retinal diseases by disturbing autophagy, increasing oxidative stress, and promoting neovascularization and fibrosis.

AKT/mTOR Signaling Pathway in RPE Cells

The AKT/mTOR pathway is a central regulator of cellular metabolism, survival, growth, and autophagy. In RPE cells, it integrates extracellular cues (e.g., nutrients, insulin, and growth factors) to maintain retinal support functions and adapt to environmental stress [26].

Activation Cascade

- Initiated by the binding of ligands such as insulin, IGF-1, VEGF, or PDGF to receptor tyrosine kinases (RTKs)
- Signal transduction sequence:
  - RTK → PI3K → PIP3 → AKT (phosphorylation at Thr308 and Ser473) → inhibition of TSC1/TSC2complex → activation of Rheb → stimulation of mTORC1

Functions in RPE Cells

(a) *Cell Survival and Anti-Apoptotic Signaling*

- AKT phosphorylates pro-apoptotic proteins (e.g., BAD and FOXO), promoting RPE survival under oxidative stress and nutrient deprivation.

(b) *Metabolic Regulation*

- mTORC1 promotes protein and lipid synthesis, glycolysis, and mitochondrial biogenesis—critical for the RPE's high metabolic demand.
- Maintains energy balance during diurnal phagocytosis of photoreceptor outer segments.

(c) *Autophagy Suppression*

- Active mTORC1 inhibits ULK1, thereby suppressing autophagy.
- Under basal conditions, this ensures anabolic activity, but chronic suppression leads to accumulation of damaged mitochondria and lipofuscin.

(d) *VEGF-A Expression and Angiogenesis*

- AKT/mTOR signaling enhances HIF-1α stability, upregulating VEGF-A transcription.
- Contributes to choroidal neovascularization in AMD and abnormal angiogenesis in diabetic retinopathy.

Dysregulation in Retinal Disease

Condition	Effect of dysregulated AKT/mTOR	Consequence
AMD	mTOR hyperactivation → impaired autophagy, oxidative stress	RPE degeneration and VEGF overproduction
Diabetic retinopathy	Chronic AKT/mTOR activation by hyperglycemia	Inflammation, angiogenesis, and metabolic dysfunction
PVR	Growth factor-driven mTOR signaling	RPE proliferation, EMT, and membrane formation

Cross Talk with Other Pathways

- *AMPK*: Acts as a counter-regulator; inhibits mTORC1 under energy stress.
- *MAPK/ERK*: Co-activated by growth factors; contributes to EMT and cell migration.
- *SIRT1/FOXO*: AKT phosphorylation suppresses FOXO3a, reducing oxidative defense gene expression.

Therapeutic Implications

- *mTOR inhibitors* (e.g., rapamycin) can restore autophagy, reduce VEGF, and alleviate oxidative damage in RPE.
- Potential for use in AMD, DR, and PVR but must be balanced to preserve RPE viability and barrier function.

Wnt Signaling Pathway

Properly regulated Wnt signaling is essential for RPE health and function, whereas its dysregulation contributes significantly to RPE dysfunction and retinal pathology. Understanding these mechanisms opens therapeutic avenues to treat and prevent diseases affecting the RPE and the retina. The central pathway is involved in regulating cell differentiation, proliferation, and migration [42].

Its function in RPE:

- Influences development and maintenance of RPE cell layers.
- Supports regeneration and cellular repair processes following injury or oxidative stress.
- Aberrant activation of Wnt signaling can lead to abnormal proliferation and pathological changes associated with proliferative vitreoretinopathy (PVR) and AMD.

Wnt signaling plays a vital and complex role in the development, homeostasis, regeneration, and pathology of the retinal pigment epithelium (RPE). It operates through several mechanisms, primarily canonical (β-catenin-dependent) and noncanonical pathways.

1. Canonical Wnt/β-catenin Pathway in RPE

   • *Mechanism*:

     – Wnt ligands bind to Frizzled (Fzd) receptors and low-density lipoprotein receptor-related proteins 5/6 (LRP5/6).
     – This binding stabilizes cytoplasmic β-catenin, allowing its nuclear translocation.
     – In the nucleus, β-catenin complexes with T-cell factor/lymphoid enhancer factor (TCF/LEF), regulating target gene transcription.

   • *Functions*:

     – *Cell proliferation and Differentiation*: Essential for proper RPE layer development during embryogenesis
     – *Barrier Integrity and Polarity*: Maintains structural integrity and polarized function of RPE cells, critical for photoreceptor support
     – *Regeneration and Repair*: Promotes cell survival and repair following injury or oxidative stress

2. Noncanonical Wnt Pathways (Planar Cell Polarity [PCP] and Calcium-Dependent Pathways)

   • *PCP Pathway*:

     – Controls cell orientation, polarization, and directional migration, essential for orderly RPE development
     – Crucial for cytoskeletal remodeling and cell junction stability

   • *Calcium-Dependent Pathway*:

     – Modulates intracellular calcium levels influencing cellular adhesion, migration, and inflammatory responses in RPE cells.

Role in Retinal Diseases

• *Age-Related Macular Degeneration (AMD)*:

  – Dysregulated Wnt signaling contributes to pathological processes such as aberrant angiogenesis (via VEGF induction), inflammation, oxidative stress, and fibrosis.

- *Proliferative Vitreoretinopathy (PVR)*:
  - Activation of canonical Wnt signaling is associated with RPE cell proliferation, epithelial–mesenchymal transition (EMT), and formation of fibrotic membranes that can lead to retinal detachment.
- *Diabetic Retinopathy*:
  - Altered Wnt signaling influences inflammatory processes, vascular permeability, and endothelial proliferation, contributing to retinal pathology.

Therapeutic Potential

- Wnt inhibitors/modulators (e.g., anti-Wnt antibodies, small-molecule antagonists, and inhibitors of β-catenin signaling):
  - Investigated for controlling fibrosis, proliferation, and pathological angiogenesis
- Wnt activators or stabilizers:
  - May enhance regeneration and repair mechanisms following injury

Interaction with Other Pathways

- Wnt signaling cross-talks extensively with other pathways in RPE:
  - *mTOR Signaling*: Cooperation in regulating cell metabolism, proliferation, and differentiation
  - *PI3K/AKT and MAPK Pathways*: Synergize or antagonize Wnt effects on cell survival and growth
  - *Notch pathway*: Coordinated regulation during differentiation and tissue repair processes

MAPK/ERK Signaling Pathway

MAPK/ERK signaling (mitogen-activated protein kinase/extracellular signal-regulated kinase pathway) is critical for maintaining normal retinal pigment epithelium (RPE) functions and is involved in cellular responses to extracellular stimuli, notably growth factors, stress signals, and cytokines. MAPK/ERK signaling is essential for RPE cellular processes including proliferation, differentiation, survival, and stress response. However, its dysregulation significantly contributes to retinal diseases like AMD, diabetic retinopathy, and PVR. Targeting MAPK/ERK signaling therapeutically could provide meaningful avenues for intervention in these retinal disorders [19].

Role of MAPK/ERK Signaling in RPE

The mitogen-activated protein kinase/extracellular signal-regulated kinase (MAPK/ERK) pathway is integral in controlling cellular growth, differentiation, survival, and apoptosis.

Mechanism of MAPK/ERK Signaling

- *Initiation*:
  - Triggered by extracellular signals such as growth factors (e.g., epidermal growth factor [EGF], fibroblast growth factor [FGF], platelet-derived growth factor [PDGF]) binding to receptor tyrosine kinases (RTKs).
  - Activation of RTKs initiates a phosphorylation cascade, beginning with the small GTPase Ras.
- *Propagation*:
  - Ras activates RAF kinases (RAF-1, B-RAF, A-RAF), which phosphorylate and activate MEK1/2.
  - Activated MEK1/2 subsequently phosphorylate and activate ERK1/2 (MAPK).
- *Transduction to Nucleus*:
  - Phosphorylated ERK1/2 translocates to the nucleus, activating various transcription factors (e.g., c-Fos, c-Jun, and Elk-1), driving the transcription of genes involved in proliferation, differentiation, and survival.

Functional Roles in RPE

- *Cell Proliferation and Survival*:
  - Essential for the proliferation of RPE cells during development and tissue regeneration.
  - Promotes cell survival under stress conditions, including oxidative stress and inflammation.
- *Differentiation and Maintenance*:
  - Supports differentiation and maturation of RPE cells, contributing to the integrity and specialized functions required for photoreceptor support and visual cycle maintenance.
- *Response to Oxidative Stress*:
  - ERK activation is part of the adaptive response against oxidative stress, helping RPE cells to resist apoptosis and maintain cellular homeostasis.
- *Cellular Migration and EMT (Epithelial–Mesenchymal Transition)*:
  - Under pathological conditions, MAPK/ERK signaling can facilitate EMT, enabling RPE cell migration, contributing to disorders such as proliferative vitreoretinopathy (PVR).

Pathological Implications

- *Age-Related Macular Degeneration (AMD)*:
  - Chronic activation of MAPK/ERK can exacerbate inflammation, oxidative damage, and abnormal proliferation of RPE cells, contributing to AMD pathogenesis.
  - ERK signaling can induce the secretion of VEGF, promoting pathological neovascularization in wet AMD.
- *Diabetic Retinopathy*:
  - Dysregulated ERK activity promotes vascular permeability, inflammation, and fibrosis, leading to retinal dysfunction.
- *Proliferative Vitreoretinopathy (PVR)*:
  - Enhanced ERK signaling contributes to the EMT of RPE cells, formation of fibrotic membranes, and retinal detachment.

Cross Talk with Other Signaling Pathways

- *PI3K/AKT Pathway*:
  - Synergizes with ERK in promoting cell survival and proliferation.
- *mTOR Signaling*:
  - ERK signaling integrates with mTOR pathways, influencing cell metabolism, autophagy, and growth.
- *Wnt Pathway*:
  - Interacts to regulate differentiation, proliferation, and cell migration.

Therapeutic Considerations

- *Inhibition of ERK Pathway*:
- Pharmacological inhibitors targeting components of the ERK pathway (MEK inhibitors, ERK inhibitors) may help control pathological proliferation, fibrosis, inflammation, and angiogenesis in retinal diseases.
- *Balancing ERK Activation*:
  - Careful modulation of ERK signaling is required, given its dual role in maintaining normal function versus driving pathology.

PI3K/AKT Signaling Pathway

The *PI3K/AKT signaling pathway* (phosphatidylinositol-3-kinase/protein kinase B pathway) is pivotal for regulating various cellular functions critical to retinal pigment epithelium (RPE) health, including cell survival, metabolism, growth, proliferation, differentiation, and protection against stress-induced apoptosis. The PI3K/AKT pathway is integral to maintaining normal RPE function by promoting cell survival, regulating metabolism, and managing autophagy. However, its chronic or uncontrolled activation significantly contributes to retinal disorders, making it a critical therapeutic target for diseases like AMD, diabetic retinopathy, and proliferative vitreoretinal disorders [26].

Mechanism of PI3K/AKT Signaling

- *Activation*:
  - Initiated by binding of growth factors (e.g., insulin-like growth factor [IGF], vascular endothelial growth factor [VEGF], epidermal growth factor [EGF]) to receptor tyrosine kinases (RTKs).
  - Activated RTKs recruit and activate PI3K, converting phosphatidylinositol-4,5-bisphosphate (PIP_2) to phosphatidylinositol-3,4,5-trisphosphate (PIP_3).
- *AKT Activation*:
  - PIP_3 binds to AKT and facilitates its phosphorylation by phosphoinositide-dependent kinase-1 (PDK1) and mTORC2, activating AKT.
  - Activated AKT phosphorylates numerous downstream targets controlling diverse biological processes.

Functions of PI3K/AKT Pathway in RPE

- *Cell Survival and Anti-Apoptotic Activity*
  - AKT promotes cell survival by phosphorylating and inhibiting apoptotic factors like BAD, caspase-9, and Forkhead box transcription factors (FOXO).
  - Protects RPE cells against apoptosis induced by oxidative stress, inflammation, and nutrient deprivation.

Cellular Metabolism

- AKT enhances metabolic functions, including glucose uptake (via GLUT transporters), lipid synthesis, and energy metabolism.
- Maintains metabolic homeostasis crucial for RPE cell function, especially under stress conditions.

Autophagy Regulation

- PI3K/AKT negatively regulates autophagy by activating mTORC1, which suppresses autophagic pathways.
- This balance is essential for maintaining protein quality control, cellular homeostasis, and preventing degeneration in RPE cells.

Proliferation and Growth

- AKT promotes proliferation and cellular growth by modulating cell-cycle regulators (cyclin D and p27^Kip1) and protein synthesis via mTORC1.
- Critical during development, tissue repair, and regeneration.

Pathological Implications in RPE

Age-Related Macular Degeneration (AMD)

- Dysregulation of PI3K/AKT contributes to chronic inflammation, oxidative stress, and impaired autophagy, increasing vulnerability to AMD.
- Sustained activation can drive pathological angiogenesis through upregulated VEGF expression.

Diabetic Retinopathy (DR)

- Hyperactivation of PI3K/AKT signaling in DR leads to increased vascular permeability, inflammation, and aberrant proliferation, exacerbating retinal injury.

Proliferative Vitreoretinopathy (PVR)

- Activation of PI3K/AKT signaling induces epithelial-mesenchymal transition (EMT), facilitating RPE migration, proliferation, and fibrotic membrane formation, characteristic of PVR.

Cross Talk with Other Pathways

- *mTOR Pathway*:
- Direct activation of mTORC1 by AKT regulates cell growth, autophagy, and metabolism.
- *MAPK/ERK Pathway*:
  - Synergistic roles in proliferation and survival, integrated to optimize cellular responses.
- *Wnt Pathway*:
  - Cross-regulation in proliferation, differentiation, EMT, and survival processes.

Therapeutic Potential

- *Inhibitors of PI3K/AKT Pathway*:
- May help control aberrant angiogenesis, proliferation, and fibrosis in retinal diseases.
- *Modulation of AKT Activity*:
  - Fine-tuning AKT signaling can balance between cell protection and pathological progression.

Bibliography

1. Amin. Metformin and retinal diseases in preclinical and clinical studies: insights and review of literature. Exp Biol Med. 2022. https://doi.org/10.1177/15353702211069986.
2. Ayten. Metabolic plasticity in a Pde6bSTOP/STOP retinitis pigmentosa mouse model following rescue. Mol Metab. 2024;88. https://doi.org/10.1016/j.molmet.2024.101994.
3. Azam. Mechanisms of rhodopsin-related inherited retinal degeneration and pharmacological treatment strategies. Cells. 2025. https://doi.org/10.3390/cells14010049.

4. Bammidi. Elevated mTORC1 and mTORC2 signaling in the retinal pigmented epithelium alters glucose metabolism, leading to a pathology resembling age-related macular degeneration. IOVS. 2024. ARVO.
5. Blitzer. Association of metformin use with age-related macular degeneration. JAMA Ophthalmol. 2021;139(3):302–9. https://doi.org/10.1001/jamaophthalmol.2020.6331.
6. Cai J. Regulation of LAMTOR1 by oxidative stress in retinal pigment epithelium: implications for age-related macular degeneration pathogenesis. Exp Eye Res. 2024. https://doi.org/10.1016/j.exer.2024.110129.
7. Cai L. Redox regulation of immunometabolism in microglia underpinning diabetic retinopathy. Antioxidants. 2024. https://doi.org/10.3390/antiox13040423.
8. Casciano. The role of the mTOR pathway in diabetic retinopathy. Front Med. 2022. https://doi.org/10.3389/fmed.2022.973856.
9. Chen Y. Metabolism dysregulation in retinal diseases and related therapies. Antioxidants. 2022. https://doi.org/10.3390/antiox11050942.
10. Chowdhury. Activated mTOR signaling in the RPE drives EMT, autophagy, and metabolic disruption, resulting in AMD-like pathology in mice. Aging Cell. 2025. https://doi.org/10.1111/acel.70018.
11. Confalonieri. Retinitis pigmentosa and therapeutic approaches: a systematic review. J Clin Med. 2024. https://doi.org/10.3390/jcm13164680.
12. Daley. Aberrant Akt2 signaling in the RPE may contribute to retinal fibrosis process in diabetic retinopathy. Cell Death Discov. 2023. https://doi.org/10.1038/s41420-023-01545-4.
13. Du Y. The Hippo signalling pathway and its impact on eye diseases. J Cell Mol Med. 2024. https://doi.org/10.1111/jcmm.18300.
14. Fleckenstein. Age-related macular degeneration a review. JAMA. 2024. https://doi.org/10.1001/jama.2023.26074.
15. Gallenga. Molecular mechanisms related to oxidative stress in retinitis pigmentosa. Antioxidants (Basel). 2021. https://doi.org/10.3390/antiox10060848.
16. Go YM. MTOR-initiated metabolic switch and degeneration in the retinal pigment epithelium. FASEB J. 2021. https://doi.org/10.1096/fj.202000612R.
17. Hurley. Retina metabolism and metabolism in the pigmented epithelium: a busy intersection. Ann Rev Vision Sci. 2021. https://doi.org/10.1146/annurev-vision-100419-115156.
18. Intartaglia. Autophagy in the retinal pigment epithelium: a new vision and future challenges. FEBS J. 2021. https://doi.org/10.1111/febs.16018.
19. Jang SY. The role of the mitogen-activated protein kinase pathway in the development of laser-induced choroidal neovascularization. Int J Mol Sci. 2025. https://doi.org/10.3390/ijms26062585.
20. Jiang F. Age-related macular degeneration: cellular and molecular signaling mechanisms. Int J Mol Sci. 2025. https://doi.org/10.3390/ijms26136174.
21. Kaplan. Metabolic rescue of cone photoreceptors in retinitis pigmentosa. Taiwan J Ophthalmol. 2021. https://doi.org/10.4103/tjo.tjo_46_21.
22. Kim J. Therapeutic potential of AAV2-shmTOR gene therapy in reducing retinal inflammation and preserving endothelial Integrity in age-related macular degeneration. Sci Rep. 2025. https://doi.org/10.1038/s41598-025-93993-4.
23. Leemput. ATM localization and gene expression in the adult mouse eye. Mol Vis. 2009. PMID: 19234633.
24. Liangliang. Role of AMPK-regulated autophagy in retinal pigment epithelial cell homeostasis: a review. Medicine. 2024. https://doi.org/10.1097/MD.0000000000038908.
25. Lu, F. mTOR activity is essential for retinal pigment epithelium regeneration in zebrafish. PLOS Genetics. 2022. https://doi.org/10.1371/journal.pgen.1009628.
26. Mebghua. ABCA4 mediated traumatic proliferative vitreoretinopathy associated with PI3K/Akt signaling pathway. Cell Symp. 2024. https://www.cell.com/heliyon/fulltext/S2405-8440(24)03055-X.
27. Merie. mTOR inhibition via rapamycin treatment partially reverts the deficit in energy metabolism caused by FH loss in RPE cells. Antioxidants. 2021. https://doi.org/10.3390/antiox10121944.

28. Moazed. Iris electron microscopy. The Iris. 2020. https://doi.org/10.1007/978-3-030-45756-3_4.
29. Pan M. Mice deficient in UXT exhibit retinitis pigmentosa-like features via aberrant autophagy activation. Autophagy. 2020. https://doi.org/10.1080/15548627.2020.1796015.
30. Pan F. Protective effects of triptolide against oxidative stress in retinal pigment epithelium cells via the PI3K/AKT/Nrf2 pathway: a network pharmacological method and experimental validation. Aging. 2024. https://doi.org/10.18632/aging.205570.
31. Rizwan. Metabolic phenotyping of healthy and diseased human RPE cells. IVOS. 2024. https://doi.org/10.1167/iovs.65.11.5.
32. Roudi. Effect of rapamycin on autophagy of retinal pigment epithelial cells under light induction. J Hainan Med Univ. 2024;30(9):p658. https://doi.org/10.13210/j.cnki.jhmu.20240024.001.
33. Ru-Xu S. ALKBH5 causes retinal pigment epithelium anomalies and choroidal neovascularization in age-related macular degeneration via the AKT/mTOR pathway. Cell Rep. 2023. https://doi.org/10.1016/j.celrep.2023.112779.
34. Song DJ. Mechanism of cone degeneration in retinitis pigmentosa. Cell Mol Neurobiol. 2022. https://doi.org/10.1007/s10571-022-01243-2.
35. Sun R. ALKBH5 causes retinal pigment epithelium anomalies and choroidal neovascularization in age-related macular degeneration via the AKT/mTOR pathway. Cell Rep. 2023. https://doi.org/10.1016/j.celrep.2023.112779.
36. Tan W. The role of inflammation in age-related macular degeneration. Int J Biol Sci. 2020. https://doi.org/10.7150/ijbs.49890.
37. Toppila. Metformin alleviates inflammation and induces mitophagy in human retinal pigment epithelium cells suffering from mitochondrial damage. Cells. 2024. https://doi.org/10.3390/cells13171433.
38. Wang C. mTORC1 signaling pathway regulates macrophages in choroidal neovascularization. Mol Immunol. 2020;121. https://doi.org/10.1016/j.molimm.2020.03.002.
39. Wigestrand. Rapamycin's impact on age-related macular degeneration—a systematic review and hormesis perspective. J Clin Transl Ophthalmol. 2024. https://doi.org/10.3390/jcto2030009.
40. Yang JL. Inhibition of mTOR signaling by rapamycin protects photoreceptors from degeneration in rd1 mice. Zool Res. 2021. https://doi.org/10.24272/j.issn.2095-8137.2021.049.
41. Zhou. Role of AMPK-regulated autophagy in retinal pigment epithelial cell homeostasis: a review. Medicine. 2024. https://doi.org/10.1097/MD.0000000000038908.
42. Zou J. Wnt inhibitory factor 1 ameliorated diabetic retinopathy through the AMPK/mTOR pathway-mediated mitochondrial function. FASEB J. 2022. https://doi.org/10.1096/fj.202200366RR.

Chapter 10
mTOR Effect on Optic Nerve

Contents

Abstract The mechanistic target of rapamycin (mTOR) signaling pathway plays a crucial role in the development, maintenance, and injury response of the human optic nerve. In retinal ganglion cells (RGCs), whose axons constitute the optic nerve, mTOR regulates axonal growth, protein synthesis, and metabolic support. During development, mTOR activity is essential for axon elongation and myelination. In the adult optic nerve, however, mTOR activity is tightly regulated, and its suppression contributes to the limited regenerative capacity of RGCs after injury. Reactivation of mTOR signaling, particularly mTORC1, has been shown in experimental models to enhance axon regeneration following optic nerve crush or glaucomatous damage. However, chronic or excessive mTOR activation may lead to maladaptive effects, including increased metabolic demand, mitochondrial dysfunction, and susceptibility to degeneration. Balancing mTOR activity appears critical

K. T. Moazed, *mTOR Signaling in Ophthalmology*,
https://doi.org/10.1007/978-3-032-05044-1_10

for promoting neuronal survival while avoiding excitotoxicity or axonal stress. Targeted modulation of mTOR may offer therapeutic potential in optic neuropathies, including glaucoma and ischemic optic neuropathy, by enhancing neuroprotection and promoting regenerative responses.

Discussion

More than 100 million individuals worldwide are affected by optic neuropathies, which collectively represent the leading cause of irreversible visual impairment. These disorders encompass a spectrum of pathological conditions, including glaucoma, traumatic optic neuropathy, optic neuritis, ischemic optic neuropathy, and optic nerve tumors. Despite extensive research, there are currently no effective therapeutic strategies for restoring visual function once significant damage to the optic nerve has occurred.

The *optic nerve*, predominantly constituted by the axons of *retinal ganglion cells (RGCs)*, lacks the intrinsic capacity to regenerate or re-establish functional connectivity following injury. As part of the central nervous system (CNS), the optic nerve is subject to multiple inhibitory mechanisms that impede axonal regeneration, including both intrinsic growth limitations of RGCs and extrinsic inhibitory signals within the CNS environment.

From a molecular biological point of view, the optic nerve is more than a simple conduit for visual signals—it is a complex, highly organized structure composed of retinal ganglion cell (RGC) axons, glial cells, myelin sheaths, and vascular components, all governed by specific molecular signals and cellular interactions.

The axons of retinal ganglion cells (RGCs) form the optic nerve, which serves as the sole conduit for transmitting visual information from the eye to the brain. Owing to their exceptional length and the spatial constraints of the optic pathway, these axons are particularly susceptible to injury. Various pathological conditions—such as glaucoma, traumatic optic neuropathy, ischemic optic neuropathy, and optic neuritis—primarily affect these axons, often resulting in irreversible visual impairment.

RGCs are essential for visual function, as they transmit visual information from the retina to higher visual centers in the brain, such as the lateral geniculate nucleus and superior colliculus. Consequently, injury-induced RGC death is a pivotal event leading to the progressive and often irreversible vision loss observed in numerous neurodegenerative optic neuropathies, including glaucoma, ischemic optic neuropathy, and optic neuritis.

In mammals, mature RGCs, similar to most central nervous system (CNS) neurons, lack the capacity to regenerate damaged axons, thereby leading to permanent vision loss following injury. To investigate the mechanisms underlying axonal regeneration, experimental models such as optic nerve crush and transection have been widely employed. Initial studies demonstrated that injured RGC axons are capable of regrowth into peripheral nervous system (PNS) grafts that provide a regeneration-permissive environment, highlighting the restrictive influence of the CNS milieu on axon regrowth [13].

Nevertheless, simply removing extrinsic inhibitory factors within the CNS has yielded limited success, enabling axon regeneration in only a small subset of injured RGCs. These findings underscore the critical role of intrinsic neuronal properties in governing the regenerative capacity. Consequently, it is now well-established that axonal regeneration in RGCs is contingent upon both intrinsic cellular programs and extrinsic environmental cues [35].

Importantly, successful axon regrowth alone is not sufficient for restoring visual function. True functional recovery requires precise reinnervation of appropriate central targets and the reformation of synaptic connections capable of supporting effective signal transmission.

The regenerative response of RGC axons following injury is governed by a tightly coordinated network of intrinsic signaling pathways. These include not only the canonical PI3K/AKT/mTOR axis but also parallel modulators and cytoskeletal regulators like GSK3 and CRMP2 [11].

Collapsin response mediator protein 2 (CRMP2) is a cytosolic phosphoprotein that plays a crucial role in neuronal development and axon guidance. It is involved in microtubule assembly by binding to tubulin heterodimers, thereby regulating axonal outgrowth and growth cone dynamics. CRMP2 is downstream of Semaphorin 3A signaling and is modulated through phosphorylation by kinases such as GSK-3β, Cdk5, and Rho kinase. In addition to its role in neurodevelopment, CRMP2 is implicated in neurodegenerative diseases, pain signaling, and epileptogenesis [31].

While the classical understanding of vision relies on electrochemical signaling, the concept of biophoton-based communication offers a provocative addition that may complement or fine-tune known mechanisms. However, this field is highly speculative, with limited empirical support. Further interdisciplinary studies involving optics, neuroscience, and quantum biology are required to clarify whether biophotons have a real functional role in signal transfer from the retina to the brain [23].

Key Molecular Biological Features of the Optic Nerve

1. *Cellular Composition*:
   - Retinal Ganglion Cell (RGC) Axons: The optic nerve comprises the bundled axons of RGCs, which originate in the inner retina and transmit action potentials to the lateral geniculate nucleus (LGN) and other visual centers.
   - Glial Cells: Oligodendrocytes (myelination), astrocytes (metabolic support and homeostasis), and microglia (immune surveillance) maintain neural integrity.
2. *Myelination*:
   - Oligodendrocytes in the post-laminar optic nerve synthesize myelin basic protein (MBP) and proteolipid protein (PLP) to form the myelin sheath, enhancing signal conduction [26].

- The lamina cribrosa marks the transition between unmyelinated (intraocular) and myelinated (retrobulbar) axons.

3. *Axonal Transport and Cytoskeleton:*

   - Microtubules and associated motor proteins (e.g., dynein and kinesin) mediate anterograde and retrograde transport of organelles, vesicles, and signaling molecules along axons [18].
   - Disruption in axonal transport is an early feature of glaucomatous optic neuropathy.

4. *Neurotrophic Factors:*

   - RGC survival and axonal integrity depend on neurotrophic support such as brain-derived neurotrophic factor (BDNF) and nerve growth factor (NGF).
   - These act through Trk receptors and downstream PI3K/AKT and MAPK pathways [34].

5. *Molecular Pathways in Injury and Degeneration*:

   - Oxidative stress, mitochondrial dysfunction, and inflammation contribute to optic nerve degeneration in diseases like glaucoma.
   - The mTOR, JNK, and NF-κB pathways regulate cell death or survival responses.
   - Axon regeneration is suppressed in the adult CNS due to inhibitory molecules interacting with Nogo receptors (NgR1) and RhoA/ROCK signaling [17].

6. *Gene Expression and Epigenetics*:

   - Gene regulatory programs, including transcription factors (e.g., Brn3, Isl1, and Klf4) and noncoding RNAs, guide RGC differentiation, axon outgrowth, and response to injury [38].
   - Epigenetic modifications such as histone acetylation and DNA methylation influence RGC survival and regenerative capacity [25].

7. *Blood–Nerve Barrier and Immune Modulation*:

   - The optic nerve has a blood–nerve barrier formed by endothelial cells and astrocytes, maintaining immune privilege and metabolic homeostasis.
   - Inflammatory responses are mediated by cytokines and complement components, with implications in autoimmune optic neuritis [22].

- *Extracellular Matrix (ECM) Composition*: Whether the ECM in the optic chiasm shares common inhibitory molecules (e.g., chondroitin sulfate proteoglycans, tenascin-C, or semaphorins) found in other nonpermissive CNS regions, or if it possesses a distinct molecular profile, is studied.
- *Glial Response*: The optic chiasm contains a dense population of specialized glial cells, including astrocytes and oligodendrocyte precursor cells. The role of these cells in shaping a regeneration-inhibitory versus permissive environment remains insufficiently defined.
- *Immune Microenvironment*: Unlike the retina or optic nerve head, the immune milieu of the optic chiasm during regeneration has not been systematically stud-

ied. Understanding the balance between proinflammatory and pro-repair immune responses could uncover new targets for intervention.

- *Axon Guidance Cues*: Developmental guidance molecules such as ephrin ligands, slits, and netrins are known to direct RGC axon trajectories at the chiasm. Whether these cues are aberrantly re-expressed or persist in the adult chiasm post-injury is not fully understood.

Biophotons and Information Transfer in Optic Nerve

There is no direct experimental evidence linking mTOR signaling to biophoton-mediated nerve conduction. However, given the shared involvement in mitochondrial regulation, redox biology, and neuronal energetics, a conceptual or indirect relationship can be reasonably proposed. Further research in quantum neuroscience and neuroenergetics may elucidate these connections in the future.

- *Quantum-biological hypothesis*: If biophotons participate in neural signaling (via coherence or tunneling), then mTOR-regulated mitochondrial function and redox states could influence the generation, modulation, or coherence of biophotons.
- *Neuroenergetics interface*: Since mTOR controls neuronal energy supply and resource allocation, it may modulate the physiological conditions under which biophoton-based mechanisms could occur.

Biophotons are spontaneously emitted photons in the visible to near-infrared range (200–800 nm) from living cells. They are not thermal radiation but result from oxidative metabolic processes, such as mitochondrial respiration and lipid peroxidation. Biophotons are coherent and of low intensity, often below the detection threshold of conventional instruments.

Indirect Links Between mTOR Signaling and Biophotonic Processes

Component	mTOR role	Link to biophotons
Mitochondria	mTORC1 regulates mitochondrial biogenesis and oxidative phosphorylation	Mitochondria are the primary sources of biophoton emission
ROS generation	mTOR influences antioxidant responses and redox balance	ROS-mediated reactions are major sources of UPE (biophotons)
Autophagy	mTOR inhibits autophagy under nutrient-rich conditions	Impaired autophagy may lead to mitochondrial dysfunction and altered biophoton output
Neuronal activity	mTOR supports synaptic transmission, axonal growth, and plasticity	Neural activity and metabolic demand may modulate biophoton emissions

Hypothesized Role in Visual Information Transfer [7]

1. Biophoton Emission by Retinal Cells
   - Photoreceptor cells (rods and cones) and retinal neurons generate endogenous photons during metabolic activity.
   - These may arise from excited molecular states (e.g., singlet oxygen, and excited flavins) returning to the ground state.
2. Optic Pathway as a Photonic Waveguide [3]
   - Some theories propose that RGC axons and myelinated optic nerve fibers may act as biological optical fibers or waveguides, allowing biophotons to travel with minimal scattering.
   - Myelin sheaths, due to their high refractive index contrast, could hypothetically enable guided light propagation, akin to silica-based optical fibers.
3. Information Encoding and Transmission
   - Biophotons may carry quantum-level information, potentially enabling high-speed or supplementary signal transmission to the brain [19].
   - This could occur in parallel with conventional electrical action potentials [8].
4. Synaptic and Mitochondrial Photonic Communication
   - Within the brain and retina, mitochondria, enriched at synaptic terminals, may emit or absorb biophotons, contributing to intra- and intercellular photonic signaling.
   - The high mitochondrial density in retinal and optic nerve tissues supports this possibility.
5. Experimental and Theoretical Support (Tentative)
   - F.A. Popp and others have proposed that biophotons play roles in cell-to-cell communication and biological coherence.
   - A few experimental models suggest photon-guiding properties in white matter tracts.
   - Quantum coherence and entanglement hypotheses are explored for their potential to explain certain aspects of neural integration and consciousness.

Quantum Energy States of Glutamate and Neural Biophotonics

Glutamate, the primary excitatory neurotransmitter in the central nervous system, may influence neural signaling not only through classical receptor-mediated pathways but also via quantum mechanisms. Specifically, studies suggest that quantum energy-level transitions of glutamate molecules—potentially involving electron rearrangements or vibrational modes—can affect the emission of biophotons (ultra-weak photon emissions in the UV to visible range) from neurons. These biophotons are proposed to function as nonclassical carriers of information, enabling an additional layer of signal transfer distinct from traditional electrochemical pathways.

This hypothesis posits that glutamate's quantum energy states can modulate neural biophotonic emissions, which in turn may participate in intra- and interneuronal communication, possibly contributing to coherence, synchronization, or long-range integration within neural networks. Though still speculative and under investigation, this paradigm suggests a quantum-based mechanism in neural processing, opening potential insights into cognition, consciousness, and neurophysiological regulation beyond classical frameworks [9].

The mTOR (mechanistic target of rapamycin) pathway has a significant role in the development, maintenance, and injury response of the optic nerve. As the optic nerve consists primarily of axons from retinal ganglion cells (RGCs), mTOR's effect on the optic nerve is closely tied to its influence on RGC survival, axonal growth, and regeneration. Dysregulation of mTOR signaling in the optic nerve is implicated in various conditions, including glaucoma, optic neuritis, and ischemic optic neuropathy.

Physiological Roles of mTOR in the Optic Nerve

Development and Maintenance

- *Axonal Growth*: During development, mTOR signaling supports axon outgrowth and guidance by regulating cytoskeletal dynamics and protein synthesis.
- *Metabolic Support*. mTOR maintains the high-energy demands of axonal function,
- *Myelination*: mTOR plays a role in the myelination of axons by oligodendrocytes, which is essential for efficient signal transmission [30].

Neuronal Survival

- mTOR promotes neuronal survival by regulating mitochondrial health, preventing oxidative stress, and supporting anti-apoptotic pathways [6].

A deeper mechanistic understanding of these interconnected pathways is vital for developing therapeutic strategies aimed at restoring vision through optic nerve regeneration.

mTOR-Related Signaling Pathways in Optic Nerve Regeneration

The *phosphoinositide 3-kinase (PI3K)/AKT/mTOR* signaling axis plays a central role in regulating mRNA translation in response to extracellular cues such as nutrients, growth factors, and various stress signals. PI3Ks catalyze the formation of phosphatidylinositol (3,4,5)-trisphosphate (PIP3), a membrane-bound lipid second messenger that is negatively regulated by the lipid phosphatase PTEN (phosphatase and tensin homolog), which functions as a crucial checkpoint in this pathway [4].

PIP3 facilitates the recruitment and activation of AKT, a serine/threonine kinase that, upon activation, promotes mTOR signaling by activating mTOR complex 1 (mTORC1) and simultaneously inhibiting glycogen synthase kinase 3 (GSK3). mTORC1, primarily localized to endomembrane compartments such as lysosomes, is activated by the small GTPase Rheb and subsequently phosphorylates key downstream effectors including 4E-binding protein 1 (4E-BP1) and ribosomal protein S6 kinase beta-1 (S6K1) [14].

Phosphorylation of 4E-BP1 results in the release of eukaryotic translation initiation factor 4E (eIF4E), allowing cap-dependent translation to proceed, while activated S6K1 promotes protein synthesis by enhancing ribosomal function. Collectively, these processes support the biosynthetic and growth demands of regenerating axons. PTEN deletion, which leads to constitutive activation of mTOR signaling, has emerged as one of the most robust interventions for promoting optic nerve regeneration in experimental models [5].

Recent studies have expanded this framework by identifying additional modulators of mTOR signaling. One such factor is Lin28, an RNA-binding protein that enhances the translation of specific mRNAs within the PI3K–mTOR axis. Lin28 has been shown to activate mTOR via phosphorylated AKT, yet it does so without directly influencing 4E-BP1 phosphorylation. Importantly, both S6K1 activation and 4E-BP1 inhibition are necessary to achieve the full regenerative effect of mTOR signaling. However, S6K1 activation alone is sufficient to promote axon regeneration, while 4E-BP1 knockdown alone is not, indicating that S6K1 may function as the dominant effector in this context [32].

Furthermore, PTEN deletion not only activates mTOR but also suppresses GSK3, leading to the activation of collapsin response mediator protein 2 (CRMP2), a microtubule-associated protein essential for axonal cytoskeletal remodeling and elongation. This dual modulation underscores the synergistic relationship between the mTOR and GSK3/CRMP2 pathways. Notably, persistent GSK3 activity severely impairs axonal regeneration even when mTOR is activated, emphasizing that mTOR-mediated protein synthesis must be accompanied by cytoskeletal reorganization for successful regenerative outcomes [31].

Neuroinflammation and the IL-33/ST2 Axis in Optic Neuropathies

A common hallmark among these diseases is the loss of retinal ganglion cells (RGCs) and their axons. To investigate the underlying mechanisms of RGC degeneration, the optic nerve crush (ONC) model has been widely adopted in experimental settings. This model closely mimics features of human optic neuropathies and serves as a valuable platform for elucidating cellular and molecular pathways involved in injury-induced neurodegeneration.

Neuroinflammation is a prominent and well-recognized feature in the ONC model and is increasingly understood to play a dual role. On one hand, a regulated inflammatory response can aid in maintaining retinal homeostasis and promoting tissue repair. On the other, excessive or chronic neuroinflammation can aggravate neuronal injury, accelerating RGC death and irreversible structural damage to the optic nerve. Thus, fine-tuning the inflammatory response following ONC is of critical importance for developing effective interventions aimed at preserving neuronal integrity and function in optic neuropathies.

Among the various molecular mediators of neuroinflammation, the interleukin-33 (IL-33)/ST2 signaling axis has recently emerged as a key pathway in the central nervous system (CNS). IL-33, originally classified as a member of the IL-1 cytokine family, functions both as a nuclear factor and an extracellular cytokine. It signals through its receptor ST2, which is primarily expressed on immune and glial cells, and plays an essential role in initiating and amplifying type II innate immune responses [28].

Although the IL-33/ST2 axis has been implicated in several CNS pathologies, including multiple sclerosis, Alzheimer's disease, and stroke, its potential role in optic nerve injury remains unexplored. The identification of IL-33/ST2 involvement in ONC could open new avenues for modulating post-injury inflammation and promoting neuroprotection. Elucidating this pathway in the context of optic neuropathies may ultimately inform the development of novel immunomodulatory therapies aimed at mitigating neuroinflammation and preserving visual function.

Developmental Decline and Barriers to Optic Nerve Regeneration: Focus on the Optic Chiasm

During early development, retinal ganglion cell (RGC) axons exhibit robust intrinsic growth potential, enabling them to extend rapidly from the retina to their synaptic targets in the brain. This capacity is tightly regulated by a network of growth-promoting signaling pathways and transcriptional programs that are active during embryogenesis. However, as RGCs mature postnatally, many of these pro-regenerative mechanisms are downregulated or silenced, leading to a sharp decline in their ability to support axon elongation. In contrast to neurons of the peripheral nervous system (PNS)—which can reactivate intrinsic growth programs following injury—central nervous system (CNS) neurons, including RGCs, generally fail to regenerate after axonal damage [20].

Understanding the mechanistic divergence between PNS and CNS regeneration remains a central challenge in neurobiology. While cell-intrinsic factors play a major role, cell-extrinsic barriers in the CNS microenvironment—particularly within key anatomical regions such as the optic chiasm—present formidable obstacles to axon regeneration.

The optic chiasm serves as a crucial midline relay station where RGC axons either cross to the contralateral hemisphere or remain ipsilateral, establishing the binocular visual field. In regenerative contexts, however, the chiasm becomes a significant point of failure. Many regenerating RGC axons stall, turn aberrantly, or fail to project beyond this region. These observations raise critical questions about the inhibitory nature of the optic chiasm microenvironment and whether it differs from other regions of the visual pathway [12].

mTOR Dysregulation and Optic Nerve Pathology (Fig. 10.1)

Optic Nerve Tumors

mTOR signaling is a central pathway in the growth and maintenance of various optic nerve tumors, particularly gliomas. Its activation supports anabolic metabolism, angiogenesis, and immune evasion. Therapeutically, mTOR inhibitors have shown promise in low-grade gliomas and tumors with genetic predispositions (e.g., NF1 and TSC), but monotherapy may be insufficient. Combination regimens and patient stratification based on molecular features hold the key to optimizing outcomes.

mTOR Signaling in Optic Nerve (ON) Tumors

Optic nerve tumors, though diverse in origin and behavior, frequently exhibit aberrant mTOR signaling, which contributes to their growth, metabolic demands, and resistance to therapy. Below is a structured overview of the general role of mTOR in optic nerve tumors, encompassing both low-grade gliomas (e.g., pilocytic astrocytoma) and high-grade malignancies (e.g., glioblastoma with optic involvement) [29].

Types of Optic Nerve Tumors

A. Primary ON Tumors

- Pilocytic astrocytoma (most common, especially in children; WHO Grade I)
- Optic glioblastoma (rare, aggressive)
- Meningioma (typically affects optic nerve sheath)
- Schwannoma (rare)

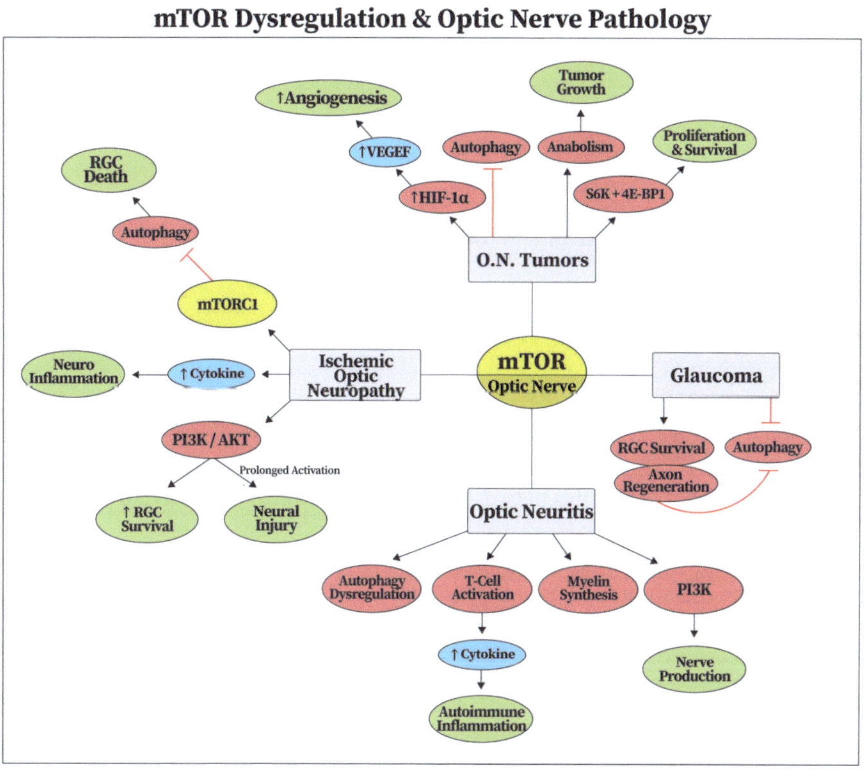

Fig. 10.1 The image presents a structural overview of how mTOR dysregulation impacts the optic nerve. It outlines four major pathological consequences: optic nerve tumors, glaucomatous nerve injury, optic neuritis, and ischemic optic neuropathy. Each condition is linked to specific downstream effects, illustrating how disrupted mTOR signaling contributes to neurodegeneration, inflammation, and impaired cellular repair processes. The diagram emphasizes the central role of mTOR in maintaining optic nerve health and how its dysregulation can lead to serious vision-threatening outcomes

B. Secondary Tumors with ON Involvement

- Chiasmatic gliomas
- Retinoblastoma extension
- Lymphoma/leukemia infiltration
- Metastases (e.g., breast, lung, melanoma)

Role of mTOR Pathway in ON Tumors

A. Cell-Autonomous Effects

1. Proliferation and Survival

- mTORC1 activation enhances ribosomal biogenesis and protein synthesis (via S6K and 4EBP1).
- Promotes tumor cell growth and survival under hypoxic and nutrient-poor conditions.

2. Angiogenesis

- mTOR upregulates HIF-1α → stimulates VEGF → enhances vascular supply to support expanding tumor.

3. Metabolism

- Supports the Warburg effect (aerobic glycolysis), sustaining high anabolic activity.

4. Autophagy Suppression

- mTORC1 suppresses autophagy, potentially allowing accumulation of damaged organelles but sustaining growth in early tumorigenesis.

B. Tumor Microenvironmental Modulation

- mTOR signaling in tumor cells influences the surrounding glial cells, microglia, macrophages, and vascular endothelial cells, contributing to:
  - Immune evasion
  - Stromal remodeling
  - Enhanced invasion/migration

Specific Tumor Contexts

Tumor type	mTOR role	Notes
Pilocytic astrocytoma	Activated via RAS/PI3K/AKT in NF1	mTOR inhibition may slow growth
Glioblastoma (optic nerve extension)	Highly upregulated	Requires dual mTORC1/2 or combo therapy
Optic nerve sheath meningioma	Variable mTOR activation	Some respond to mTOR inhibitors in TSC context
Lymphoma	Less mTOR-driven	mTOR targeting plays a minor role
Metastases	mTOR activation depends on primary	Breast cancer brain metastases may respond to mTOR inhibitors

mTOR plays a critical role in the pathogenesis and progression of optic nerve gliomas (ONGs), especially those associated with neurofibromatosis type 1 (NF1).

Optic Nerve Glioma in NF1

Optic pathway gliomas (OPGs) are typically low-grade pilocytic astrocytomas (WHO grade I) arising in the optic nerve, chiasm, or tract. They occur in up to 15–20% of children, often presenting before age 6. These tumors are associated with mutations in the NF1 gene, which encodes neurofibromin, a Ras GTPase-activating protein [37].

In NF1-associated optic nerve gliomas, mTOR signaling is a central driver of tumor growth, metabolic activation, and visual pathway dysfunction. Pharmacologic inhibition of mTOR, particularly in combination strategies, represents a promising avenue for preserving visual function and controlling tumor progression. However, challenges such as resistance mechanisms and microenvironmental complexity necessitate further investigation.

NF1, RAS Pathway, and mTOR Activation

NF1 Loss and RAS Hyperactivation

- Neurofibromin negatively regulates RAS, a key upstream activator of:
  - PI3K → AKT → mTORC1
  - RAF → MEK → ERK (MAPK pathway)

mTORC1 Upregulation

- In NF1-deficient astrocytes, constitutive RAS activation leads to persistent activation of mTORC1.
- This promotes:
  - *Cell growth*
  - *Protein synthesis*
  - *Angiogenesis*
  - *Suppression of autophagy*
  - *Resistance to apoptosis*

mTOR in Optic Pathway Glioma Pathophysiology

A. Role in Tumor Growth

- mTORC1 promotes proliferation and metabolic activity of glioma cells.
- Encourages astrocytic lineage expansion, characteristic of pilocytic glioma.

B. Microenvironment Modulation

- mTOR activation affects tumor-associated microglia and immune signaling, particularly through:
  - CXCL12/CXCR4 axis
  - TGF-β and IL-6 production
- This supports a pro-tumorigenic, inflammatory niche.

C. Impact on Visual Function

- mTOR-driven glioma growth along the optic nerve compresses axons and impairs retinal ganglion cell (RGC) conduction.
- Visual impairment in NF1-OPG patients is linked not only to tumor burden but also to mTOR-mediated neuroinflammatory mechanisms.

Optic Nerve Damage in Glaucoma

RGC Loss In glaucoma, as described in Chap. 6 of this book, the elevated intraocular pressure and other stressors lead to axonal injury and RGC death. mTOR dysregulation contributes to this process [34]:

1. Neuroprotective Role of mTOR in RGCs
   - mTORC1 activation promotes protein synthesis, mitochondrial biogenesis, and cellular metabolism, supporting the survival of RGCs under glaucomatous stress.
   - It upregulates the expression of anti-apoptotic and prosurvival proteins, helping RGCs resist mechanical stress, oxidative damage, and ischemia induced by elevated intraocular pressure (IOP).
   - mTORC2 contributes by activating Akt and maintaining cytoskeletal integrity and cell polarity.
2. mTOR and Axonal Regeneration
   - mTOR signaling is essential for RGC axon regeneration, which is normally suppressed in adult CNS neurons.
   - After optic nerve injury (as occurs in glaucoma), reactivation of mTOR (e.g., via PTEN deletion or growth factor stimulation) can restore regenerative competence.
   - mTOR enhances the synthesis of axonal growth-associated proteins and supports cytoskeletal remodeling.
3. Autophagy Regulation—A Double-Edged Sword
   - mTORC1 inhibits autophagy by phosphorylating ULK1 (Unc-51-like kinase 1), which may be detrimental in chronic glaucoma where autophagy is needed to remove damaged organelles and proteins.

- Impaired autophagy due to mTOR overactivity may exacerbate RGC degeneration in later stages.
- Therapeutic strategies sometimes aim to modulate mTOR to restore autophagic flux, especially in the aged or stressed retina.

Optic Neuritis (ON)

The Role of mTOR Signaling in Optic Neuritis

Optic neuritis (ON) is an inflammatory demyelinating disorder of the optic nerve, often associated with autoimmune conditions such as multiple sclerosis (MS), neuromyelitis optica spectrum disorder (NMOSD), and myelin oligodendrocyte glycoprotein antibody-associated disease (MOGAD). The disease is characterized by inflammation, demyelination, axonal injury, and retinal ganglion cell (RGC) degeneration, resulting in acute or subacute vision loss. Emerging evidence implicates the mechanistic target of rapamycin (mTOR) pathway as a significant regulator of neuroinflammation, axonal integrity, and neuroprotection in optic neuritis and related neuroinflammatory conditions.

mTOR signaling plays a multifaceted role in optic neuritis, regulating immune activation, neuroinflammation, oligodendrocyte function, autophagy, and RGC survival. While mTOR activation may support cellular resilience, its dysregulation contributes to inflammation and axonal degeneration. Targeted modulation of the mTOR pathway holds significant potential for preserving visual function and limiting neurodegeneration in optic neuritis and related demyelinating diseases.

1. mTOR in Immune Regulation and Neuroinflammation

   mTOR, particularly mTORC1, plays a pivotal role in T-cell activation, differentiation, and cytokine production. In the context of optic neuritis and experimental autoimmune encephalomyelitis (EAE, a model of MS), hyperactivation of mTOR in peripheral immune cells contributes to the expansion of pathogenic Th1 and Th17 cells, while inhibition of mTOR has been shown to promote regulatory T-cell (Treg) differentiation, leading to suppression of autoimmune inflammation. Thus, mTOR modulation may influence the severity and recurrence of optic neuritis by regulating adaptive immune responses.
2. mTOR and Demyelination/Remyelination

   mTOR signaling is also critical in oligodendrocyte lineage progression and myelin synthesis. While excessive mTOR activity may exacerbate inflammation, it is also necessary for remyelination, as it regulates protein and lipid synthesis required for myelin membrane formation. Studies suggest that temporal and cell-type-specific modulation of mTOR may support remyelination following demyelinating insults in the optic nerve.
3. mTOR and RGC Survival

   RGC loss is a major consequence of optic neuritis and is closely associated with irreversible vision impairment. mTOR regulates cell survival, metabolism, and axonal transport in neurons. Activation of the PI3K/AKT/mTOR axis has been associated with neuroprotection in RGCs under various injury paradigms. In optic neuritis, mTOR activity may support neuronal resilience, although excessive activation can inhibit autophagy, leading to cellular stress and degeneration.

4. Autophagy, mTOR, and Optic Nerve Injury

   mTOR is a negative regulator of autophagy, a cellular process that clears damaged organelles and proteins. During optic neuritis, dysregulated autophagy may exacerbate axonal and glial damage. mTOR inhibition, through agents like rapamycin, can restore autophagic flux, reduce neuroinflammation, and mitigate optic nerve damage in preclinical models. However, the effects appear to be context-dependent and vary with the disease stage.

Ischemic Optic Neuropathy (ION)

The Role of mTOR Signaling in Ischemic Optic Neuropathy

Ischemic optic neuropathy (ION)—a leading cause of sudden, irreversible vision loss in adults—results from vascular insufficiency to the optic nerve head. It is classified into non-arteritic (NAION) and arteritic (AION) forms. The pathogenesis of ION involves complex interactions between vascular compromise, inflammation, oxidative stress, and axonal degeneration. Recent studies suggest that the (mTOR) pathway may play a critical role in modulating these pathological processes.

mTOR plays a context-dependent role in ischemic optic neuropathy, balancing cellular survival, metabolic regulation, autophagy, and inflammation. Strategic modulation of the mTOR pathway may represent a promising therapeutic avenue to mitigate RGC loss and preserve visual function in ION.

1. mTOR and RGC Survival

   mTOR is a central regulator of cell growth, metabolism, and survival. In models of optic nerve ischemia, activation of the PI3K/AKT/mTOR pathway has been associated with enhanced retinal ganglion cell (RGC) survival. mTORC1 promotes protein synthesis and cellular bioenergetics, which are essential for RGC resilience following ischemic insult. However, prolonged or dysregulated mTOR activation may exacerbate injury by increasing metabolic demand and suppressing protective autophagy pathways.

2. mTOR and Autophagy in ION

   Autophagy plays a dual role in ION: It can be protective by removing damaged organelles, but excessive or insufficient autophagy may contribute to RGC death. mTORC1 acts as a negative regulator of autophagy, and studies indicate that transient inhibition of mTOR using rapamycin can enhance autophagic flux and reduce optic nerve damage in ischemic models. Fine-tuning mTOR activity may therefore help maintain a beneficial autophagic response during the acute phase of ION.

3. mTOR in Inflammation and Glial Reactivity

    Ischemia triggers glial activation and neuroinflammation, which contribute to secondary damage. mTOR signaling is involved in the polarization of microglia and astrocytes, and its modulation affects the balance between proinflammatory (M1) and anti-inflammatory (M2) states. Inhibition of mTOR has been shown to suppress proinflammatory cytokine release and limit glial scar formation, potentially improving axonal preservation.

mTOR and Optic Nerve Regeneration

mTOR is a key regulator of axonal regeneration, In the central nervous system (CNS), including the optic nerve, mTOR activity declines with age and injury, limiting the intrinsic capacity for axonal regeneration. Enhancing mTOR activity in RGCs has been shown to promote axonal regeneration after optic nerve injury in animal models.

The *mTOR* pathway impacts the optic nerve by regulating retinal ganglion cell (RGC) survival, axonal growth, and regeneration. This involves multiple interconnected pathways that modulate cell metabolism, protein synthesis, cytoskeletal dynamics, and stress responses. Dysregulation of these pathways contributes to optic nerve pathologies, such as glaucoma, optic neuritis, and ischemic optic neuropathy.

The optic nerve, predominantly composed of the axons of retinal ganglion cells (RGCs), is part of the central nervous system (CNS) and, as such, exhibits limited intrinsic regenerative capacity. Following injury, RGCs fail to regenerate axons across the lesion site or re-establish functional synaptic connections with central targets such as the lateral geniculate nucleus. The irreversible loss of RGCs is a hallmark of several debilitating and progressive optic neuropathies, including glaucoma, ischemic optic neuropathy, and optic neuritis. These conditions collectively represent major causes of permanent visual impairment and blindness.

Given the lack of spontaneous regeneration, significant research efforts are focused on elucidating the molecular barriers to axonal regrowth and developing therapeutic strategies to overcome them. Emerging treatment approaches aim to promote RGC survival, enhance axon regeneration, and restore functional connectivity along the visual pathway [39].

Strategies for Optic Nerve Regeneration

Neurotrophic Factor Delivery Administration of growth factors such as brain-derived neurotrophic factor (BDNF), ciliary neurotrophic factor (CNTF), and nerve growth factor (NGF) supports RGC survival and can modestly promote axonal outgrowth [24].

Modulation of Intracellular Signaling Pathways [36]

- Activation of PI3K/AKT/mTOR signaling enhances axonal regeneration and cellular survival.
- Inhibition of PTEN (a negative regulator of mTOR) and SOCS3 (a suppressor of cytokine signaling) has shown robust regenerative effects in experimental models.
- Targeting the JAK/STAT, MAPK/ERK, and Hippo/YAP pathways is under investigation for promoting regeneration and combating neuroinflammation.

Manipulation of Transcriptional and Epigenetic Programs [2]

- Reprogramming RGCs using transcription factors such as KLF family members, SOX11, and c-MYC has demonstrated regenerative potential.
- Histone deacetylase inhibitors (HDACi) and DNA methyltransferase inhibitors are explored for modulating gene expression favoring regeneration.

Stem Cell-Based Therapies [21]

- Transplantation of RGC precursors or induced pluripotent stem cell (iPSC)-derived neurons aims to replace lost cells and reconnect with central targets.
- Challenges remain in axonal guidance, integration, and immune rejection.

Gene Therapy [16]

- Viral vectors (e.g., AAV) are used to deliver genes that enhance regenerative signaling or suppress inhibitory cues.
- Examples include overexpression of BDNF, mTOR activators, or CRISPR-mediated gene editing to remove regeneration inhibitors.

Neutralization of Extrinsic Inhibitory Molecules [15]

- The CNS environment contains myelin-associated inhibitors such as Nogo-A, MAG, and OMgp, which activate RhoA/ROCK signaling to block axonal extension.
- Pharmacological or antibody-mediated inhibition of these molecules may create a more permissive environment for regrowth.

Key Pathways Involving mTOR in the Optic Nerve (Fig. 10.2)

1. PI3K/Akt/mTOR Pathway

   - *Overview*: This is the primary upstream pathway activating mTOR, with phosphoinositide 3-kinase (PI3K) and Akt being key intermediates.
   - *Mechanism*:

     – PI3K phosphorylates PIP2 to PIP3, leading to Akt activation.
     – Akt phosphorylates and inhibits TSC2 (tuberous sclerosis complex 2), relieving its suppression on mTORC1.
     – mTORC1 activation promotes protein synthesis, cell survival, and axonal regeneration.

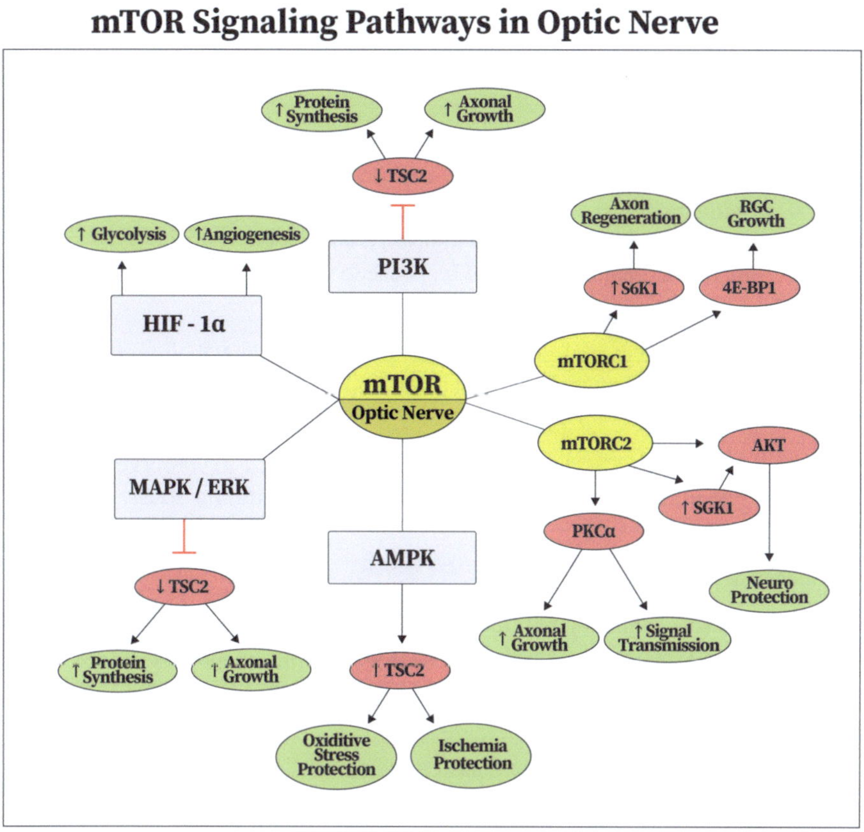

Fig. 10.2 The image illustrates four primary signaling pathways involved in regulating optic nerve function: PI3K, HIF-1α, MAPK/ERK, and AMPK. These pathways play critical roles in processes such as cell survival, metabolism, angiogenesis, and inflammation. Additionally, the image highlights how these signals converge through the two distinct mTOR complexes—mTORC1 and mTORC2—which serve as central hubs for integrating environmental and cellular cues. Through these complexes, mTOR modulates downstream effects that influence neuronal growth, energy homeostasis, and stress responses, underscoring its vital role in maintaining optic nerve integrity and function

- *Relevance to the Optic Nerve:*
  - Promotes RGC survival under stress (e.g., in glaucoma or ischemia).
  - Stimulates axonal regeneration after optic nerve injury.

2. mTORC1 and mTORC2 Pathways

- *mTORC1:*
  - Regulates protein synthesis through downstream effectors like S6K1 (ribosomal protein S6 kinase) and 4E-BP1 (eukaryotic translation initiation factor-binding protein 1)

  - Controls mitochondrial biogenesis and energy production to support RGC and axonal function
  - Inhibits autophagy under normal conditions but is required for sufficient energy and material turnover

- *mTORC2:*
  - Modulates cytoskeletal dynamics through effectors like Akt, SGK1 (serum and glucocorticoid-regulated kinase 1), and PKCα
  - Supports axonal integrity and response to injury

AMPK/mTOR Pathway

- *Overview*: AMP-activated protein kinase (AMPK) is a metabolic regulator that inhibits mTOR under energy-deprived conditions.
- *Mechanism*:
  - AMPK activates TSC2 and directly inhibits mTORC1 to conserve energy.
  - This balances cellular metabolism and autophagy during stress, promoting optic nerve survival.
- *Relevance to the Optic Nerve:*
  - Protects RGCs under conditions of oxidative stress or ischemia.
  - A balance between AMPK and mTOR activity is crucial for neuronal homeostasis.

MAPK/mTOR Pathway

- *Overview*: The mitogen-activated protein kinase (MAPK) pathway interacts with mTOR to regulate growth and stress responses.
- *Mechanism*:
  - Growth factors activate ERK1/2 (extracellular signal-regulated kinases), which can enhance mTORC1 activity via the inhibition of TSC2.
  - Enhances protein synthesis and axonal growth.
- *Relevance to the Optic Nerve*:
  - Promotes regeneration and survival in RGCs after injury.
  - Aberrant activation can lead to maladaptive responses, including inflammation and fibrosis.

HIF-1α/mTOR Pathway

- *Overview*: Hypoxia-inducible factor 1-alpha (HIF-1α) is regulated by mTORC1 and supports cellular adaptation to hypoxia.
- *Mechanism*:
  - mTORC1 increases HIF-1α expression, promoting glycolysis and angiogenesis.
  - Enhances cellular survival in low-oxygen environments, such as ischemic optic neuropathy.

- *Relevance to the Optic Nerve*:
  - Helps RGCs and axons adapt to ischemic stress.
  - Excessive activation may contribute to pathological neovascularization.

mTOR and Autophagy in Optic Nerve

mTOR inhibits autophagy through suppression of ULK1 (Unc-51-like kinase 1), a key autophagy initiator [33].

- *Mechanism*:
  - Active mTORC1 suppresses autophagy, maintaining a balance between degradation and synthesis of cellular components.
  - During stress, reduced mTOR activity enables autophagy, clearing damaged organelles and proteins.
- *Relevance to the Optic Nerve*:
  - Essential for clearing damaged axonal components after injury.
  - Dysregulated autophagy contributes to RGC death in glaucoma.

Axonal Regeneration Pathways

- *Intrinsic Growth Pathways* [27]
  - mTORC1 reactivation is necessary for RGC axonal regeneration.
  - Works synergistically with cAMP, JAK/STAT3, and neurotrophic factor signaling (e.g., CNTF).
- *RhoA/ROCK and Cytoskeletal Dynamics* [1]
  - mTORC2 regulates cytoskeletal remodeling via RhoA/ROCK signaling.
  - Supports axonal elongation and guidance.

Bibliography

1. Akram. Axonal regeneration: underlying molecular mechanisms and potential therapeutic targets. Biomedicines. 2022. https://doi.org/10.3390/biomedicines10123186.
2. Ashok. Epigenetic regulation of optic nerve development, protection, and repair. Int J Mol Sci. 2022. https://doi.org/10.3390/ijms23168927.
3. Casey. Exploring ultraweak photon emissions as optical markers of brain activity. J ISCI. 2025. https://doi.org/10.1016/j.isci.2025.112019.
4. Chen H. PTEN and AKT/GSK-3β/CRMP-2 signaling pathway are involved in neuronal apoptosis and axonal injury in early brain injury after SAH in rats. Genes Dis. 2022;9(1) https://doi.org/10.1016/j.gendis.2020.05.002.
5. Eaton. Unwanted axon growth: PTEN and the suppression of axon plasticity In ADULT nerves. bioRxiv. 2025. https://doi.org/10.1101/2025.06.04.657750.

6. Espinosa. Role of mitochondrial dysfunction in neuropathy. Int J Mol Sci. 2025. https://doi.org/10.3390/ijms26073195.
7. Findik. Exploring a novel hypothesis: could the eye function as a radar or ultrasound device in depth and distance perception? Neurophysiological Insights. Life. 2025. https://doi.org/10.3390/life15040536.
8. Frede. Optical polarization evolution and transmission in multi-ranvier-node axonal myelin-sheath waveguides. IEEE Trans Mol Biol Multi-Scale Commun. 2024;10 https://doi.org/10.1109/TMBMC.2024.3464415.
9. Han Z. Quantum energy levels of glutamate modulate neural biophotonic signals. Photochem Photobiol Sci. 2021. https://doi.org/10.1007/s43630-021-00022-0.
10. Homaira. Translational machinery and translation regulation in axon regeneration. Neural Regen Res. 2025. https://doi.org/10.4103/NRR.NRR-D-24-00313.
11. Hottin. GSK3 is a central player in retinal degenerative diseases but a challenging therapeutic target. Cells. 2022. https://doi.org/10.3390/cells11182898.
12. Lee J. Optic nerve regeneration: Potential treatment approaches. Curr Opin Pharmacol. 2024;74 https://doi.org/10.1016/j.coph.2023.102428.
13. Jagrit. Bioengineered scaffolds for axonal regeneration. Transl Neurosci. 2025. https://doi.org/10.1007/978-3-031-89307-0_24.
14. Jikuan. Phosphorylated S6K1 and 4E-BP1 play different roles in constitutively active Rheb-mediated retinal ganglion cell survival and axon regeneration after optic nerve injury. Neural Regen Res. 2023. https://doi.org/10.4103/1673-5374.371372.
15. Kalafatakis. Nogo-A and LINGO-1: two important targets for remyelination and regeneration. Int J Mol Sci. 2023. https://doi.org/10.3390/ijms24054479.
16. Kharisova. Looking to the future of viral vectors in ocular gene therapy: clinical review. Biomedicines. 2025. https://doi.org/10.3390/biomedicines13020365.
17. Lin L. YAP signaling in glia: pivotal roles in neurological development, regeneration and diseases. Neurosci Bull. 2024; https://doi.org/10.1007/s12264-024-01308-w.
18. Liu D. Optineurin-facilitated axonal mitochondria delivery promotes neuroprotection and axon regeneration. Nat Commun. 2025. https://doi.org/10.1038/s41467-025-57135-8.
19. Liu N. Intracellular simulated biophoton stimulation and transsynaptic signal transmission. Appl Phys Lett. 2022. https://doi.org/10.1063/5.0128956.
20. Liu ZG. Unlocking the potential for optic nerve regeneration over long distances: a multi-therapeutic intervention. Front Neurol. 2025. https://doi.org/10.3389/fneur.2024.1526973.
21. Lu Y. Human induced pluripotent stem cell-derived extracellular vesicles promote neuroprotection effects in rat optic nerve crush model. Exp Eye Res. 2025;258. https://doi.org/10.1016/j.exer.2025.110505.
22. Ma SK. Risk of autoimmune diseases following optic neuritis: a nationwide population-based cohort study. Front Med. 2022. https://doi.org/10.3389/fmed.2022.903608.
23. Moazed. Quantum biology of the eye. Cham: Springer; 2023. https://doi.org/10.1007/978-3-031-32060-6_7.
24. Nguyen. Co-delivery of neurotrophic factors and a zinc chelator substantially increases retinal ganglion cell survival and axon protection in the optic nerve crush model. Acta Biomaterialia. 2025. https://doi.org/10.1016/j.actbio.2025.06.007.
25. Palomés-Borrajo. Histone acetylation in central and peripheral nervous system injuries and regeneration: epigenetic dynamics and therapeutic perspectives. Int J Mol Sci. 2025. https://doi.org/10.3390/ijms26136277.
26. Pieczonka. Role of oligodendrocyte lineage cells in white matter injury. Cham: Springer; 2025. https://doi.org/10.1007/978-3-031-87919-7_11.
27. Poitras. Unleashing intrinsic growth pathways in regenerating peripheral neurons. Int J Mol Sci. 2022. https://doi.org/10.3390/ijms232113566.
28. Qian Z. The IL-33/ST2 axis protects retinal ganglion cells by modulating the astrocyte response after optic nerve injury. Neurosci Bull. 2024. https://doi.org/10.1007/s12264-024-01279-y.
29. Renzi. Precision medicine for pediatric glioma and NF1-associated tumors: the role of small molecule inhibitors. Curr Oncol. 2025. https://doi.org/10.3390/curroncol32050280.

30. Shi XY. Gastrodin promotes CNS myelinogenesis and alleviates demyelinating injury by activating the PI3K/AKT/mTOR signaling. Acta Pharmacol Sin. 2025. https://doi.org/10.1038/s41401-025-01492-z.
31. Takizawa. CRMP2 and its phosphorylation prevent axonal misrouting of the corticospinal tract. Neurosci Lett. 2025. https://doi.org/10.1016/j.neulet.2025.138231.
32. Thevarajan. LIN28-mediated gene regulatory loops synchronize developmental transitions throughout organogenesis. bioRxiv. 2025. https://doi.org/10.1101/2025.01.22.634324.
33. Vahsen. ULK1 as a novel therapeutic target in neurodegeneration. Neural Regen Res. 2021. https://doi.org/10.4103/1673-5374.300442.
34. Wang X. The molecular mechanisms underlying retinal ganglion cell apoptosis and optic nerve regeneration in glaucoma (Review). Int J Mol Med. 2025. https://doi.org/10.3892/ijmm.2025.5504.
35. Wang Y. Unraveling neurodevelopment: synergistic effects of intrinsic genetic programs and extrinsic environmental cues. Adv Sci. 2025. https://doi.org/10.1002/advs.202414890.
36. Wong K. Retinal ganglion cell survival and axon regeneration after optic nerve injury: role of inflammation and other factors. Int J Mol Sci. 2022. https://doi.org/10.3390/ijms231710179.
37. Tang Y. Neurofibromatosis Type 1-associated optic pathway gliomas: current challenges and future prospects. Cancer Manag Res. 2023. https://doi.org/10.2147/CMAR.S362678.
38. Yuan. Advances in regeneration of retinal ganglion cells and optic nerves. Int J Mol Sci. 2021. https://doi.org/10.3390/ijms22094616.
39. Zhang Q. Emerging therapeutic strategies for optic nerve regeneration. Trends Pharmacol Sci. 2025;46(1). https://doi.org/10.1016/j.tips.2024.11.008.

Chapter 11
mTOR Effect on the Optic Radiation and Visual Cortex

Contents

Abstract The mechanistic target of rapamycin (mTOR) is a master regulator of neuronal growth, synaptic plasticity, and energy metabolism in the human brain, with critical roles in the development and function of the visual cortex. During neurodevelopment, mTOR signaling governs cortical neuron differentiation, dendritic arborization, and synapse formation—processes essential for establishing functional visual pathways. In the mature visual cortex, mTOR activity modulates experience-dependent synaptic remodeling, visual learning, and memory consolidation. Dysregulation of mTOR, particularly hyperactivation of mTORC1, has been implicated in a range of cortical pathologies including focal cortical dysplasia, tuberous sclerosis complex, and epilepsy—all of which may involve visual processing deficits. Moreover, aberrant mTOR signaling can disrupt the balance of excitation and inhibition within the visual cortex, impairing visual perception and higher-order integration. Therapeutic modulation of mTOR has shown promise in preserving cortical function and plasticity, highlighting its potential as a target in both neurodevelopmental and neurodegenerative disorders affecting the visual system.

K. T. Moazed, *mTOR Signaling in Ophthalmology*,
https://doi.org/10.1007/978-3-032-05044-1_11

Discussion

The *mTOR (mechanistic target of rapamycin)* pathway is a key regulator of cellular metabolism, growth, protein synthesis, and autophagy in the brain. Its activity influences brain development, synaptic plasticity, cognitive functions, and responses to injury or disease. Dysregulation of mTOR signaling has been implicated in various neurological disorders, including neurodevelopmental disorders, neurodegenerative diseases, and brain cancers.

In this chapter, we examine the role of mTOR signaling in the terminal components of the visual system—focusing on the lateral geniculate nucleus (LGN) of the thalamus, the optic radiations, and the primary visual cortex. We explore how mTOR regulates the development, synaptic plasticity, metabolic homeostasis, and disease-related alterations in these central visual processing regions.

The mechanistic target of rapamycin (mTOR) pathway plays a significant role in the lateral geniculate nucleus (LGN) and optic radiations, the critical components of the visual pathway responsible for relaying and processing visual information between the retina and the visual cortex.

mTORC1's Effect on the Lateral Geniculate Nucleus (LGN)

mTORC1 (mechanistic target of rapamycin complex 1) is a master regulator of key cellular processes, including protein synthesis, metabolism, autophagy, proliferation, and survival. In the lateral geniculate nucleus (LGN)—a primary thalamic relay center for visual information—mTORC1 signaling plays an essential role in the development and functional organization of the visual system. During early postnatal development, mTORC1 activity supports neuronal growth, dendritic arborization, and synaptogenesis, processes that are crucial for establishing the topographically precise retinogeniculate projections from retinal ganglion cells (RGCs).

Furthermore, mTORC1 contributes to the laminar refinement and segregation of ON and OFF pathways within the LGN, ensuring accurate relay of contrast-sensitive visual signals to the primary visual cortex (V1). Disruptions in mTORC1 signaling during critical periods of development can impair synaptic plasticity and circuit refinement, potentially contributing to visual processing deficits such as amblyopia. Additionally, aberrant mTORC1 activation has been implicated in neurodevelopmental disorders and may influence LGN vulnerability to neurodegenerative processes [22].

A. mTOR Role in Development and Synaptic Refinement [6]

- The *LGN* is the main thalamic relay center for visual information from the retina to the cortex.

- During development, mTOR (especially mTORC1) supports:
  - *Synaptogenesis* of retinal ganglion cell (RGC) inputs
  - *Dendritic arborization* and maturation of relay neurons
  - *Segregation of eye-specific layers*, a process driven by visual activity and requiring activity-dependent mTOR signaling

B. Activity-Dependent Plasticity [12]

- Visual input activates mTOR through BDNF-TrkB, NMDAR, and Ca2+/Akt pathways in LGN neurons.
- mTORC1 promotes translation of synaptic proteins such as Arc, PSD-95, and eEF2, which are essential for:
  - *Strengthening synapses*
  - *Experience-driven refinement* of receptive fields
- This is critical during the critical period for visual development.

C. mTOR Dysregulation in LGN [3]

- *Hyperactivation* (e.g., in TSC and PTEN loss):
  - Leads to abnormal connectivity, increased excitability, and possible epileptogenicity in thalamocortical circuits
- *Inhibition* (e.g., prolonged rapamycin exposure):
  - Can impair plasticity and reduce visual acuity, especially if administered during critical developmental windows

Retinal Development and Retinogeniculate Connections [1]

- Studies show that disruption of mTORC1 signaling in retinal progenitor cells can lead to aberrant retinogeniculate termination topographies, meaning the axons from the retina do not connect properly to the LGN.
- Specifically, loss of mTORC1 activity can cause:
  - Decreased proliferation and increased apoptosis of retinal progenitor cells during development, affecting retinal lamination and stratification.
  - Irregular segregation of retinal ganglion cell axons at the optic chiasm, leading to overlapping projections in the LGN instead of the typical organized, binocular pattern.
  - This ultimately leads to visually mediated behavioral deficits, suggesting the importance of mTORC1 in establishing the correct wiring of the visual system.

Potential Role in Modulating Neuronal Excitability and Plasticity [6]

- mTORC1 is involved in regulating protein synthesis in neurons, which is critical for synaptic plasticity, long-term potentiation, and long-term memory formation.
- While direct research on mTORC1's role in the LGN's excitability is limited, studies on other brain regions suggest it can influence:
  - The expression of ionotropic glutamate receptors (like NMDA receptors) and voltage-gated potassium channels which control postsynaptic excitability
  - The balance of protein synthesis of specific receptors and ion channels, potentially affecting how the LGN filters and transmits information from the retina to the visual cortex

mTOR Effect on Optic Radiations

The optic radiation, also known as the geniculocalcarine tract, is a key component of the post-thalamic visual pathway that conveys visual information from the lateral geniculate nucleus (LGN) to the primary visual cortex (V1). This long-range, myelinated white matter tract is essential for the conscious perception of visual stimuli. mTOR signaling, particularly via mTORC1, plays a vital role in regulating the cellular and molecular processes that underlie the development, maturation, and maintenance of the optic radiation.

During brain development, mTORC1 promotes neuronal growth, axonal elongation, cytoskeletal remodeling, and target-specific axon guidance—all of which are critical for the correct topographical organization of the optic radiation. In addition, mTORC1 supports the energy-intensive process of myelination by enhancing protein and lipid synthesis in oligodendrocytes. This ensures efficient saltatory conduction along the optic radiation, enabling the rapid and accurate transmission of visual signals [8].

mTOR activity also influences axon–glial interactions, which are crucial for axonal stability and myelin sheath integrity. Dysregulation of mTOR signaling—either due to genetic mutations, metabolic stress, or inflammation—can lead to impaired myelination, axonal misrouting, or neurodegeneration. Such abnormalities have been observed in conditions like tuberous sclerosis complex (TSC), where hyperactivation of mTORC1 results in cortical tubers, white matter abnormalities, and disrupted visual processing. Diffusion tensor imaging (DTI) studies in TSC and other neurodevelopmental disorders have revealed alterations in the structural integrity of the optic radiation, correlating with visual perceptual deficits [16].

Moreover, in neurodegenerative conditions, such as multiple sclerosis (MS) and traumatic brain injury (TBI), aberrant mTOR signaling contributes to axonal damage, demyelination, and glial scarring within visual pathways, including the optic radiation. Therapeutic modulation of mTOR, especially using inhibitors like rapamycin (sirolimus), is under investigation for its potential to restore white matter homeostasis, reduce neuroinflammation, and support remyelination.

A. Structural and Functional Support [19]

- *Optic radiations* are white matter tracts transmitting visual signals from the LGN to the primary visual cortex.
- mTOR regulates:
  - *Axonal growth* and *pathfinding* during development via downstream effectors like *S6K1* and *4E-BP1*
  - *Oligodendrocyte differentiation* and myelination, particularly via mTORC1
  - mTORC1 is necessary for neural regeneration, but mTORC2 and GSK3β are inhibitory for AKT-induced axon regeneration in the central nervous system.

B. Myelination and Metabolic Support [27]

- mTOR signaling in *oligodendrocyte progenitor cells (OPCs)*:
  - Promotes maturation into myelinating oligodendrocytes
  - Enhances *lipid biosynthesis* required for myelin production
  - Coordinates energy metabolism in long-range axons of the optic radiations

C. mTOR Dysregulation in Optic Radiations [24]

- *mTOR Hyperactivity* (e.g., TSC and NF1):
  - Leads to dysmyelination, ectopic axonal sprouting, and thalamocortical miswiring
  - Correlated with white matter abnormalities seen on DTI MRI in neurodevelopmental disorders
- *mTOR Inhibition*:
  - Excessive suppression may impair remyelination in demyelinating diseases (e.g., MS affecting optic radiations)
  - Controlled inhibition may reduce gliosis and axonal loss post-injury

mTOR Effect in the Visual Cortex

The *primary visual cortex (V1)*, located in the occipital lobe, is the cortical endpoint of the visual pathway and is responsible for processing fundamental aspects of visual information, such as orientation, spatial frequency, motion, and binocular disparity. mTOR signaling, predominantly through mTORC1, is critically involved in the regulation of neuronal growth, synaptic development, metabolic support, and plasticity within the visual cortex throughout development and into adulthood.

During early postnatal life, the visual cortex undergoes intense structural and functional remodeling driven by both intrinsic genetic programs and sensory experience. mTORC1 supports this process by regulating protein synthesis, cytoskeletal organization, and mitochondrial biogenesis, all of which are vital for dendritic arborization, axon elongation, and synapse formation. mTORC1 activity is necessary for the proper formation of ocular dominance columns and orientation-selective circuits, particularly during the critical period—a window of heightened plasticity when the visual cortex is highly sensitive to environmental stimuli. Experimental inhibition of mTOR during this time has been shown to disrupt binocular alignment, cortical layer formation, and the refinement of thalamocortical projections.

Physiological Roles of mTOR in the Brain

Neurodevelopment [23]

- *Neural Stem Cell Proliferation and Differentiation:*
  - mTOR controls the proliferation and differentiation of neural progenitor cells during brain development.
  - It supports the growth of neurons and glial cells by regulating protein and lipid synthesis.
- *Axonal and Dendritic Growth:*
  - mTOR regulates cytoskeletal remodeling and synaptic formation, crucial for proper neuronal connectivity.

Synaptic Plasticity and Memory [9]

mTORC1 integrates upstream signals from neurotrophins (e.g., BDNF), neurotransmitters (e.g., glutamate via NMDA and metabotropic receptors), and intracellular energy sensors (e.g., AMPK) to regulate activity-dependent synaptic plasticity, including long-term potentiation (LTP) and long-term depression (LTD). These mechanisms underlie the cortex's ability to adapt to changing sensory inputs and are critical for visual learning, perceptual adaptation, and rehabilitation after injury. mTORC1 modulates the local translation of key synaptic proteins such as PSD-95, GluR1, and eEF2, contributing to changes in synaptic strength and dendritic spine remodeling.

Metabolic Regulation [10]

mTOR maintains brain energy homeostasis by integrating signals from nutrients, growth factors, and cellular energy levels.

Autophagy [4]

mTOR inhibits autophagy under nutrient-rich conditions to focus on growth. During stress, reduced mTOR activity enhances autophagy, aiding in the clearance of damaged organelles and aggregated proteins.

Pathological mTOR Dysregulation

Aberrant mTOR signaling in the visual cortex has been implicated in a range of neurodevelopmental and neuropsychiatric disorders.

mTOR in the Adult Visual Cortex and Disease

In the adult visual cortex, mTORC1 maintains neuronal viability, supports ongoing synaptic remodeling, and regulates glial support functions.

However, under pathological conditions such as traumatic brain injury (TBI), ischemia, or neurodegenerative disorders, mTOR signaling can become maladaptive:

- Hyperactivation may contribute to excitotoxicity, gliosis, and synaptic dysfunction.
- Conversely, mTOR inhibition, particularly with agents like rapamycin, has demonstrated neuroprotective effects by promoting autophagy, reducing oxidative stress, and limiting inflammation.

Neurodevelopment and Circuit Formation [18]

- During early postnatal development, mTORC1 promotes:
  - *Neuronal growth* and *dendritic branching*
  - *Formation and maturation of synapses*
  - *Myelination* of cortical axons

mTOR-driven translation of local proteins at synapses is critical for shaping visual cortical maps, particularly during the critical period (early postnatal weeks in rodents and infancy in humans).

Synaptic Plasticity [9]

mTOR regulates long-term synaptic changes that underlie visual learning and memory:

- Long-Term Potentiation (LTP):
  - Requires mTOR-dependent translation of proteins like Arc, PSD-95, and CaMKII
  - Enhanced by visual stimuli and light exposure
- Ocular Dominance Plasticity (ODP):
  - In the developing cortex, deprivation of input from one eye leads to structural and functional shifts toward the open eye.
  - mTOR facilitates this activity-dependent remodeling.
- Critical period reopening in adulthood:
  - Activating mTOR signaling pharmacologically may restore plasticity in the adult cortex, offering therapeutic potential for amblyopia.

Visual Experience and Activity-Dependent mTOR Activation [20]

- Visual stimuli enhance calcium influx through NMDA receptors and BDNF-TrkB signaling, both of which activate the PI3K–Akt–mTOR axis.
- This drives local translation of synaptic proteins at dendritic spines, reinforcing active circuits.

mTOR Dysregulation and Visual Cortex Pathology (Fig. 11.1)

Tuberous Sclerosis Complex (TSC) [30]

Tuberous sclerosis complex (TSC) is a genetic disorder caused by mutations in the *TSC1* or *TSC2* genes, which encode hamartin and tuberin, respectively—key negative regulators of mTORC1 signaling. Loss of function in both genes leads to constitutive hyperactivation of mTORC1, resulting in widespread neurodevelopmental abnormalities. In the visual cortex, this dysregulation manifests as:

- *Cortical malformations (tubers)*: Disorganized cortical lamination and aberrant neuronal differentiation give rise to characteristic cortical tubers, often affecting the occipital lobes.

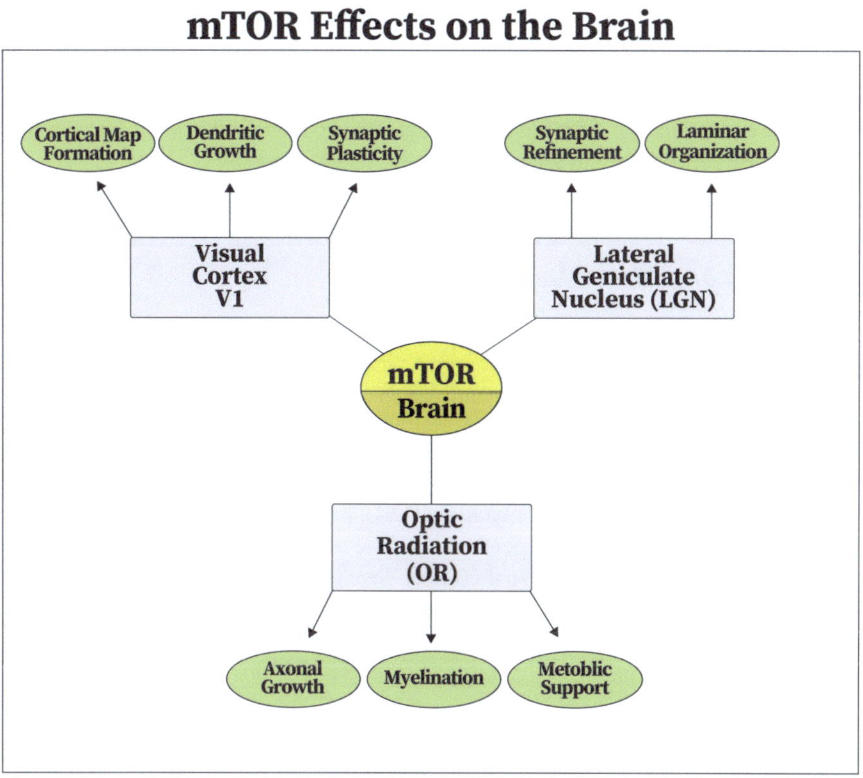

Fig. 11.1 The image depicts the impact of mTOR signaling across three key stages of the visual pathway: from the lateral geniculate nucleus (LGN), through the optic radiation, and finally to the visual cortex. Each mTOR-mediated effect is highlighted in green, illustrating its role in modulating neural processing at these critical junctures

- *Visual evoked potential (VEP) abnormalities*: Altered synaptic connectivity and myelination impair the integrity of visual signal processing, reflected in delayed or diminished VEP responses.
- *Increased susceptibility to seizures and ASD features*: Hyperexcitable cortical networks predispose individuals to epilepsy, while disrupted synaptic pruning and neuronal connectivity contribute to the high prevalence of autism spectrum features in TSC.
- *Disruption of inhibitory/excitatory* balance and impairment of visual processing and attention.

Autism Spectrum Disorders (ASD) [13]

In autism spectrum disorder (ASD), neuroglial dysfunction contributes significantly to neural circuit abnormalities. Microglia exhibit atypical synaptic pruning, astrocytes demonstrate impaired regulation of extracellular glutamate levels, and oligodendrocytes show deficiencies in myelination processes. Together, these glial abnormalities compromise the structural and functional integrity of neuronal networks.

- Hyperactive mTOR signaling in cortical circuits is implicated in ASD.
- mTOR dysregulation affects cortical connectivity, including in visual processing networks, contributing to abnormal sensory responses.

Amblyopia and Visual Deprivation [29]

Amblyopia, commonly referred to as "lazy eye," is a neurodevelopmental disorder characterized by reduced visual acuity in one eye due to abnormal visual experience during early critical periods. While the primary deficit originates from imbalanced visual input, the underlying pathology is deeply rooted in altered synaptic plasticity within the visual cortex.

The mechanistic target of rapamycin (mTOR), particularly mTORC1, plays a pivotal role in regulating activity-dependent synaptic remodeling, dendritic growth, and protein synthesis essential for visual cortical development. Dysregulation of mTOR signaling—either through genetic mutations or aberrant upstream signaling (e.g., excessive PI3K/AKT or insufficient AMPK input)—can disrupt these processes, thereby impeding normal binocular integration and ocular dominance plasticity.

- *Hyperactivation of mTORC1* leads to excessive synaptic stabilization, reducing the capacity for activity-dependent synaptic refinement essential for correcting imbalanced input.
- *Inhibition of mTORC1*, particularly during critical periods, has been shown to enhance synaptic plasticity and rescue visual function in amblyopic models.
- *mTOR-mediated translational control* of synaptic proteins such as 4E-BP1 and S6K1 modulates cortical responsiveness and may determine the threshold for visual cortical reorganization.

Thus, aberrant mTOR signaling contributes to the persistence of amblyopia by impairing the plasticity of cortical circuits necessary for functional recovery. Therapeutic modulation of mTOR pathways, including low-dose rapalogs, represents a promising avenue for enhancing visual cortical plasticity and extending the window for amblyopia treatment beyond early childhood.

Age-Related Cortical Decline and Neurodegeneration [26]

mTOR Dysregulation and Visual Cortex Involvement in Age-Related Cortical Decline and Neurodegeneration

With aging, dysregulation of mTOR signaling contributes to progressive decline in cortical function and heightened vulnerability to neurodegeneration.

- Impaired autophagic clearance: Chronic hyperactivation of mTORC1 suppresses autophagy, leading to the accumulation of dysfunctional mitochondria, misfolded proteins, and lipofuscin within cortical neurons. These changes contribute to cellular stress and reduced neuronal resilience.
- Reduced synaptic plasticity: mTOR dysregulation disrupts the balance of protein synthesis and degradation needed for experience-dependent synaptic remodeling. This impairs visual learning, contrast sensitivity, and adaptive responses to changing visual stimuli.
- Neuroinflammation and glial reactivity: Elevated mTOR activity in aging astrocytes and microglia enhances the production of proinflammatory cytokines and impairs neuroprotective functions, exacerbating cortical degeneration.
- Oxidative stress and energy imbalance: mTOR-driven suppression of AMPK signaling hampers cellular energy sensing and mitochondrial biogenesis, further contributing to cortical metabolic decline [2].

In neurodegenerative diseases such as Alzheimer's and Parkinson's, mTOR hyperactivation in the visual cortex has been linked to early visual processing deficits, including impaired motion detection and contrast sensitivity. These visual symptoms may precede cognitive decline and reflect early cortical involvement.

Therapeutic modulation of mTOR signaling—particularly through low-dose rapamycin or calorie restriction mimetics—has shown potential in preserving visual cortical function by restoring autophagy, reducing neuroinflammation, and enhancing synaptic adaptability in aging models.

- Chronic mTORC1 overactivation in aging may impair:
  - *Autophagy* (leading to toxic protein accumulation)
  - *Mitochondrial homeostasis*
  - *Cognitive and visual cortical function*
- Conversely, partial mTOR inhibition may enhance autophagy and protect against age-related cognitive and visual decline.

Traumatic brain injury (TBI) frequently results in enduring axonal damage and persistent neurological deficits. Although PTEN (phosphatase and tensin homolog) is a known inhibitor of neuronal growth, the long-term alterations in its activity following TBI and its specific impact on sensory–motor circuit recovery remain insufficiently characterized. In this context, neuronal-specific deletion of PTEN (PTEN-nKO) has been shown to significantly enhance both structural and functional recovery over an extended period post-injury. Mechanistically, PTEN exerts its inhibitory influence on axonal regeneration by antagonizing the Akt/mTOR signaling pathway—specifically through the suppression of Akt activation, which in turn inhibits mTOR signaling. Importantly, raptor, an essential scaffolding protein of mTORC1, plays a critical role in promoting axonal regeneration; thus, its inhibition further compromises regenerative processes [28].

Experiments following unilateral optic nerve crush (ONC) cause bilateral retinal thinning accompanied by astrocyte and microglial activation in the contralateral primary visual cortex (V1). The upregulation of genes associated with neuroinflammation and apoptosis in both hemispheres of the V1 region is detected which indicates involvement of critical signaling pathways, including MAPK, TNF, and apoptosis pathways.

This study explores the heterogeneity of astrocytes and microglia, identifying distinct subpopulations and key branching points along inflammatory trajectories. The specific subsets of glial cells play dominant roles in orchestrating the neuroinflammatory response following optic nerve injury, offering potential cellular targets for therapeutic modulation [17].

mTOR Signaling Pathways in the Brain

The mechanistic target of rapamycin (mTOR) is a serine/threonine kinase that plays a central role in regulating brain development, plasticity, and homeostasis through its two major complexes (Fig. 11.2).

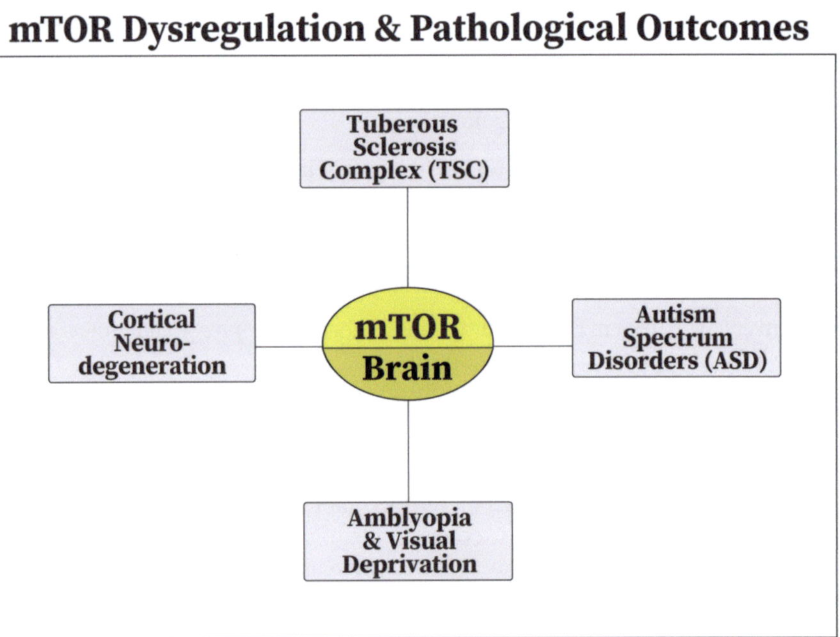

Fig. 11.2 The image illustrates the most common pathological conditions associated with dysregulation of the mTOR signaling pathway in the brain. These include neurodevelopmental disorders such as tuberous sclerosis complex (TSC) and autism spectrum disorders (ASD), as well as sensory processing impairments like amblyopia and visual deprivation. Additionally, dysregulated mTOR activity contributes to cortical neurodegeneration

PI3K/Akt/mTOR Pathway [14]

- *Overview*: This is the primary upstream activator of mTOR, responding to growth factors such as insulin and BDNF (brain-derived neurotrophic factor).
- *Mechanism*:
  - PI3K activates Akt, which phosphorylates TSC2 (tuberous sclerosis complex 2), relieving its inhibition on mTORC1.
  - mTORC1 promotes protein synthesis, lipid metabolism, and cell growth.
- *Relevance to the Brain:*
  - Supports neuronal survival and synaptic plasticity.
  - Dysregulation is implicated in neurodevelopmental disorders like autism spectrum disorders (ASD) and epilepsy [25].

AMPK/mTOR Pathway [21]

- *Overview*: AMP-activated protein kinase (AMPK) inhibits mTORC1 under conditions of energy stress.
- *Mechanism*:
  - AMPK activates TSC2 or phosphorylates raptor, directly suppressing mTORC1 activity.
- *Relevance to the Brain*:
  - Protects neurons during metabolic stress by enhancing autophagy and conserving energy.
  - Dysregulated AMPK–mTOR interaction is linked to neurodegenerative diseases.

MAPK/mTOR Pathway [15]

- *Overview*: The mitogen-activated protein kinase (MAPK) pathway interacts with mTOR to regulate growth and stress responses.
- *Mechanism*:
  - Activation of ERK1/2 enhances mTORC1 activity by inhibiting TSC2.
- *Relevance to the Brain:*
  - Promotes synaptic plasticity and memory.
  - Hyperactivation is associated with gliomas and other brain cancers.

mTORC1 and mTORC2 [5]

mTORC1 is more involved in growth and metabolism, while mTORC2 is critical for cytoskeletal organization and survival (Fig. 11.3).

- *mTORC1:*

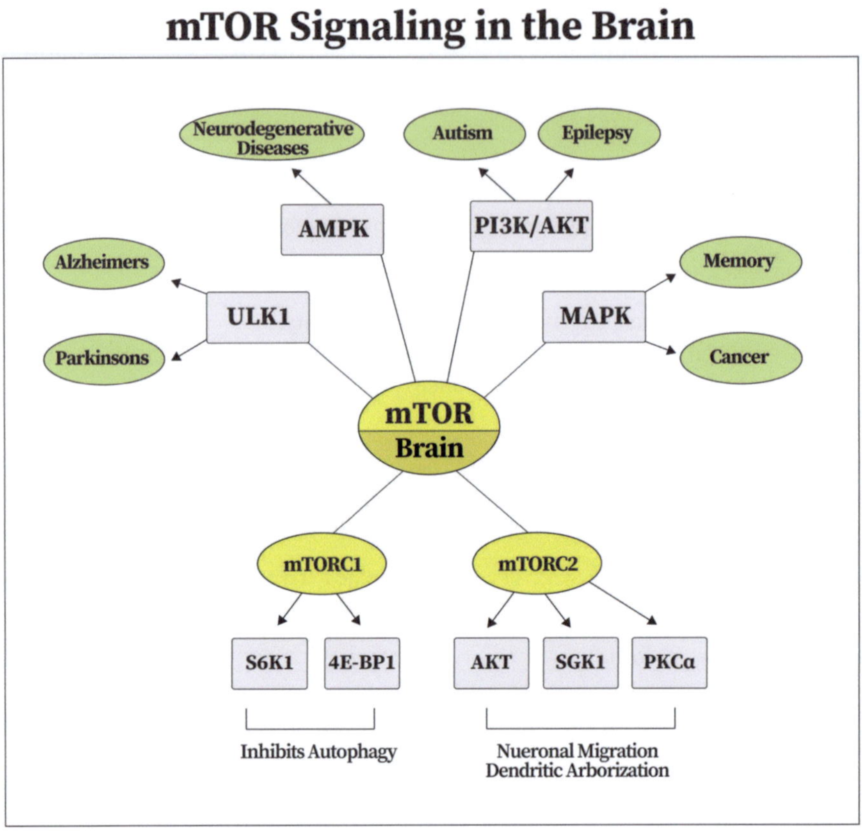

Fig. 11.3 The image illustrates the mTOR signaling pathways mediated by mTORC1 and mTORC2, along with their downstream effectors in the brain. Each complex regulates distinct pathological processes, as indicated above, through key signaling molecules such as ULK1 (autophagy regulation via mTORC1), AMPK (energy sensing), PI3K/AKT (cell growth and survival), and MAPK (proliferation and differentiation)

  - Regulates protein synthesis via effectors like S6K1 and 4E-BP1
  - Inhibits autophagy under normal conditions

- *mTORC2:*
  - Modulates cytoskeletal dynamics through Akt, SGK1, and PKCα
  - Plays a role in neuronal migration and dendritic arborization

mTOR and Autophagy [7]

- Inhibition of Autophagy:
  - Active mTORC1 suppresses autophagy by phosphorylating ULK1 (a key initiator of autophagy).
- Relevance to the Brain:

- Autophagy is essential for clearing damaged proteins and organelles, particularly in neurons.
- Impaired mTOR–autophagy balance contributes to protein aggregation diseases like Alzheimer's and Parkinson's.

Bibliography

1. Bohlson. Complement in the brain: contributions to neuroprotection, neuronal plasticity, and neuroinflammation. Ann Rev Immunol. 2023. https://doi.org/10.1146/annurev-immunol-101921-035639.
2. Buonfiglio. Oxidative stress: a suitable therapeutic target for optic nerve diseases? Antioxidants. 2023. https://doi.org/10.3390/antiox12071465.
3. Chen Y. Mechanisms and functions of activity-regulated cytoskeleton-associated protein in synaptic plasticity. Mol Neurobiol. 2023. https://doi.org/10.1007/s12035-023-03442-4.
4. Deleyto-Seldas. The mTOR–autophagy axis and the control of metabolism. Front Cell Dev Biol. 2021. https://doi.org/10.3389/fcell.2021.655731.
5. Dhaliwal. mTORC1 and mTORC2 synergy in human neural development, disease, and regeneration. Neural Regen Res. 2026. https://doi.org/10.4103/NRR.NRR-D-24-00961.
6. Duménieu. Mechanisms of plasticity in subcortical visual areas. Cells. 2021. https://doi.org/10.3390/cells10113162.
7. Festa. Microglial-to-neuronal CCR5 signaling regulates autophagy in neurodegeneration. Neuron. 2023. https://doi.org/10.1016/j.neuron.2023.04.006.
8. Figlia. Myelination and mTOR. NIH. 2017. https://doi.org/10.1002/glia.23273.
9. Gao. Role of mTOR-regulated autophagy in synaptic plasticity related proteins downregulation and the reference memory deficits induced by anesthesia/surgery in aged mice. Front Aging Neurosci. 2021. https://doi.org/10.3389/fnagi.2021.628541.
10. Goul. The molecular basis of nutrient sensing and signalling by mTORC1 in metabolism regulation and disease. Nat Rev Mol Cell Biol. 2023. https://doi.org/10.1038/s41580-023-00641-8.
11. Gupta. Autophagy and apoptosis cascade: which is more prominent in neuronal death? Cell Mol Life Sci. 2021. https://doi.org/10.1007/s00018-021-04004-4.
12. Gupta. Exploring the connection between BDNF/TrkB and AC/cAMP/PKA/CREB signaling pathways: potential for neuroprotection and therapeutic targets for neurological disorders. Mol Neurobiol. 2025. https://doi.org/10.1007/s12035-025-05001-5.
13. Ilic. Neuroglial dysregulation in autism spectrum disorder: pathogenetic insights, genetic threads, and therapeutic horizons. Neuroglia. 2025. https://doi.org/10.3390/neuroglia6010011.
14. Iranpanah. The exosome-mediated PI3K/Akt/mTOR signaling pathway in neurological diseases. Pharmaceutics. 2023. https://doi.org/10.3390/pharmaceutics15031006.
15. Iroegbu. ERK/MAPK signalling in the developing brain: perturbations and consequences. Neurosci Biobehav Rev. 2021;131 https://doi.org/10.1016/j.neubiorev.2021.10.009.
16. Karalis. The role of TSC1 and TSC2 proteins in neuronal axons. Mol Psychiatry. 2024. https://doi.org/10.1038/s41380-023-02402-7.
17. Li D. Single-cell rna sequencing of the primary visual cortex in mice with optic nerve injury. IVOS. 2025;66:31. https://doi.org/10.1167/iovs.66.5.31.
18. Litwa. Shared mechanisms of neural circuit disruption in tuberous sclerosis across lifespan: bridging neurodevelopmental and neurodegenerative pathology. Front Genet. 2022. https://doi.org/https://doi.org/10.3389/fgene.2022.997461
19. Miao L. mTORC1 is necessary but mTORC2 and GSK3β are inhibitory for AKT3-induced axon regeneration in the central nervous system. Neuroscience. 2016. https://doi.org/https://doi.org/10.7554/eLife.14908.

20. Moya-Alvarado. BDNF/TrkB signaling endosomes in axons coordinate CREB/mTOR activation and protein synthesis in the cell body to induce dendritic growth in cortical neurons. Neuroscience. 2023. https://doi.org/10.7554/eLife.77455.
21. Muraleedharan. AMPK in the brain: its roles in glucose and neural metabolism. FEBS J. 2021. https://doi.org/10.1111/febs.16151.
22. Nord. Reduced mTORC1-signaling in progenitor cells leads to retinal lamination deficits. Dev Dyn. 2024. https://doi.org/https://doi.org/10.1002/dvdy.707.
23. Nussinov. Neurodevelopmental disorders, like cancer, are connected to impaired chromatin remodelers, PI3K/mTOR, and PAK1-regulated MAPK. Biophys Rev. 2023. https://doi.org/https://doi.org/10.1007/s12551-023-01054-9.
24. Payne. Brain volumes in genetic syndromes associated with mTOR dysregulation: a systematic review and meta-analysis. Mol Psychiatry. 2024. https://doi.org/10.1038/s41380-024-02863-4.
25. Ravizza. mTOR and neuroinflammation in epilepsy: implications for disease progression and treatment. Nat Rev Neurosci. 2024. https://doi.org/10.1038/s41583-024-00805-1.
26. Reed. Neuroprotective effects of metformin through the modulation of neuroinflammation and oxidative stress. Cells. 2025. https://doi.org/10.3390/cells14141064.
27. Schumacher. Peripheral myelin: from development to maintenance. J Neurochem. 2024. https://doi.org/https://doi.org/10.1111/jnc.16268.
28. Shi Z. Reversing persistent PTEN activation after traumatic brain injury fuels long-term axonal regeneration via Akt/mTORC1 signaling cascade. Adv Sci. 2024:16. https://doi.org/10.1002/advs.202410136.
29. Wang G. Activation of p38 MAPK hinders the reactivation of visual cortical plasticity in adult amblyopic mice. Exp Eye Res. 2023;236 https://doi.org/10.1016/j.exer.2023.109651.
30. Wang S. Unraveling the function of TSC1-TSC2 complex: implications for stem cell fate. Stem Cell Res Ther. 2025. https://doi.org/https://doi.org/10.1186/s13287-025-04170-3.
31. Xie P-L. Pharmacological mTOR inhibitors in ameliorating Alzheimer's disease: current review and perspectives. Front Pharmacol. 2024. https://doi.org/10.3389/fphar.2024.1366061.

Chapter 12
mTOR Pharmacological Alterations

Contents

Abstract Pharmacological targeting of the mechanistic target of rapamycin (mTOR) has emerged as a promising strategy in ophthalmology, given mTOR's central role in regulating cellular growth, metabolism, autophagy, and survival across various ocular tissues. mTOR inhibitors, such as rapamycin (sirolimus) and its analogs (rapalogs), have demonstrated therapeutic potential in modulating pathological angiogenesis, inflammation, fibrosis, and neurodegeneration in multiple ophthalmic disorders. In the anterior segment, mTOR inhibition has shown benefit in delaying cataractogenesis and modulating fibrosis in corneal wound healing and glaucoma surgery. In the posterior segment, mTOR modulators are under investigation for their roles in suppressing choroidal neovascularization in age-related macular degeneration (AMD), preserving photoreceptors in retinitis pigmentosa, and enhancing retinal ganglion cell survival in glaucomatous optic neuropathy. Systemic and intraocular formulations are being evaluated to optimize tissue specificity, minimize adverse effects, and overcome barriers related to ocular bioavailability. As our understanding of mTOR's tissue-specific roles deepens, its pharmacological manipulation offers a versatile platform for targeted interventions in both anterior and posterior segment diseases.

K. T. Moazed, *mTOR Signaling in Ophthalmology*,
https://doi.org/10.1007/978-3-032-05044-1_12

Discussion

The mTOR (mechanistic target of rapamycin) pathway is central to cellular homeostasis, integrating signals from nutrients, growth factors, energy status, and stress to regulate protein synthesis, lipid metabolism, mitochondrial function, autophagy, and cytoskeletal dynamics. Because of its wide-reaching physiological roles, pharmacological manipulation of mTOR has become a major area of clinical and translational research. Both inhibition and controlled activation of mTOR signaling are being explored for therapeutic benefits across a broad spectrum of diseases [16].

Pharmacological manipulation of mTOR represents a powerful but double-edged tool. While inhibitors such as rapamycin and ATP-competitive agents offer therapeutic benefits across multiple disciplines, their systemic effects necessitate precise dose modulation, temporal control, and tissue targeting. Emerging strategies aim to fine-tune mTOR signaling rather than fully inhibit it, offering new hope in treating complex diseases involving aberrant cell growth, metabolism, and neurodegeneration [14].

mTOR plays a central role in integrating signals from upstream pathways like PI3K/Akt, AMPK, and MAPK. Pharmacological modulation of mTOR using rapalogs, dual mTORC1/2 inhibitors, and pathway-specific modulators has shown therapeutic promise across diverse diseases, including cancer, metabolic disorders, and neurodegeneration. Future directions aim to refine these therapies by improving specificity, overcoming resistance, and minimizing systemic side effects [9].

To better understand mTOR modulators, a concise review of mTOR structure and its key signaling pathways is essential, especially in relation to how these pathways govern distinct cellular functions.

The mechanistic target of rapamycin (mTOR) is a serine/threonine kinase that regulates cellular growth, metabolism, protein synthesis, and autophagy. Two of its catalytic subunit distinct complexes: *mTORC1* (mTOR Complex 1) and *mTORC2* (mTOR Complex 2) are mostly investigated. These complexes interact with multiple signaling pathways, influencing physiology and pathology. Pharmacological modulation of mTOR is critical in treating cancers, metabolic disorders, neurodegenerative diseases, and other conditions [29].

mTOR Complexes and Their Roles

mTORC1

- *Regulates*: Protein synthesis, lipid biosynthesis, autophagy inhibition, and metabolic processes.
- *Key Effectors*:
  - *S6K1 (Ribosomal Protein S6 Kinase 1)*: Promotes mRNA translation and ribosome biogenesis.

- *4E-BP1 (Eukaryotic Translation Initiation Factor 4E-Binding Protein 1)*: Regulates cap-dependent translation.
- *ULK1 (Unc-51-like kinase 1)*: Inhibition suppresses autophagy.

mTORC2

- *Regulates:* Cytoskeletal organization, cell survival, and metabolism
- *Key Effectors:*
  - *Akt (Protein Kinase B)*: Enhances cell survival and growth
  - *SGK1 (Serum- and Glucocorticoid-Induced Kinase 1)*: Regulates ion transport and cell survival
  - *PKCα (Protein Kinase C alpha)*: Influences cytoskeletal dynamics

Upstream and Downstream Pathways

PI3K/Akt/mTOR Pathway

- *Activation*: Growth factors (e.g., insulin, IGF) activate PI3K, generating PIP3, which recruits Akt.
- *Mechanism:*
  - Akt phosphorylates TSC2, relieving its inhibition of mTORC1.
  - mTORC1 stimulates protein synthesis and inhibits autophagy.

AMPK/mTOR Pathway

- *Inhibition by AMPK*: Low energy levels activate AMPK, which inhibits mTORC1 via TSC2 or raptor phosphorylation.
- *Function*: Conserves energy by reducing anabolic processes and enhancing autophagy.

MAPK/mTOR Pathway

- *Activation by ERK1/2:* Growth factor signaling through MAPK can activate mTORC1 by inhibiting TSC2.
- *Function*: Supports cellular growth and proliferation.

Summarized Pharmacological Modulation of mTOR and Its Targets

mTOR Inhibitors

- *Rapalogs (mTORC1 Inhibitors)*:
  - *Examples*: Sirolimus (rapamycin), everolimus, and temsirolimus
  - *Mechanism*: Bind FKBP12 (FK506-binding protein 12), which interacts with mTORC1 to inhibit its activity
  - *Applications:*
    - Immunosuppression (e.g., in organ transplantation)
    - Cancer treatment (e.g., renal cell carcinoma)
    - Tuberous sclerosis complex (TSC)
    - Neuroprotection (investigational for neurodegenerative diseases)
- *ATP-Competitive Inhibitors (Dual mTORC1/2 Inhibitors):*
  - *Examples*: Torin1 and MLN0128
  - *Mechanism*: Directly inhibit the kinase activity of mTOR, affecting both mTORC1 and mTORC2
  - *Applications*: Advanced cancers, overcoming resistance to rapalogs
- *PI3K/mTOR Dual Inhibitors*:
  - *Examples*: BEZ235 and BGT226.
  - *Mechanism*: Target both PI3K and mTOR kinase activity
  - *Applications*: Cancers with hyperactive PI3K/Akt signaling

Pathway-Specific Modulators

- *AMPK Activators* (e.g., Metformin, AICAR) [31]
  - Indirectly inhibit mTORC1 by activating AMPK
  - Used for type 2 diabetes and metabolic disorders: under investigation for cancer and neuroprotection
- *Akt Inhibitors* (e.g., MK-2206) [17]
  - Prevent mTORC1 activation downstream of PI3K signaling
  - Target cancer and conditions involving excessive mTOR activation
- *ERK Pathway Inhibitors*: (e.g., Trametinib) [8]
  - Indirectly affect mTOR by targeting MAPK signaling
  - Applications in cancers with activated MAPK/mTOR pathways

Pharmacologic modulators of mTOR (mechanistic target of rapamycin) can also be categorized based on their mode of action into *activators, inhibitors* (direct and indirect), and *others* (e.g., dual modulators or context-dependent agents) (Table 12.1).

Below is a structured categorization:

Table 12.1 The table provides a comparative overview of mTORC modulators, categorizing them by agent/class, mechanism of action, and selectivity for mTORC1 versus mTORC2

Comparative table of mTOR modulators			
Agent/class	Category	Mechanism	Selectivity
Rapamycin (Sirolimus)	Allosteric inhibitor	Binds FKBP12, inhibits mTORC1	mTORC1
Everolimus	Allosteric inhibitor	Binds FKBP12, inhibits mTORC1	mTORC1
Temsirolimus	Allosteric inhibitor	Binds FKBP12, inhibits mTORC1	mTORC1
Ridaforolimus	Allosteric inhibitor	Binds FKBP12, inhibits mTORC1	mTORC1
Torin-1	ATP-competitive inhibitor	Blocks mTOR kinase domain (C1/C2)	mTORC1/ mTORC2
Torin-2	ATP-competitive inhibitor	Blocks mTOR kinase domain (C1/C2)	mTORC1/ mTORC2
PP242	ATP-competitive inhibitor	Blocks mTOR kinase domain (C1/C2)	mTORC1/ mTORC2
AZD8055	ATP-competitive inhibitor	Blocks mTOR kinase domain (C1/C2)	mTORC1/ mTORC2
INK128 (Sapanisertib)	ATP-competitive inhibitor	Blocks mTOR kinase domain (C1/C2)	mTORC1/ mTORC2
KU-0063794	ATP-competitive inhibitor	Blocks mTOR kinase domain (C1/C2)	mTORC1/ mTORC2
BEZ235 (Dactolisib)	Dual PI3K/mTOR inhibitor	Blocks PI3K and mTOR kinases	PI3K + mTORC1/ mTORC2
PI-103	Dual PI3K/mTOR inhibitor	Blocks PI3K and mTOR kinases	PI3K + mTORC1/ mTORC2
GDC-0980 (Apitolisib)	Dual PI3K/mTOR inhibitor	Blocks PI3K and mTOR kinases	PI3K + mTORC1/ mTORC2
PF-04691502	Dual PI3K/mTOR inhibitor	Blocks PI3K and mTOR kinases	PI3K + mTORC1/ mTORC2
Metformin	Indirect inhibitor	Activates AMPK, inhibits mTOR indirectly	Indirect
Resveratrol	Indirect inhibitor	Activates AMPK, inhibits mTOR indirectly	Indirect
AICAR	Indirect inhibitor	Activates AMPK, inhibits mTOR indirectly	Indirect
Berberine	Indirect inhibitor	Activates AMPK, inhibits mTOR indirectly	Indirect
Sestrins	Indirect inhibitor	Endogenous regulator of AMPK/ mTOR	Indirect

(continued)

Table 12.1 (continued)

Comparative table of mTOR modulators			
Agent/class	Category	Mechanism	Selectivity
Leucine	Activator	Activates mTORC1 via Rag GTPases	mTORC1
Insulin	Activator	Activates PI3K/Akt/mTOR	mTORC1
IGF-1	Activator	Activates PI3K/Akt/mTOR	mTORC1
MHY1485	Activator	Promotes mTORC1 activity	mTORC1
Phosphatidic acid	Activator	Promotes lysosomal mTORC1 localization	mTORC1
Curcumin	Context-dependent	Inhibits PI3K/Akt/mTOR (dose/context dependent)	Variable
Quercetin	Context-dependent	AMPK activation; indirect mTOR inhibition	Variable
Fisetin	Context-dependent	Senotherapeutic, mTOR modulation	Variable
Spermidine	Context-dependent	Autophagy inducer, indirect mTOR modulation	Variable
EGCG	Context-dependent	PI3K/Akt/mTOR inhibition	Variable
Ketogenic diet	Context-dependent	Suppresses insulin/IGF-1, indirectly mTOR inhibition	Variable
RapaLink-1	Hybrid inhibitor	Fusion of rapamycin and kinase inhibitor	mTORC1/mTORC2
CC-223	Experimental inhibitor	ATP-competitive mTOR inhibitor	mTORC1/mTORC2
Vistusertib	Experimental inhibitor	ATP-competitive mTOR inhibitor	mTORC1/mTORC2
OSI-027	Experimental inhibitor	ATP-competitive mTOR inhibitor	mTORC1/mTORC2
DS-7423	Experimental inhibitor	Dual PI3K/mTOR inhibitor	PI3K + mTORC1/mTORC2
GSK1059615	Experimental inhibitor	Dual PI3K/mTOR inhibitor	PI3K + mTORC1/mTORC2

I. mTOR Inhibitors

A. *Allosteric Inhibitors (Rapalogs)—mTORC1-Specific* [20]

These bind FKBP12 and inhibit mTORC1 incompletely:

- *Rapamycin (Sirolimus)*
- *Everolimus*
- *Temsirolimus*
- *Ridaforolimus*

These primarily inhibit S6K1 activity and show minimal effect on 4E-BP1 or mTORC2.

B. *ATP-Competitive Inhibitors—Dual mTORC1/mTORC2 Inhibitors* [15]

Block the kinase domain of mTOR:

- *Torin-1/Torin-2*
- *PP242*
- *AZD8055*
- *INK128 (Sapanisertib)*
- *MLN0128*
- *KU-0063794*

More complete inhibition, including 4E-B P1 and mTORC2/Akt signaling.

C. *Dual PI3K/mTOR Inhibitors* [11]

Target both PI3K and mTOR:

- *BEZ235 (Dactolisib)*
- *PI-103*
- *GDC-0980 (Apitolisib)*
- *PF-04691502*

Used in cancer therapy due to simultaneous inhibition of upstream and downstream nodes.

D. *Indirect Inhibitors (Upstream Signaling Modifiers)* [1]

Modulate upstream pathways that influence mTOR:

- *Metformin*—via AMPK activation
- *Resveratrol*—activates AMPK
- *AICAR*—AMPK activator
- *Berberine*—AMPK activation
- *Sestrins*—endogenous AMPK/mTOR modulators
- *STAT3 inhibitors*, *TSC2 enhancers*, etc.

II. mTOR Activators

Less common and typically work by inhibiting upstream negative regulators [7]:

- *Leucine and other BCAAs*—directly activate mTORC1 via Rag GTPases
- *Insulin*—via PI3K/Akt pathway
- *IGF-1 (Insulin-like growth factor 1)*—activates PI3K/Akt
- *MHY1485*—synthetic mTOR activator (blocks lysosomal mTOR inactivation)
- *Phosphatidic acid (PA)*—promotes mTORC1 localization to lysosome
- *Glucose, ATP, growth factors*—indirectly activate mTOR
- *TSC1/TSC2 inhibitors* promote Rheb-mediated mTORC1 activation

III. Other/Context-Dependent Agents

These may have dual or modulatory effects depending on cellular context or dose [19]:

- *Curcumin*—mTOR inhibition via PI3K/Akt suppression (context-dependent)
- *Quercetin*—AMPK activation; indirect mTOR inhibition
- *Fisetin*—senotherapeutic with partial mTOR modulation
- *Spermidine*—promotes autophagy and mTOR modulation indirectly
- *EGCG (Green tea catechin)*—inhibits PI3K/Akt/mTOR axis
- *Ketogenic diet*—reduces insulin and IGF-1; indirectly suppresses mTOR

Detailed Specific Pharmacological Alterations of mTOR Signaling

Pharmacological agents that alter mTOR signaling have shown utility in diverse fields including oncology, neurology, immunology, ophthalmology, and aging biology. These interventions primarily act on the two major mTOR complexes: mTORC1and mTORC2.

The following is an expanded description of some of the more important mTOR modulators.

mTOR Inhibitors

A. Rapamycin and Rapalogs (Allosteric Inhibitors of mTORC1)

Rapamycin (sirolimus), the prototype mTOR inhibitor, forms a complex with the immunophilin FKBP12, which then binds to mTORC1 and inhibits its activity allosterically. While highly effective at suppressing mTORC1, it does not directly inhibit mTORC2 at conventional doses.

- *Clinical Applications* [21]:
  - *Tuberous sclerosis complex (TSC)*: Used to reduce tumor size in subependymal giant cell astrocytomas (SEGAs) and renal angiomyolipomas by suppressing hyperactive mTORC1 due to TSC1/TSC2 loss.
  - *Organ transplantation*: Prevents rejection by inhibiting T-cell proliferation.
  - *Cancer therapy*: Approved for renal cell carcinoma, breast cancer, and other malignancies.
  - *Age-related disorders*: Low-dose, intermittent rapamycin (or analogs) is under investigation for immune rejuvenation, reduction of age-related inflammation, and lifespan extension.

  - *Ophthalmology*: Investigational for diseases involving abnormal proliferation and neovascularization (e.g., AMD, PVR, and diabetic retinopathy) and to modulate corneal, retinal, or optic nerve degeneration, as discussed in previous chapters.
- *Limitations*:
  - Side effects include impaired wound healing, hyperlipidemia, mouth ulcers, and insulin resistance.
  - Prolonged use can suppress adaptive immunity and increase infection risk.
  - Chronic use may disrupt mTORC2 with metabolic consequences.

B. Second-Generation mTOR Inhibitors (ATP-Competitive Inhibitors)

These molecules inhibit both *mTORC1 and mTORC2* by targeting the ATP-binding site of the mTOR kinase domain [2].

- *Examples: Torin1/Torin2, PP242, AZD8055, INK128 (Sapanisertib), MLN0128*
- *Mechanism of action:* Prevent phosphorylation of all mTOR downstream targets, including 4E-BP1 (translation repressor) and AKT (Ser473 site via mTORC2)
- *Advantages*: More complete inhibition of mTOR pathway; greater efficacy in some resistant cancers
- *Limitations*: Greater risk of toxicity due to suppression of mTORC2, which regulates AKT-mediated survival and metabolism

C. Dual PI3K/mTOR Inhibitors

Since mTOR lies downstream of the *PI3K/AKT pathway*, dual inhibitors block both nodes to prevent compensatory feedback loops that often limit the efficacy of single-agent therapies [3].

- *Examples: BEZ235 (Dactolisib), PI-103, GDC-0980 (Apitolisib), and PF-04691502*
- *Applications*: Being evaluated in solid tumors and hematologic malignancies; some preclinical exploration in retinal and neurodegenerative diseases
- *Challenges*: Narrow therapeutic index, gastrointestinal toxicity, insulin resistance, and poor long-term tolerability and have limited clinical adoption

D. Indirect Modulators of mTOR Signaling

AMPK Activators (mTOR Suppressors) [27]

- *Examples: Metformin, AICAR.*
- *Mechanism*: Activate AMPK, which phosphorylates and activates TSC2, thereby suppressing mTORC1.
- *Applications*:
  - *Metabolic disease*: Metformin suppresses hepatic mTORC1 activity and improves insulin sensitivity.
  - *Neuroprotection and longevity*: Both agents are being explored for age-related cognitive decline, Alzheimer's disease, and retinal protection through enhanced autophagy and reduced oxidative stress.
  - *Ophthalmology*: Metformin use has been associated with reduced risk of glaucoma and AMD progression in observational studies.

ULK1 Agonists and Autophagy Enhancers [22]

- ULK1 is the autophagy-initiating kinase suppressed by mTORC1.
- *Pharmacological activation of ULK1* or enhancement of autophagic flux (e.g., with *trehalose* or *spermidine*) may bypass mTORC1 inhibition and provide neuroprotection without full pathway suppression.

C. S6K and 4E-BP1 Modulators [5]

- Targeting mTORC1 downstream effectors offers more selective intervention in protein synthesis, especially in conditions involving synaptic plasticity, such as amblyopia or cognitive disorders.
- *Potential agents* are under development to fine-tune translational control without broadly suppressing mTOR.

Potential mTOR Activators

Though pharmacological activation of mTOR is less common, controlled enhancement of mTOR activity may benefit certain neurodegenerative, hypometabolic, or injury-repair contexts where anabolic and regenerative processes are impaired.

- *Approaches include:*
  - Inhibition of upstream repressors such as PTEN or TSC1/2 (limited by oncogenic potential)
  - Nutritional stimulation (e.g., leucine and arginine) or use of anabolic agents (e.g., IGF-1)
  - AMPK inhibition (e.g., Compound C) to indirectly relieve mTORC1 suppression—currently restricted to experimental models

Therapeutic Implications Across Systems

- *Cancer:* mTOR inhibitors impair cell growth and angiogenesis.
- *Neurology:* In TSC, ASD, epilepsy, and cognitive decline, mTOR modulation may correct synaptic overgrowth or underactivity.
- *Ophthalmology:* Targeting mTOR in retinal diseases modulates autophagy, VEGF production, and oxidative stress.
- *Aging:* Rapalogs are promising geroprotectors; trials (e.g., PEARL and Dog Aging Project) are ongoing.
- *Immunology:* Dose-dependent immunosuppressive or immunostimulatory effects are exploited in transplantation and vaccines.

Rapamycin

In 1964, a Canadian expedition departed Halifax aboard the HMCS *Cape Scott* for Easter Island (Rapa Nui), a remote Chilean territory in the southeastern Pacific Ocean. The purpose was to study the island's isolated population. During this expedition, soil samples were collected that ultimately led to the discovery of a groundbreaking compound: Rapamycin [10].

Rapamycin is a highly specific allosteric inhibitor of mTORC1, with profound effects on cellular growth, metabolism, autophagy, and inflammation. Its clinical and experimental applications span oncology, immunology, neurobiology, ophthalmology, and aging. In the visual system, rapamycin demonstrates protective roles in the retina, optic nerve, thalamus, and cortex, making it a candidate for diseases involving neurodegeneration, dysregulated growth, and inflammation.

Its use, however, requires careful modulation, as dose, timing, and tissue specificity determine whether it exerts protective or deleterious effects. Advances in targeted delivery, combination therapies, and biomarker-guided applications may broaden its therapeutic impact while minimizing adverse effects.

Rapamycin Key Uses and Benefits

The role of rapamycin in regulating mTOR signaling encompasses its molecular mechanisms, systemic physiological effects, involvement in various disease states, and relevance to the visual system. While its ophthalmic effects have been thoroughly addressed in earlier chapters, its broader systemic impacts also warrant attention.

- Organ Transplant Rejection Prevention: Rapamycin is an FDA-approved drug used to prevent organ rejection in transplant patients. It works by suppressing the immune system to reduce the likelihood of the body attacking the transplanted organ [13].

- Cancer Treatment: Due to its ability to inhibit cell growth and proliferation, rapamycin is used in the treatment of certain cancers, particularly those where the mTOR pathway is overactive. Some of its analogs, such as everolimus and temsirolimus, are also used in cancer therapy [30].
- Tuberous Sclerosis Complex (TSC) Treatment: Rapamycin shows promise in treating TSC, a genetic disorder causing benign tumor growth in various organs. It has been shown to reduce seizures in some TSC patients, and studies are ongoing to evaluate its effectiveness against TSC-related tumors like subependymal giant cell astrocytomas (SEGAs) [4].
- Lymphangioleiomyomatosis (LAM) Treatment: Rapamycin can also be beneficial in the treatment of LAM, a rare lung disease characterized by the abnormal proliferation of muscle-like cells. It can help stabilize lung function and improve the quality of life in LAM patients [6].
- Potential for Life Extension and Anti-Aging: Rapamycin's ability to inhibit the mTOR pathway, which plays a role in aging, has sparked interest in its potential to promote longevity. Studies in various organisms, including mice, have shown that rapamycin can extend the lifespan and delay the onset of age-related diseases. However, more research is needed to establish its long-term safety and effectiveness in humans for this purpose [25].
- Epilepsy and focal cortical dysplasia type 2 (FCD2): Dysregulated mTOR pathway is implicated in the pathogenesis of seizures associated with genetic variants in mTOR pathway components. mTOR inhibitors are approved for the treatment of epilepsy in patients with tuberous sclerosis complex (TSC), the prototypical mTORopathy. Increasing evidence indicates that mTOR inhibitors may also have therapeutic potential in other mTORopathies, including DEPDC5-related epilepsy and focal cortical dysplasia type II (FCD2) [18].

Rapamycin Side Effects and Considerations

While rapamycin offers numerous benefits, it is crucial to acknowledge its potential side effects:

- Immunosuppression: Rapamycin weakens the immune system, increasing the risk of infections and potentially certain cancers.
- Metabolic Side Effects: Some studies have shown that chronic use of rapamycin may lead to glucose intolerance, insulin resistance, and hyperlipidemia.
- Other Side Effects: Other common side effects include mouth sores, fatigue, constipation, diarrhea, high blood pressure, and swelling.
- Wound Healing Problems: Rapamycin can also impair or slowdown wound healing.

Important Notes

- Not a Universal Anti-Aging Solution: Despite the promising research on rapamycin and aging, it is important to understand that it is not a magical cure for aging, and its effects are likely complex and context-dependent.
- Clinical Trials and Research: While rapamycin is FDA-approved for specific uses, research into its potential applications, particularly in the fields of aging and longevity, is ongoing.
- Ethical Concerns: The off-label use of rapamycin for anti-aging purposes and the emergence of online clinics offering the drug with minimal oversight raise ethical concerns about patient safety and the potential for misuse (Table 12.2).

Clinical Applications and Research Uses

1. Oncology [28]
   - Inhibits tumor cell proliferation and angiogenesis
   - Used in *renal cell carcinoma, breast cancer, and pancreatic neuroendocrine tumors*
   - Often combined with other agents (e.g., *PI3K or MEK inhibitors*) due to resistance via feedback loops
2. Neurodevelopmental Disorders [23]
   - In *Tuberous Sclerosis Complex (TSC)*: mTORC1 is hyperactivated due to *TSC1/2 mutations.*
   - Rapamycin and *everolimus* reduce cortical tubers, subependymal giant cell astrocytomas (SEGA), and seizure burden.
   - May normalize aberrant synaptogenesis and thalamocortical connectivity.

Table 12.2 The table summarizes the biological effects of rapamycin across multiple physiological systems, including its impacts on the immune system, metabolism, cardiovascular function, digestive processes, nervous system activity, and aging

System	Effects of rapamycin
Immune system	Suppresses T cell activation; used in organ transplantation
Metabolism	Alters insulin signaling; may cause glucose intolerance
Cardiovascular	Reduces vascular smooth muscle proliferation; used in drug-eluting stents
Liver	Modulates lipid metabolism; potential hepatic steatosis
Nervous system	Enhances autophagy; neuroprotective effects in models of Alzheimer's, Parkinson's, and epilepsy
Aging	Increases lifespan in model organisms by reducing cellular senescence and preserving stem cell function

3. Age-Related Disorders [26]

   - In models of *age-related macular degeneration (AMD)* and *retinal degeneration*, rapamycin improves:

     – *Autophagic clearance*
     – *Photoreceptor survival*
     – *Anti-inflammatory signaling* [12]

4. Autoimmunity and Transplantation [24]

   - Inhibits T-cell proliferation without affecting IL-2 production
   - Used to prevent rejection in *kidney and liver transplants*

Emerging Therapeutics and Research Directions

Brain-Specific mTOR Modulators: Targeting mTOR in specific brain regions to treat neurodegenerative and psychiatric disorders.

mTORC2-Specific Inhibitors: Developing selective inhibitors for mTORC2, which plays a role in cytoskeletal dynamics and metabolism.

Resistance Mechanisms: Studying feedback loops and cross talk with other pathways (e.g., PI3K and AMPK) to overcome resistance in cancer therapy.

Combination Therapies: Pairing mTOR inhibitors with checkpoint inhibitors, anti-angiogenic drugs, or metabolic modulators.

Bibliography

1. Ali. Recent advances and limitations of mTOR inhibitors in the treatment of cancer. Cancer Cell Int. 2022. https://doi.org/https://doi.org/10.1186/s12935-022-02706-8.
2. Anubhav. Targeting the mTOR pathway using novel ATP-competitive inhibitors, Torin1, Torin2 and XL388, in the treatment of glioblastoma. Int J Oncol. 2021. https://doi.org/10.3892/ijo.2021.5263.
3. Ayvaz. All-trans retinoic acid enhances anti-proliferative effect of dual PI3K and mTOR inhibitor NVP-BEZ235 in triple negative breast cancer. Naunyn-Schmiedeberg's Arch Pharmacol. 2025. https://doi.org/10.1007/s00210-025-03981-8.
4. Becker. Long-term efficacy and safety of mammalian target of rapamycin inhibitor treatment for subependymal giant cell astrocytoma in tuberous sclerosis. Pediatric Neurol. 2025;168 https://doi.org/10.1016/j.pediatrneurol.2025.04.007.
5. Böhm. The dynamic mechanism of 4E-BP1 recognition and phosphorylation by mTORC1. Mol Cell. 2021. https://doi.org/10.1016/j.molcel.2021.03.031.
6. Evans. The bi-steric inhibitor RMC-5552 reduces mTORC1 signaling and growth in lymphangioleiomyomatosis. ATS J. 2024. https://doi.org/10.1165/rcmb.2024-0242OC.
7. Gerasimenko. mTOR pathway: insights into an established pathway for brain mosaicism in epilepsy. Neurobiol Dis. 2023. https://doi.org/10.1016/j.nbd.2023.106144.
8. Han H. Trametinib and M17, a novel small molecule inhibitor of AKT, display a synergistic antitumor effect in triple negative breast cancer cells through the AKT/mTOR and MEK/ERK pathways. Bioorganic Chem. 2025;154 https://doi.org/10.1016/j.bioorg.2024.107981.

9. Hao. PI3K/AKT/mTOR inhibitors for hormone receptor-positive advanced breast cancer. Cancer Treat Rev. 2025;132 https://doi.org/10.1016/j.ctrv.2024.102861.
10. Hobby. A treasure from a barren island: the discovery of rapamycin. Clin Kid J. 2022. https://doi.org/10.1093/ckj/sfac116.
11. Ihlamur. The mTOR signaling pathway and mTOR inhibitors in cancer: next-generation inhibitors and approaches. Curr Mol Med. 2024. https://doi.org/10.2174/1566524023666230509161645.
12. Jiande L. Rapamycin inhibits corneal inflammatory response and neovascularization in a mouse model of corneal alkali burn. Exp Eye Res. 2023;233 https://doi.org/10.1016/j.exer.2023.109539.
13. Jiang SM, Li XJ, Wang ZL, Chen ZW, Liu ZL, Li Q, Chen XL. Role of autophagy in rejection after solid organ transplantation: a systematic review of the literature. World J Transplant. 2025. https://doi.org/10.5500/wjt.v15.i3.103163.
14. Lipton. The Neurology of mTOR. Neuron. 2014. https://doi.org/10.1016/j.neuron.2014.09.034.
15. Lisi. mTOR kinase: a possible pharmacological target in the management of chronic pain. BioMed Res Int. 2015. https://doi.org/10.1155/2015/394257.
16. Mao B. Overview of research into mTOR inhibitors. Molecules. 2022. https://doi.org/10.3390/molecules27165295.
17. Martorana. AKT inhibitors: new weapons in the fight against breast cancer? Front Pharmacol. 2021. https://doi.org/10.3389/fphar.2021.662232.
18. Moloney. An overview of the value of mTOR inhibitors to the treatment of epilepsy: the evidence to date. Expert Rev Neurother. 2025. https://doi.org/10.1080/14737175.2025.2462280.
19. Narci. Context dependent isoform specific PI3K inhibition confers drug resistance in hepatocellular carcinoma cells. BMC Cancer. 2022. https://doi.org/10.1186/s12885-022-09357-y.
20. Parada. Effect of FKBP12-derived intracellular peptides on rapamycin-induced FKBP–FRB interaction and autophagy. Cells. 2022. https://doi.org/10.3390/cells11030385.
21. Paschalidou. Efficacy and safety of topical sirolimus for the treatment of angiofibromas in tuberous sclerosis: a systematic review and meta-analysis. Curr Pharmacol Rep. 2023. https://doi.org/10.1007/s40495-023-00350-y.
22. Pupyshev. Multiple mechanisms of the therapeutic effect of trehalose in inhibition of experimental neurodegeneration. Neurochem Journal. 2024. https://doi.org/10.1134/S1819712423040190.
23. Querfurth. Mammalian/mechanistic target of rapamycin (mTOR) complexes in neurodegeneration. Mol Neurodegener. 2021. https://doi.org/10.1186/s13024-021-00428-5.
24. Reyes. Association between immunosuppressive therapy utilized in the treatment of autoimmune disease or transplant and cancer progression. Biomedicines. 2022. https://doi.org/10.3390/biomedicines11010099.
25. Roark. Rapamycin for longevity: the pros, the cons, and future perspectives. Front Aging. 2025. https://doi.org/10.3389/fragi.2025.1628187.
26. Selvarani. Effect of rapamycin on aging and age-related diseases—past and future. GeroScience. 2020. https://doi.org/10.1007/s11357-020-00274-1.
27. Strang. Small molecule modulators of AMP-activated protein kinase (AMPK) activity and their potential in cancer therapy. J Med Chem. 2025. https://doi.org/10.1021/acs.jmedchem.4c02354.
28. Sun L. Rapamycin targets STAT3 and impacts c-Myc to suppress tumor growth. Cell Chem Biol. 2021. https://doi.org/10.1016/j.chembiol.2021.10.006.
29. Szwed. Regulation and metabolic functions of mTORC1 and mTORC2. Physiol Rev. 2021. https://doi.org/10.1152/physrev.00026.2020.
30. Thaker. Advancements in mTOR inhibitors for non-small-cell lung cancer: mechanisms, efficacy, and future perspectives. Small Mol Med Chem. 2025. https://doi.org/10.1055/a-2507-3598.
31. Zhang T. The anti-aging mechanism of metformin: from molecular insights to clinical applications. Molecules. 2025. https://doi.org/10.3390/molecules30040816.

Index

K. T. Moazed, *mTOR Signaling in Ophthalmology*,
https://doi.org/10.1007/978-3-032-05044-1

S

MIX
Papier aus verantwortungsvollen Quellen
Paper from responsible sources
FSC® C105338

If you have any concerns about our products,
you can contact us on
ProductSafety@springernature.com

In case Publisher is established outside the EU,
the EU authorized representative is:
Springer Nature Customer Service Center GmbH
Europaplatz 3, 69115 Heidelberg, Germany

Printed by Libri Plureos GmbH
in Hamburg, Germany